Cardiovascular Disorders

SOURCEBOOK

Fifth Edition

Health Reference Series

Fifth Edition

Cardiovascular Disorders
SOURCEBOOK

Basic Consumer Health Information about Heart and Blood Vessel Disorders, Such as Cardiomyopathy, Heart Attack, Heart Failure, Heart Rhythm Disorders, Heart Valve Disease, Aneurysms, Atherosclerosis, Stroke, Peripheral Arterial Disease, Varicose Veins, and Deep Vein Thrombosis, with Details about Risk Factors, Prevention, Diagnosis, and Treatment

Along with Information about Cardiovascular Concerns of Special Significance to Children, Men, Women, and Minority Populations, a Glossary of Related Medical Terms, and a Directory of Resources for Further Help and Information

Edited by
Sandra J. Judd

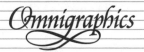

155 W. Congress, Suite 200, Detroit, MI 48226

Bibliographic Note

Because this page cannot legibly accommodate all the copyright notices, the Bibliographic
Note portion of the Preface constitutes an extension of the copyright notice.

Edited by Sandra J. Judd

Health Reference Series
Karen Bellenir, *Managing Editor*
David A. Cooke, MD, FACP, *Medical Consultant*
Elizabeth Collins, *Research and Permissions Coordinator*
EdIndex, Services for Publishers, *Indexers*

* * *

Omnigraphics, Inc.
Matthew P. Barbour, *Senior Vice President*
Kevin M. Hayes, *Operations Manager*

* * *

Peter E. Ruffner, *Publisher*
Copyright © 2014 Omnigraphics, Inc.
ISBN 978-0-7808-1309-0
E-ISBN 978-0-7808-1310-6

Lbrary of Congress Cataloging-in-Publication Data

Cardiovascular disorders sourcebook : basic consumer health information about heart and
blood vessel disorders, such as cardiomyopathy, heart attack, heart failure, heart rhythm
disorders, heart valve disease, aneurysms, atherosclerosis, stroke, peripheral arterial
disease, varicose veins, and deep vein thrombosis, with details about risk factors,
prevention, diagnosis, and treatment : along with information about cardiovascular
concerns of special significance ... -- Fifth edition / edited by Sandra J. Judd.
    pages cm. -- (Health reference series)
  Includes bibliographical references and index.
  Summary: "Provides basic consumer health information about risk factors, symptoms,
diagnosis, and treatment of disorders of the heart and blood vessels, along with prevention
strategies and concerns specific to men, women, children, and minority populations.
Includes index, glossary of related terms, and directory of resources"-- Provided by
publisher.
  ISBN 978-0-7808-1309-0 (hardcover : alk. paper) 1. Cardiovascular system--
Diseases--Popular works. I. Judd, Sandra J., editor of compilation.

  RC672.C35 2014
  616.1--dc23
                                                              2013044021

Table of Contents

Visit www.healthreferenceseries.com to view *A Contents Guide to the Health Reference Series*, a listing of more than 16,000 topics and the volumes in which they are covered.

Part V: Diagnosing Cardiovascular Disorders

Part VI: Treating Cardiovascular Disorders

Part VII: Preventing Cardiovascular Disorders

Part VIII: Additional Help and Information

Preface

About This Book

Cardiovascular disease is the leading cause of death in the United States. According to the Centers for Disease Control and Prevention, 715,000 Americans suffer a heart attack and 600,000 people die of heart disease in the United States every year. Additionally, stroke kills almost 130,000 Americans annually and is a leading cause of long-term disability. Yet cardiovascular disease is often preventable. With careful attention to diet, an active lifestyle, and control of contributing factors such as diabetes, cholesterol levels, blood pressure, tobacco use, and weight, Americans can reduce their chances of facing heart disease, stroke, or other blood vessel disorders. Furthermore, advances in our understanding of how to treat cardiovascular conditions make it possible to reduce the disabling health consequences frequently associated with these disorders.

Cardiovascular Disorders Sourcebook, Fifth Edition provides information about the symptoms, diagnosis, and treatment of disorders of the heart and blood vessels, including cardiomyopathy, heart attack, heart rhythm disorders, heart valve disease, atherosclerosis, stroke, peripheral arterial disease, and deep vein thrombosis. It offers details about the conditions associated with increased risks, explains the methods used to diagnose and treat them, and offers suggestions for steps men and women can take to decrease their likelihood of developing these disorders. The book also includes a discussion of cardiovascular concerns specific to men, women, children, and minority populations, and it concludes with a glossary and a directory of resources for further help and information.

How to Use This Book

This book is divided into parts and chapters. Parts focus on broad areas of interest. Chapters are devoted to single topics within a part.

Part I: Understanding Cardiovascular Risks and Emergencies describes how the heart works, explains the known risk factors for cardiovascular disease, and offers details about the conditions that make it more likely that a person will develop a cardiovascular disorder. It describes recent research regarding the genetic links and risk factors for cardiovascular disease, and it explains how to recognize a cardiac emergency and what to do when one occurs.

Part II: Heart Disorders provides basic information about the types of disorders that affect the heart. These include problems with the heart's blood supply, problems with the heart's rhythm, heart valve disease, and certain infectious diseases, as well as heart attack, sudden cardiac arrest, cardiomyopathy, and heart failure. Individual chapters include information about the development, symptoms, diagnosis, and treatment of each disorder.

Part III: Blood Vessel Disorders discusses the types of disorders that affect the arteries and veins, including atherosclerosis, carotid artery disease, stroke, disorders of the peripheral arteries and veins, and aortic disorders. It explains how these disorders arise, what their symptoms are, how they are diagnosed, and how they are treated.

Part IV: Cardiovascular Disorders in Specific Populations describes the unique ways that cardiovascular disease affects men, women, and children. It also offers some statistics on the occurrence of cardiovascular disorders in each of these populations, and it concludes with a discussion of cardiovascular disease among minority populations in the United States.

Part V: Diagnosing Cardiovascular Disorders explains the methods used to diagnose disorders of the heart and blood vessels. It describes diagnostic tests, including blood tests, electrocardiography and echocardiography, angiography, stress testing, and Holter and event monitors, and it explains how to prepare, what to expect, and which risks are associated with each test.

Part VI: Treating Cardiovascular Disorders discusses medications and procedures used to treat these disorders, including antiarrhythmic and anticoagulant medications, catheterization, coronary artery bypass grafting, stenting, pacemakers, and valvuloplasty. It also includes a discussion of aneurysm and heart defect repair, heart transplant, and the use of the total artificial heart. The section concludes with a discussion of cardiac and stroke rehabilitation techniques.

Part VII: Preventing Cardiovascular Disorders describes the things that can be done to help prevent heart and blood vessel disease. It explains how to control risk factors such as high blood pressure, high cholesterol, diabetes, and stress, and it offers suggestions for increasing healthy behaviors, such as maintaining a heart-healthy diet, managing weight, incorporating physical activity into a daily routine, and quitting smoking.

Part VIII: Additional Help and Information includes a glossary of terms related to cardiovascular disease and a directory of resources offering additional help and support.

Bibliographic Note

This volume contains documents and excerpts from publications issued by the following U.S. government agencies: Centers for Disease Control and Prevention (CDC); Genetics Home Reference; National Center for Complementary and Alternative Medicine; National Diabetes Education Program; National Heart, Lung, and Blood Institute; National Institute of Arthritis and Musculoskeletal and Skin Diseases; National Institute of Neurological Disorders and Stroke; National Institutes of Health; Office of Minority Health; Office on Women's Health (www.womenshealth.gov and www.hearthealthywomen.org); and the U.S. Food and Drug Administration.

In addition, this volume contains copyrighted documents from the following organizations: A.D.A.M., Inc.; American Association for Clinical Chemistry; American College of Cardiology; American College of Rheumatology; American Heart Association; Cleveland Clinic; Concordia University; Congenital Heart Information Network; Dartmouth-Hitchcock Medical Center; HealthDay/ScoutNews LLC; Heart Rhythm Society; March of Dimes; Massachusetts General Hospital; National Jewish Health; National Stroke Association; Nemours Foundation; New Zealand Dermatological Society; Ohio State University Extension; Ohio State University Medical Center; Queen Mary, University of London;

Society for Cardiovascular Angiography and Interventions; Sudden Cardiac Arrest Foundation; University of Iowa/IowaNow; University of Washington School of Medicine; Virtual Medical Centre; Wellcome Trust Centre for Human Genetics; and the World Heart Federation.

Full citation information is provided on the first page of each chapter or section. Every effort has been made to secure all necessary rights to reprint the copyrighted material. If any omissions have been made, please contact Omnigraphics to make corrections for future editions.

Acknowledgements

Thanks go to the many organizations, agencies, and individuals who have contributed materials for this *Sourcebook* and to medical consultant Dr. David Cooke and prepress services provider WhimsyInk. Special thanks go to managing editor Karen Bellenir and permissions coordinator Liz Collins for their help and support.

About the Health Reference Series

The *Health Reference Series* is designed to provide basic medical information for patients, families, caregivers, and the general public. Each volume takes a particular topic and provides comprehensive coverage. This is especially important for people who may be dealing with a newly diagnosed disease or a chronic disorder in themselves or in a family member. People looking for preventive guidance, information about disease warning signs, medical statistics, and risk factors for health problems will also find answers to their questions in the *Health Reference Series*. The *Series*, however, is not intended to serve as a tool for diagnosing illness, in prescribing treatments, or as a substitute for the physician/patient relationship. All people concerned about medical symptoms or the possibility of disease are encouraged to seek professional care from an appropriate healthcare provider.

A Note about Spelling and Style

Health Reference Series editors use *Stedman's Medical Dictionary* as an authority for questions related to the spelling of medical terms and the *Chicago Manual of Style* for questions related to grammatical structures, punctuation, and other editorial concerns. Consistent adherence is not always possible, however, because the individual volumes within the *Series* include many documents from a wide variety of different producers and copyright holders, and the editor's primary goal is to present material from each source as accurately as is possible following the terms specified by each document's producer. This sometimes means that information in different chapters or sections may follow other guidelines and alternate spelling authorities. For example, occasionally a copyright holder may require that eponymous terms be shown in possessive forms (Crohn's disease *vs.* Crohn disease) or that British spelling norms be retained (leukaemia *vs.* leukemia).

Locating Information within the Health Reference Series

The *Health Reference Series* contains a wealth of information about a wide variety of medical topics. Ensuring easy access to all the fact sheets, research reports, in-depth discussions, and other material contained within the individual books of the series remains one of our highest priorities. As the *Series* continues to grow in size and scope, however, locating the precise information needed by a reader may become more challenging.

A Contents Guide to the Health Reference Series was developed to direct readers to the specific volumes that address their concerns. It presents an extensive list of diseases, treatments, and other topics of general interest compiled from the Tables of Contents and major index headings. To access *A Contents Guide to the Health Reference Series*, visit www.healthreferenceseries.com.

Medical Consultant

Medical consultation services are provided to the *Health Reference Series* editors by David A. Cooke, MD, FACP. Dr. Cooke is a graduate of Brandeis University, and he received his M.D. degree from the University of Michigan. He completed residency training at the University of Wisconsin Hospital and Clinics. He is board-certified in Internal Medicine. Dr. Cooke currently works as part of the University of Michigan Health System and practices in Ann Arbor, MI. In his free time, he enjoys writing, science fiction, and spending time with his family.

Our Advisory Board

We would like to thank the following board members for providing guidance to the development of this series:

Dr. Lynda Baker, Associate Professor of Library and
Information Science, Wayne State University, Detroit, MI

Nancy Bulgarelli, William Beaumont Hospital Library,
Royal Oak, MI

Karen Imarisio, Bloomfield Township Public Library,
Bloomfield Township, MI

Karen Morgan, Mardigian Library,
University of Michigan-Dearborn, Dearborn, MI

Rosemary Orlando, St. Clair Shores Public Library,
St. Clair Shores, MI

Health Reference Series *Update Policy*

The inaugural book in the *Health Reference Series* was the first edition of *Cancer Sourcebook* published in 1989. Since then, the *Series* has been enthusiastically received by librarians and in the medical community. In order to maintain the standard of providing high-quality health information for the layperson the editorial staff at Omnigraphics felt it was necessary to implement a policy of updating volumes when warranted.

Medical researchers have been making tremendous strides, and it is the purpose of the *Health Reference Series* to stay current with the most recent advances. Each decision to update a volume is made on an individual basis. Some of the considerations include how much new information is available and the feedback we receive from people who use the books. If there is a topic you would like to see added to the update list, or an area of medical concern you feel has not been adequately addressed, please write to:

Editor
Health Reference Series
Omnigraphics, Inc.
155 W. Congress, Suite 200
Detroit, MI 48226
E-mail: editorial@omnigraphics.com

Part One

Understanding Cardiovascular Risks and Emergencies

Chapter 1

How the Heart Works

What Is the Heart?

Your heart is a muscular organ that pumps blood to your body. Your heart is at the center of your circulatory system. This system consists of a network of blood vessels, such as arteries, veins, and capillaries. These blood vessels carry blood to and from all areas of your body.

An electrical system controls your heart and uses electrical signals to contract the heart's walls. When the walls contract, blood is pumped into your circulatory system. Inlet and outlet valves in your heart chambers ensure that blood flows in the right direction.

Your heart is vital to your health and nearly everything that goes on in your body. Without the heart's pumping action, blood can't move throughout your body.

Your blood carries the oxygen and nutrients that your organs need to work well. Blood also carries carbon dioxide (a waste product) to your lungs so you can breathe it out.

A healthy heart supplies your body with the right amount of blood at the rate needed to work well. If disease or injury weakens your heart, your body's organs won't receive enough blood to work normally.

Excerpted from "What Is the Heart?" National Heart, Lung, and Blood Institute, National Institutes of Health, November 17, 2011.

Anatomy of the Heart

Your heart is located under your rib cage in the center of your chest between your right and left lungs. Its muscular walls beat, or contract, pumping blood to all parts of your body.

The size of your heart can vary depending on your age, size, and the condition of your heart. A normal, healthy, adult heart usually is the size of an average clenched adult fist. Some diseases can cause the heart to enlarge.

The Exterior of the Heart

The heart has four chambers, the right and left atria and the right and left ventricles.

Some of the main blood vessels (arteries and veins) that make up your circulatory system are directly connected to the heart.

The right side of your heart: The superior and inferior vena cavae are to the left of the heart muscle. These veins are the largest veins in your body.

After your body's organs and tissues have used the oxygen in your blood, the vena cavae carry the oxygen-poor blood back to the right atrium of your heart.

The superior vena cava carries oxygen-poor blood from the upper parts of your body, including your head, chest, arms, and neck. The inferior vena cava carries oxygen-poor blood from the lower parts of your body.

The oxygen-poor blood from the vena cavae flows into your heart's right atrium and then to the right ventricle. From the right ventricle, the blood is pumped through the pulmonary arteries to your lungs.

Once in the lungs, the blood travels through many small, thin blood vessels called capillaries. There, the blood picks up more oxygen and transfers carbon dioxide to the lungs—a process called gas exchange.

The oxygen-rich blood passes from your lungs back to your heart through the pulmonary veins.

The left side of your heart: Oxygen-rich blood from your lungs passes through the pulmonary veins. The blood enters the left atrium and is pumped into the left ventricle.

From the left ventricle, the oxygen-rich blood is pumped to the rest of your body through the aorta. The aorta is the main artery that carries oxygen-rich blood to your body.

Like all of your organs, your heart needs oxygen-rich blood. As blood is pumped out of your heart's left ventricle, some of it flows into the coronary arteries.

Your coronary arteries are located on your heart's surface at the beginning of the aorta. They carry oxygen-rich blood to all parts of your heart.

The Interior of the Heart

Heart chambers: Your heart is divided into four chambers. The two upper chambers of your heart are called the atria. They receive and collect blood.

The two lower chambers of your heart are called ventricles. The ventricles pump blood out of your heart to other parts of your body.

The septum: An internal wall of tissue divides the right and left sides of your heart. This wall is called the septum.

The area of the septum that divides the atria is called the atrial or interatrial septum. The area of the septum that divides the ventricles is called the ventricular or interventricular septum.

Heart valves: Your heart has four valves. The valves include the aortic valve, the tricuspid valve, the pulmonary valve, and the mitral valve.

Blood flow: Blood enters the right atrium of your heart from the superior and inferior vena cavae.

From the right atrium, blood is pumped into the right ventricle. From the right ventricle, blood is pumped to your lungs through the pulmonary arteries.

Oxygen-rich blood comes in from your lungs through the pulmonary veins into your heart's left atrium. From the left atrium, the blood is pumped into the left ventricle. The left ventricle pumps the blood to the rest of your body through the aorta.

For the heart to work well, your blood must flow in only one direction. Your heart's valves make this possible. Both of your heart's ventricles have an "in" (inlet) valve from the atria and an "out" (outlet) valve leading to your arteries.

Healthy valves open and close in exact coordination with the pumping action of your heart's atria and ventricles. Each valve has a set of flaps called leaflets or cusps that seal or open the valve. This allows blood to pass through the chambers and into your arteries without backing up or flowing backward.

Heart Contraction and Blood Flow

Heartbeat

Almost everyone has heard the real or recorded sound of a heartbeat. When your heart beats, it makes a "lub-DUB" sound. Between the time you hear "lub" and "DUB," blood is pumped through your heart and circulatory system.

A heartbeat may seem like a simple, repeated event. However, it's a complex series of very precise and coordinated events. These events take place inside and around your heart.

Each side of your heart uses an inlet valve to help move blood between the atrium and ventricle. The tricuspid valve does this between the right atrium and ventricle. The mitral valve does this between the left atrium and ventricle. The "lub" is the sound of the tricuspid and mitral valves closing.

Each of your heart's ventricles also has an outlet valve. The right ventricle uses the pulmonary valve to help move blood into the pulmonary arteries. The left ventricle uses the aortic valve to do the same for the aorta. The "DUB" is the sound of the aortic and pulmonary valves closing.

Each heartbeat has two basic parts: diastole and systole.

During diastole, the atria and ventricles of your heart relax and begin to fill with blood. At the end of diastole, your heart's atria contract (atrial systole) and pump blood into the ventricles.

The atria then begin to relax. Next, your heart's ventricles contract (ventricular systole) and pump blood out of your heart.

Pumping Action

Your heart uses its four valves to ensure your blood flows in only one direction. Healthy valves open and close in coordination with the pumping action of your heart's atria and ventricles.

Each valve has a set of flaps called leaflets or cusps that seal or open the valve. The cusps allow pumped blood to pass through the chambers and into your blood vessels without backing up or flowing backward.

Oxygen-poor blood from the vena cavae fills your heart's right atrium. The atrium contracts (atrial systole). The tricuspid valve located between the right atrium and ventricle opens for a short time and then shuts. This allows blood to enter the right ventricle without flowing back into the right atrium.

When your heart's right ventricle fills with blood, it contracts (ventricular systole). The pulmonary valve located between your right ventricle and pulmonary artery opens and closes quickly.

This allows blood to enter into your pulmonary arteries without flowing back into the right ventricle. This is important because the right ventricle begins to refill with more blood through the tricuspid valve. Blood travels through the pulmonary arteries to your lungs to pick up oxygen.

Oxygen-rich blood returns from the lungs to your heart's left atrium through the pulmonary veins. As your heart's left atrium fills with blood, it contracts. This event is called atrial systole.

The mitral valve located between the left atrium and left ventricle opens and closes quickly. This allows blood to pass from the left atrium into the left ventricle without flowing backward.

As the left ventricle fills with blood, it contracts. This event is called ventricular systole. The aortic valve located between the left ventricle and aorta opens and closes quickly. This allows blood to flow into the aorta. The aorta is the main artery that carries blood from your heart to the rest of your body.

The aortic valve closes quickly to prevent blood from flowing back into the left ventricle, which already is filling up with new blood.

Circulation and Blood Vessels

Your heart and blood vessels make up your overall blood circulatory system. Your blood circulatory system is made up of four subsystems.

Arterial Circulation

Arterial circulation is the part of your circulatory system that involves arteries, like the aorta and pulmonary arteries. Arteries are blood vessels that carry blood away from your heart. (The exception is the coronary arteries, which supply your heart muscle with oxygen-rich blood.)

Healthy arteries are strong and elastic (stretchy). They become narrow between heartbeats, and they help keep your blood pressure consistent. This helps blood move through your body.

Arteries branch into smaller blood vessels called arterioles. Arteries and arterioles have strong, flexible walls that allow them to adjust the amount and rate of blood flowing to parts of your body.

Venous Circulation

Venous circulation is the part of your circulatory system that involves veins, like the vena cavae and pulmonary veins. Veins are blood vessels that carry blood to your heart.

Veins have thinner walls than arteries. Veins can widen as the amount of blood passing through them increases.

Capillary Circulation

Capillary circulation is the part of your circulatory system where oxygen, nutrients, and waste pass between your blood and parts of your body.

Capillaries are very small blood vessels. They connect the arterial and venous circulatory subsystems.

The importance of capillaries lies in their very thin walls. Oxygen and nutrients in your blood can pass through the walls of the capillaries to the parts of your body that need them to work normally.

Capillaries' thin walls also allow waste products like carbon dioxide to pass from your body's organs and tissues into the blood, where it's taken away to your lungs.

Pulmonary circulation: Pulmonary circulation is the movement of blood from the heart to the lungs and back to the heart again. Pulmonary circulation includes both arterial and venous circulation.

Oxygen-poor blood is pumped to the lungs from the heart (arterial circulation). Oxygen-rich blood moves from the lungs to the heart through the pulmonary veins (venous circulation).

Pulmonary circulation also includes capillary circulation. Oxygen you breathe in from the air passes through your lungs into your blood through the many capillaries in the lungs. Oxygen-rich blood moves through your pulmonary veins to the left side of your heart and out of the aorta to the rest of your body.

Capillaries in the lungs also remove carbon dioxide from your blood so that your lungs can breathe the carbon dioxide out into the air.

Your Heart's Electrical System

Your heart's electrical system controls all the events that occur when your heart pumps blood. The electrical system also is called the cardiac conduction system. If you've ever seen the heart test called an electrocardiogram (EKG), you've seen a graphical picture of the heart's electrical activity.

Your heart's electrical system is made up of three main parts:

- The sinoatrial (SA) node, located in the right atrium of your heart

- The atrioventricular (AV) node, located on the interatrial septum close to the tricuspid valve

- The His-Purkinje system, located along the walls of your heart's ventricles

A heartbeat is a complex series of events. These events take place inside and around your heart. A heartbeat is a single cycle in which your heart's chambers relax and contract to pump blood. This cycle includes the opening and closing of the inlet and outlet valves of the right and left ventricles of your heart.

Each heartbeat has two basic parts: diastole and systole. During diastole, the atria and ventricles of your heart relax and begin to fill with blood.

At the end of diastole, your heart's atria contract (atrial systole) and pump blood into the ventricles. The atria then begin to relax. Your heart's ventricles then contract (ventricular systole), pumping blood out of your heart.

Each beat of your heart is set in motion by an electrical signal from within your heart muscle. In a normal, healthy heart, each beat begins with a signal from the SA node. This is why the SA node sometimes is called your heart's natural pacemaker. Your pulse, or heart rate, is the number of signals the SA node produces per minute.

The signal is generated as the vena cavae fill your heart's right atrium with blood from other parts of your body. The signal spreads across the cells of your heart's right and left atria.

This signal causes the atria to contract. This action pushes blood through the open valves from the atria into both ventricles.

The signal arrives at the AV node near the ventricles. It slows for an instant to allow your heart's right and left ventricles to fill with blood. The signal is released and moves along a pathway called the bundle of His, which is located in the walls of your heart's ventricles.

From the bundle of His, the signal fibers divide into left and right bundle branches through the Purkinje fibers. These fibers connect directly to the cells in the walls of your heart's left and right ventricles.

The signal spreads across the cells of your ventricle walls, and both ventricles contract. However, this doesn't happen at exactly the same moment.

The left ventricle contracts an instant before the right ventricle. This pushes blood through the pulmonary valve (for the right ventricle) to your lungs, and through the aortic valve (for the left ventricle) to the rest of your body.

As the signal passes, the walls of the ventricles relax and await the next signal.

This process continues over and over as the atria refill with blood and more electrical signals come from the SA node.

Chapter 2

Risk Factors for Cardiovascular Disorders

Chapter Contents

Section 2.1

Coronary Heart Disease Risk Factors

Excerpted from "What Are Coronary Heart Disease Risk Factors?"
National Heart, Lung, and Blood Institute, National Institutes of Health,
February 1, 2011.

What Are Coronary Heart Disease Risk Factors?

Overview

There are many known CHD risk factors. You can control some risk factors, but not others. Risk factors you can control include the following:

- High blood cholesterol and triglyceride levels (a type of fat found in the blood)
- High blood pressure
- Diabetes and prediabetes
- Overweight and obesity
- Smoking
- Lack of physical activity
- Unhealthy diet
- Stress

The risk factors you can't control are age, gender, and family history of CHD.

Many people have at least one CHD risk factor. Your risk of CHD and heart attack increases with the number of risk factors you have and their severity. Also, some risk factors put you at greater risk of CHD and heart attack than others. Examples of these risk factors include smoking and diabetes.

Many CHD risk factors start during childhood. This is even more common now because many children are overweight and don't get enough physical activity. Some CHD risk factors can even develop within the first ten years of life.

Researchers continue to study and learn more about CHD risk factors.

Outlook

CHD is the number one killer of both women and men in the United States. Following a healthy lifestyle can help you and your children prevent or control many CHD risk factors.

Because many lifestyle habits begin during childhood, parents and families should encourage their children to make heart healthy choices. For example, you and your children can lower your risk of CHD if you maintain a healthy weight, follow a healthy diet, do physical activity regularly, and don't smoke.

On average, people at low risk of CHD live nearly ten years longer than people at high risk of CHD.

If you already have CHD, lifestyle changes can help you control your risk factors. This may prevent CHD from worsening. Even if you're in your seventies or eighties, a healthy lifestyle can lower your risk of dying from CHD.

If lifestyle changes aren't enough, your doctor may recommend other treatments to help control your risk factors.

Your doctor can help you find out whether you have CHD risk factors. He or she also can help you create a plan for lowering your risk of CHD, heart attack, and other heart problems.

If you have children, talk with their doctors about their heart health and whether they have CHD risk factors. If they do, ask your doctor to help create a treatment plan to reduce or control these risk factors.

Coronary Heart Disease Risk Factors

High Blood Cholesterol and Triglyceride Levels

Cholesterol: High blood cholesterol is a condition in which your blood has too much cholesterol—a waxy, fat-like substance. The higher your blood cholesterol level, the greater your risk of coronary heart disease (CHD) and heart attack.

Cholesterol travels through the bloodstream in small packages called lipoproteins. Two major kinds of lipoproteins carry cholesterol throughout your body:

- *Low-density lipoproteins (LDL):* LDL cholesterol sometimes is called "bad" cholesterol. This is because it carries cholesterol to tissues, including your heart arteries. A high LDL cholesterol level raises your risk of CHD.

- *High-density lipoproteins (HDL):* HDL cholesterol sometimes is called "good" cholesterol. This is because it helps remove cholesterol from your arteries. A low HDL cholesterol level raises your risk of CHD.

Many factors affect your cholesterol levels. For example, after menopause, women's LDL cholesterol levels tend to rise, and their HDL cholesterol levels tend to fall. Other factors—such as age, gender, diet, and physical activity—also affect your cholesterol levels.

Healthy levels of both LDL and HDL cholesterol will prevent plaque from building up in your arteries. Routine blood tests can show whether your blood cholesterol levels are healthy. Talk with your doctor about having your cholesterol tested and what the results mean.

Children also can have unhealthy cholesterol levels, especially if they're overweight or their parents have high blood cholesterol. Talk with your child's doctor about testing your child' cholesterol levels.

Triglycerides: Triglycerides are a type of fat found in the blood. Some studies suggest that a high level of triglycerides in the blood may raise the risk of CHD, especially in women.

High Blood Pressure

"Blood pressure" is the force of blood pushing against the walls of your arteries as your heart pumps blood. If this pressure rises and stays high over time, it can damage your heart and lead to plaque buildup.

Blood pressure is measured as systolic and diastolic pressures. "Systolic" refers to blood pressure when the heart beats while pumping blood. "Diastolic" refers to blood pressure when the heart is at rest between beats.

You most often will see blood pressure numbers written with the systolic number above or before the diastolic number, such as 120/80 mmHg. (The mmHg is millimeters of mercury—the units used to measure blood pressure.)

All levels above 120/80 mmHg raise your risk of CHD. This risk grows as blood pressure levels rise. Only one of the two blood pressure numbers has to be above normal to put you at greater risk of CHD and heart attack.

Often, high blood pressure has no signs or symptoms. However, the condition can be detected using a simple test that involves placing a blood pressure cuff around your arm.

Most adults should have their blood pressure checked at least once a year. If you have high blood pressure, you'll likely need to be checked

14

more often. Talk with your doctor about how often you should have your blood pressure checked.

Children also can develop high blood pressure, especially if they're overweight. Your child's doctor should check your child's blood pressure at each routine checkup.

In children, blood pressure normally rises with age and body size. Newborns often have very low blood pressure numbers, while older teens have numbers similar to adults. The ranges for normal blood pressure and high blood pressure generally are lower for youth than for adults.

Your child should have routine blood pressure checks starting at three years of age. To find out whether a child has high blood pressure, a doctor will compare the child's blood pressure numbers to average numbers for his or her age, gender, and height.

Both children and adults are more likely to develop high blood pressure if they're overweight or have diabetes.

Diabetes and Prediabetes

Diabetes is a disease in which the body's blood sugar level is too high. The two types of diabetes are type 1 and type 2.

In type 1 diabetes, the body's blood sugar level is high because the body doesn't make enough insulin. Insulin is a hormone that helps move blood sugar into cells, where it's used for energy. In type 2 diabetes, the body's blood sugar level is high mainly because the body doesn't use its insulin properly.

Over time, a high blood sugar level can lead to increased plaque buildup in your arteries. Having diabetes doubles your risk of CHD.

Prediabetes is a condition in which your blood sugar level is higher than normal, but not as high as it is in diabetes. If you have prediabetes and don't take steps to manage it, you'll likely develop type 2 diabetes within ten years. You're also at higher risk of CHD.

Being overweight or obese raises your risk of type 2 diabetes. With modest weight loss and moderate physical activity, people who have prediabetes may be able to delay or prevent type 2 diabetes. They also may be able to lower their risk of CHD and heart attack. Weight loss and physical activity also can help control diabetes.

Even children can develop type 2 diabetes. Most children who have type 2 diabetes are overweight.

Type 2 diabetes develops over time and sometimes has no symptoms. Go to your doctor or local clinic to have your blood sugar levels tested regularly to check for diabetes and prediabetes.

Overweight and Obesity

The terms "overweight" and "obesity" refer to body weight that's greater than what is considered healthy for a certain height. More than two-thirds of American adults are overweight, and almost one-third of these adults are obese.

The most useful measure of overweight and obesity is body mass index (BMI). BMI is calculated from your height and weight. In adults, a BMI of 18.5 to 24.9 is considered normal. A BMI of 25 to 29.9 is considered overweight. A BMI of 30 or more is considered obese.

You can use the National Heart, Lung, and Blood Institute's (NHLBI's) online BMI calculator to figure out your BMI, or your doctor can help you.

Overweight is defined differently for children and teens than it is for adults. Children are still growing, and boys and girls mature at different rates. Thus, BMIs for children and teens compare their heights and weights against growth charts that take age and gender into account. This is called BMI-for-age percentile.

Being overweight or obese can raise your risk of CHD and heart attack. This is mainly because overweight and obesity are linked to other CHD risk factors, such as high blood cholesterol and triglyceride levels, high blood pressure, and diabetes.

Smoking

Smoking tobacco or long-term exposure to secondhand smoke raises your risk of CHD and heart attack.

Smoking triggers a buildup of plaque in your arteries. Smoking also increases the risk of blood clots forming in your arteries. Blood clots can block plaque-narrowed arteries and cause a heart attack.

Some research shows that smoking raises your risk of CHD in part by lowering HDL cholesterol levels.

The more you smoke, the greater your risk of heart attack. Studies show that if you quit smoking, you cut your risk of heart attack in half within a year. The benefits of quitting smoking occur no matter how long or how much you've smoked.

Most people who smoke start when they're teens. Parents can help prevent their children from smoking by not smoking themselves. Talk with your child about the health dangers of smoking and ways to overcome peer pressure to smoke.

Lack of Physical Activity

Inactive people are nearly twice as likely to develop CHD as those who are active. A lack of physical activity can worsen other CHD risk factors, such as high blood cholesterol and triglyceride levels, high blood pressure, diabetes and prediabetes, and overweight and obesity.

It's important for children and adults to make physical activity part of their daily routines. One reason many Americans aren't active enough is because of hours spent in front of TVs and computers doing work, schoolwork, and leisure activities.

Some experts advise that children and teens should reduce screen time because it limits time for physical activity. They recommend that children aged two and older should spend no more than two hours a day watching TV or using a computer (except for schoolwork).

Being physically active is one of the most important things you can do to keep your heart healthy. The good news is that even modest amounts of physical activity are good for your health. The more active you are, the more you will benefit.

Unhealthy Diet

An unhealthy diet can raise your risk of CHD. For example, foods that are high in saturated and trans fats and cholesterol raise LDL cholesterol. Thus, you should try to limit these foods.

Saturated fats are found in some meats, dairy products, chocolate, baked goods, and deep-fried and processed foods. Trans fats are found in some fried and processed foods. Cholesterol is found in eggs, many meats, dairy products, commercial baked goods, and certain types of shellfish.

It's also important to limit foods that are high in sodium (salt) and added sugars. A high-salt diet can raise your risk of high blood pressure.

Added sugars will give you extra calories without nutrients like vitamins and minerals. This can cause you to gain weight, which raises your risk of CHD. Added sugars are found in many desserts, canned fruits packed in syrup, fruit drinks, and nondiet sodas.

You also should try to limit how much alcohol you drink. Too much alcohol will raise your blood pressure. It also will add calories, which can cause weight gain.

Stress

Stress and anxiety may play a role in causing CHD. Stress and anxiety also can trigger your arteries to tighten. This can raise your blood pressure and your risk of heart attack.

The most commonly reported trigger for a heart attack is an emotionally upsetting event, especially one involving anger. Stress also may indirectly raise your risk of CHD if it makes you more likely to smoke or overeat foods high in fat and sugar.

Age

As you get older, your risk of CHD and heart attack rises. This is in part due to the slow buildup of plaque inside your heart arteries, which can start during childhood.

In men, the risk of CHD increases faster after age forty-five. In women, the risk of CHD increases faster after age fifty-five.

Most people have some plaque buildup in their heart arteries by the time they're in their seventies. However, only about 25 percent of those people have chest pain, heart attacks, or other signs of CHD.

Gender

Before age fifty-five, women have a lower risk of CHD than men. This is because before menopause, estrogen provides women some protection against CHD. After age fifty-five, however, the risk of CHD increases similarly in both women and men.

Some risk factors may affect CHD risk differently in women than in men. For example, diabetes raises the risk of CHD more in women.

Also, some risk factors for heart disease only affect women, such as preeclampsia. Preeclampsia is a condition that can develop during pregnancy. The two main signs of preeclampsia are a rise in blood pressure and excess protein in the urine.

Preeclampsia is linked to an increased lifetime risk of heart disease, including CHD, heart attack, heart failure, and high blood pressure. (Likewise, having heart disease risk factors, such as diabetes or obesity, increases your risk of preeclampsia.)

Family History

Family history plays a role in CHD risk. Your risk increases if your father or a brother was diagnosed with CHD before fifty-five years of age, or if your mother or a sister was diagnosed with CHD before sixty-five years of age.

However, having a family history of CHD doesn't mean that you will have it too. This is especially true if your affected family member smoked or had other CHD risk factors that were not well treated.

Making lifestyle changes and taking medicines to treat other risk factors often can lessen genetic influences and stop or slow the progress of CHD.

Section 2.2

Risk Factors for Stroke

Knowing your risk factors is the first step in preventing stroke. You can change or treat some risk factors, but others you can't. By having regular medical checkups and knowing your risk, you can focus on what you can change and lower your risk of stroke.

What risk factors can I change or treat?

High blood pressure: This is the single most important risk factor for stroke because it's the number one cause of stroke. Know your blood pressure and have it checked at least once every two years. If it's consistently 140/90 or above, it's high. Talk to your doctor about how to manage it.

Tobacco use: Tobacco use damages blood vessels. Don't smoke and avoid secondhand smoke.

Diabetes mellitus: Having diabetes increases your risk of stroke because it can cause disease of blood vessels in the brain. Work with your doctor to manage diabetes.

High blood cholesterol: High blood cholesterol increases the risk of blocked arteries. If an artery leading to the brain becomes blocked, a stroke can result.

Physical inactivity and obesity: Being inactive, obese, or both, can increase your risk of cardiovascular disease.

Carotid or other artery disease: The carotid arteries in your neck supply most of the blood to your brain. A carotid artery damaged by a fatty buildup of plaque inside the artery wall may become blocked by a blood clot, causing a stroke.

Transient ischemic attacks (TIAs): Recognizing and treating TIAs can reduce the risk of a major stroke. TIAs produce stroke-like symptoms but have no lasting effects. Know the warning signs of a TIA and seek emergency medical treatment immediately.

Atrial fibrillation or other heart disease: In atrial fibrillation the heart's upper chambers quiver rather than beating effectively. This causes the blood to pool and clot, increasing the risk of stroke. People with other types of heart disease have a higher risk of stroke, too.

Certain blood disorders: A high red blood cell count makes clots more likely, raising the risk of stroke. Sickle cell anemia increases stroke risk because the "sickled" cells stick to blood vessel walls and may block arteries.

Excessive alcohol intake: Drinking an average of more than one drink per day for women or more than two drinks a day for men raises blood pressure. Binge drinking can lead to stroke.

Illegal drug use: Intravenous drug use carries a high stroke risk. Cocaine use also has been linked to stroke. Illegal drugs commonly cause hemorrhagic strokes.

What are the risk factors I can't control?

Increasing age: Stroke affects people of all ages. But the older you are, the greater your stroke risk.

Gender: In most age groups, more men than women have stroke, but more women die from stroke.

Heredity and race: People whose close blood relations have had a stroke have a higher risk of stroke. African Americans have a higher risk of death and disability from stroke than whites, because they have high blood pressure more often. Hispanic Americans are also at higher risk of stroke.

Prior stroke: Someone who has had a stroke is at higher risk of having another one.

Chapter 3

Conditions that Increase the Risk of Cardiovascular Disorders

Chapter Contents

Section 3.1

Depression and Heart Disease

Depression may have more far-reaching consequences than previously believed. Recent data suggests that individuals who suffer from a mood disorder could be twice as likely to have a heart attack compared to individuals who are not depressed.

This process has been poorly understood—until now. A new study led by Concordia University has found that depressed individuals have a slower recovery time after exercise compared to those who are nondepressed.

These findings suggest that a dysfunctional biological stress system is at play among depressed individuals. Published in the journal *Psychophysiology*, the research warns of the importance of testing for cardiovascular disease among people suffering from major depression.

"There have been two competing theories as to why depression is linked to cardiovascular disease," says first author Jennifer Gordon, who is a Ph.D. candidate at McGill University. "Depressed people may have poorer health behaviors, which may in turn lead to heart problems. The other possibility is physiological: a problem with the stress system known as the fight or flight response. Our study was the first to examine the role of a dysfunctional fight or flight response in depression in a large population."

Heart Rate Recovery Is a Powerful Diagnostic Tool

A total of 886 participants, who were on average sixty years old, took part in the study conducted by Concordia in association with the Montreal Heart Institute, McGill University, the Hôpital Sacré-Coeur de Montréal, the Université du Québec à Montréal and the University of Calgary.

Approximately 5 percent of participants were diagnosed with a major depressive disorder. All individuals were asked to undergo a stress test after which their heart rate and blood pressure were recorded.

Recovery heart rates and blood pressure levels were compared between depressed and nondepressed individuals.

"We found that it took longer for the heart rate of depressed individuals to return to normal," says senior author, Simon Bacon, a professor in the Concordia University Department of Exercise Science and a researcher at the Montreal Heart Institute. "Heart rate recovery from exercise is one way to measure the fight or flight stress response. The delayed ability to establish a normal heart rate in the depressed individuals indicates a dysfunctional stress response. We believe that this dysfunction can contribute to their increased risk for heart disease."

"The take-home message of this study is that health care professionals should not only address the mental disorder, but also the potential for heart disease in patients who are suffering from major depression," adds Bacon. "Both of these health issues should be treated to minimize risk of severe consequences."

Section 3.2

Diabetes and Cardiovascular Disease

Diabetes as a Risk Factor for Cardiovascular Disease

If you have diabetes you are two to four times more likely to develop cardiovascular disease than people without diabetes. Cardiovascular disease is the leading cause of mortality for people with diabetes.

If you have diabetes your risk of cardiovascular disease rises for a number of reasons. Hypertension, abnormal blood lipids, and obesity, all risk factors in their own right for cardiovascular disease, occur more frequently in people with diabetes.

Diabetes and Heart Disease

Uncontrolled diabetes causes damage to your body's blood vessels, making them more prone to damage from atherosclerosis and hypertension. People with diabetes develop atherosclerosis at a younger age and more severely than people without diabetes.

Hypertension is more than twice as common in people with diabetes as in people with normal blood glucose levels.

People who have diabetes are more likely to have a heart attack or stroke than people who do not, and their prognosis is worse.

If you have diabetes you can have a heart attack without realizing it. Diabetes can damage nerves as well as blood vessels so a heart attack can be "silent," that is, lacking the typical chest pain.

Premenopausal women who have diabetes have an increased risk of heart disease because diabetes cancels out the protective effects of estrogen.

If you have diabetes you have a two- to threefold greater risk of heart failure compared to people without diabetes.

Diabetes and Stroke

If you have diabetes and hypertension you are about twice as likely to have a stroke as somebody with hypertension alone. Your risk of transient ischemic attacks is between two and six times higher than somebody who does not have diabetes.

Diabetes and Peripheral Arterial Disease

Diabetes can damage the blood vessels and over time. This puts people with diabetes at far greater risk of intermittent claudication and lower-limb amputation compared to the general population. Intermittent claudication occurs three times more often in men with diabetes and almost nine times more often in women with diabetes than in their counterparts without diabetes.

Protecting Yourself from Cardiovascular Disease If You Have Diabetes

If you control your blood glucose you can reduce your risk of a cardiovascular disease event by 42 percent and the risk of heart attack, stroke, or death from cardiovascular disease by 57 percent.

If you control your blood glucose levels you reduce your risk of cardiovascular disease by between 33 percent and 50 percent.

If you control your blood lipids you can reduce cardiovascular disease complications by 20 percent to 50 percent.

Losing weight and maintaining a healthy diet will improve your diabetes status.

If you have impaired glucose tolerance and lose weight, you can prevent the onset of diabetes.

Stopping smoking will reduce your cardiovascular disease risk.

Risk Factors for Diabetes

The risk factors for Type 1 diabetes have not been proven yet. It is thought that environmental triggers like viruses, toxins in the food chain, and dietary components may play a role.

The most significant modifiable risk factor for Type 2 diabetes is being overweight or obese. Smoking doubles the risk of cardiovascular disease if you have diabetes.

The most important nonmodifiable risk factor is ethnicity, with Hispanics, Asians, Arabs, Africans, Pacific Islanders, and indigenous (American, Canadian, and Australian) populations at particular risk.

Increasing age and a family history of diabetes also places you at greater risk.

Section 3.3

High Blood Pressure and Heart Disease

The information in this chapter is from "Blood Pressure and Heart Disease" and "Pregnancy and High Blood Pressure," U.S. Department of Health and Human Services, Office on Women's Health, 2013. For additional information, visit www.womenshealth.gov or www.hearthealthywomen.org.

What is blood pressure?

Blood pressure is a measure of the force of blood against the walls of your arteries (or blood vessels) as blood flows through the body. Blood pressure is given as two numbers. The first or top number is the systolic pressure—the pressure of the blood in the vessels as the heart beats. The second or bottom number is the diastolic pressure—the pressure in the vessels as the heart relaxes between beats. Blood pressure is measured in millimeters of mercury (mm Hg), reflecting how much the pressure in your arteries would raise a column of mercury. A blood pressure of 120 mm Hg systolic and 80 mm Hg diastolic is written 120/80 ("120 over 80").

What is high blood pressure?

Normal blood pressure is less than 120 mm Hg systolic and 80 mm Hg diastolic. For adults, high blood pressure (hypertension) is when blood pressure is higher than 140 mm Hg systolic and/or 90 mm Hg diastolic. High blood pressure is dangerous because it makes the heart work too hard and leads to hardening of the arteries, increasing your risk of heart disease and stroke.

What is prehypertension?

If your blood pressure is higher than 120/80 but lower than 140/90, you have prehypertension. This means that you don't have high blood pressure yet, but are very likely to develop it in the future.

Table 3.1. Classification of Blood Pressure For Adults[1]

Category	Systolic (mm Hg)		Diastolic (mm Hg)
Normal	Less than 120	and	Less than 80
Prehypertension	120–139	or	80–89
Stage 1 High BP	140–159	or	90–99
Stage 2 High BP	160 or higher	or	100 or higher

How does high blood pressure affect heart disease risk?

High blood pressure increases your risk of dying early or having a heart attack, stroke, or heart failure. For each rise in blood pressure of 20 mm Hg systolic (top) or 10 mm Hg diastolic (bottom), your risk of heart disease doubles. It is estimated that controlling blood pressure could prevent one-third of heart disease problems in women.[2] Women and men with high blood pressure at age fifty develop heart disease seven years earlier and die on average five years earlier than people with normal blood pressure at this age.[3]

High blood pressure damages your heart in a number of ways. It can cause your heart to become enlarged as a result of being overworked. Eventually, the heart gets weaker and cannot pump blood as effectively through your body. An enlarged, thickened heart can cause irregular heartbeats (arrhythmia). High blood pressure also contributes to the buildup of fatty plaque in the arteries. It makes your arteries stiffer and less flexible, making it harder for blood to flow through them easily.

High blood pressure that is not controlled affects not only your heart and blood vessels, but other organs as well. It can cause impaired vision and blindness, and kidney damage that may require dialysis or a kidney transplant.

What is "white coat hypertension"?

Many people become anxious when visiting their healthcare provider, causing their blood pressure to temporarily rise. This condition is called white coat hypertension (the name refers to the white coats that doctors usually wear) and is more common in women than men.[4]

If your healthcare provider thinks you may have white coat hypertension, you may be asked to wear a device called an ambulatory blood pressure monitor, or Holter monitor. It is usually worn for twenty-four hours in order to see what your blood pressure is like outside of the hospital, office, or clinic and in a more relaxed environment.

Women with white coat hypertension are not at the same increased risk for heart disease as women with traditional high blood pressure.[5,6] However, they may have a slightly higher risk than women who don't have white coat hypertension.[7]

What other types of hypertension are there?

Many older people develop a form of high blood pressure called isolated systolic hypertension (ISH). This occurs when the top (systolic) number is high but the bottom (diastolic) number is normal.

There are also specific types of high blood pressure that can develop during pregnancy (gestational hypertension and preeclampsia) that are risky for both the mother and baby, and require careful monitoring and treatment. However, these conditions do not increase the risk of heart disease or stroke.

References

1. Chobanian AV, Bakris GL, Black HR, et al. The Seventh Report of the Joint National Committee on Prevention, Detection, Evaluation, and Treatment of High Blood Pressure: The JNC 7 Report. *JAMA*. 2003;289:2560–71.

2. Wong ND, Thakral G, Franklin SS, et al. Preventing heart disease by controlling hypertension: impact of hypertensive subtype, stage, age, and sex. *Am Heart J*. 2003;145:888–95.

3. Franco OH, Peeters A, Bonneux L, de Laet C. Blood Pressure in Adulthood and Life Expectancy With Cardiovascular

Disease in Men and Women. Life Course Analysis. *Hypertension*. 2005.

4. Dolan E, Stanton A, Atkins N, et al. Determinants of white-coat hypertension. *Blood Press Monit*. 2004;9:307–9.

5. Celis H, Staessen JA, Thijs L, et al. Cardiovascular risk in white-coat and sustained hypertensive patients. *Blood Press*. 2002;11:352–56.

6. Pierdomenico SD, Cipollone F, Lapenna D, Bucci A, Cuccurullo F, Mezzetti A. Endothelial function in sustained and white coat hypertension. *Am J Hypertens*. 2002;15:946–52.

7. Gustavsen PH, Hoegholm A, Bang LE, Kristensen KS. White coat hypertension is a cardiovascular risk factor: a 10-year follow-up study. *J Hum Hypertens*. 2003;17:811–17.

Section 3.4

High Cholesterol and Heart Disease

High cholesterol is one of the major controllable risk factors for coronary heart disease, heart attack, and stroke. As your blood cholesterol rises, so does your risk of coronary heart disease. If you have other risk factors (such as high blood pressure or diabetes) as well as high cholesterol, this risk increases even more. The more risk factors you have, the greater your chance of developing coronary heart disease. Also, the greater the level of each risk factor, the more that factor affects your overall risk.

When too much low-density lipoprotein (LDL, or bad) cholesterol circulates in the blood, it can slowly build up in the inner walls of the arteries that feed the heart and brain. Together with other substances, it can form plaque, a thick, hard deposit that can narrow the arteries and make them less flexible. This condition is known as atherosclerosis.

If a clot forms and blocks a narrowed artery, a heart attack or stroke can result.

High blood cholesterol: As blood cholesterol rises, so does risk of coronary heart disease. When other risk factors (such as high blood pressure and tobacco smoke) are present, this risk increases even more. Your cholesterol level can be affected by your age, gender, family health history, and diet.

Section 3.5

Metabolic Syndrome and Cardiovascular Disease

"Metabolic Syndrome," © 2013 A.D.A.M., Inc. Reprinted with permission.

Metabolic syndrome is a name for a group of risk factors that occur together and increase the risk for coronary artery disease, stroke, and type 2 diabetes.

Causes

Metabolic syndrome is becoming more and more common in the United States. Researchers are not sure whether the syndrome is due to one single cause, but all of the risks for the syndrome are related to obesity.

The two most important risk factors for metabolic syndrome are:

- extra weight around the middle and upper parts of the body (central obesity). The body may be described as "apple-shaped."

- insulin resistance. The body uses insulin less effectively than normal. Insulin is needed to help control the amount of sugar in the body. As a result, blood sugar and fat levels rise.

Other risk factors include:

- aging;

- genes that make you more likely to develop this condition;

- hormone changes;
- lack of exercise.

People who have metabolic syndrome often have two other problems that can either cause the condition or make it worse:

- excess blood clotting;
- increased levels of blood substances that are a sign of inflammation throughout the body.

Exams and Tests

Metabolic syndrome is present if you have three or more of the following signs:

- Blood pressure equal to or higher than 130/85 mmHg
- Fasting blood sugar (glucose) equal to or higher than 100 mg/dL
- Large waist circumference (length around the waist):
  - Men: 40 inches or more
  - Women: 35 inches or more
- Low high-density lipoprotein (HDL) cholesterol:
  - Men: Under 40 mg/dL
  - Women: Under 50 mg/dL
- Triglycerides equal to or higher than 150 mg/dL

Treatment

The goal of treatment is to reduce your risk of heart disease and diabetes.

Your doctor will recommend lifestyle changes or medicines to help reduce your blood pressure, LDL cholesterol, and blood sugar:

- Lose weight: The goal is to lose between 7 percent and 10 percent of your current weight. You will probably need to eat five hundred to one thousand fewer calories per day.
- Get thirty minutes of moderate intensity exercise, such as walking, five to seven days per week.
- Lower your cholesterol using weight loss, exercise, and cholesterol-lowering medicines, if needed.

- Lower your blood pressure using weight loss, exercise, and medicine, if needed.

Some people may benefit from daily low-dose aspirin.
People who smoke should quit.

Outlook (Prognosis)

People with metabolic syndrome have an increased long-term risk for developing heart disease, type 2 diabetes, stroke, kidney disease, and poor blood supply to the legs.

When to Contact a Medical Professional

Call your health care provider if you have signs or symptoms of this condition.

Alternative Names

Insulin resistance syndrome; syndrome X

References

Inzucchi SE, Sherwin RS. Type 2 diabetes mellitus. In: Goldman L, Schafer AI, eds. *Cecil Medicine. 24th ed*. Philadelphia, PA: Saunders Elsevier; 2011:chap 237.

Alberti KG, Eckel RH, Grundy SM, Zimmet PZ, Cleeman JI, Donato KA, et al. Harmonizing the metabolic syndrome: a joint interim statement of the International Diabetes Federation Task Force on Epidemiology and Prevention: National Heart, Lung, and Blood Institute; American Heart Association; World Heart Federation; International Atherosclerosis Society; and International Association for the Study of Obesity. *Circulation*. 2009;120:1640–45.

Rosenzweig JL, Ferrannini E, Grundy SM, Haffner SM, Heine RJ, Horton ES, et al. Primary prevention of cardiovascular disease and type 2 diabetes in patients at metabolic risk: an Endocrine Society clinical practice guideline. *J Clin Endocrinol Metab*. 2008; 93:3671–89.

Section 3.6

Sleep Apnea and Cardiovascular Disease

"Sleep Apnea and Heart Disease, Stroke," reprinted with permission from www.heart.org. © 2013 American Heart Association, Inc. All rights reserved.

Plain old snoring can get a little annoying, especially for someone listening to it. But when a snorer repeatedly stops breathing for brief moments, it can lead to cardiovascular problems and potentially be life-threatening.

It's a condition known as sleep apnea, in which the person may experience pauses in breathing five to thirty times per hour or more during sleep. These episodes wake the sleeper as he or she gasps for air. It prevents restful sleep and is associated with high blood pressure, arrhythmia, stroke, and heart failure.

Heart disease is the leading cause of death in America, and stroke is the number four cause and a leading cause of disability. High blood pressure is a major risk factor for both.

"The evidence is very strong for the relationship between sleep apnea and hypertension and cardiovascular disease generally, so people really need to know that," said Donna Arnett, Ph.D., chair and professor of epidemiology at the School of Public Health at the University of Alabama at Birmingham and the incoming president of the American Heart Association.

A Common Problem

One in five adults suffers from at least mild sleep apnea, and it afflicts more men than women, Dr. Arnett said. The most common type is obstructive sleep apnea in which weight on the upper chest and neck contributes to blocking the flow of air. (Another type, called central sleep apnea, is far less prevalent.)

Obstructive sleep apnea is associated with obesity, which is also a major risk factor for heart disease and stroke. Besides obesity contributing to sleep apnea, sleep deprivation caused by sleep apnea can, in an ongoing unhealthy cycle, lead to further obesity, Dr. Arnett explained.

Listen to Those Snoring Complaints

Often a roommate or sleeping partner of someone with sleep apnea notices it. "It's really hard to detect if you live alone, unless you go through a sleep study," Dr. Arnett said. People with sleep apnea may be more tired during the day, she said, and therefore prone to accidents or falling asleep.

Dr. Arnett told of her own family's experience with sleep apnea. She accompanied her seventy-three-year-old mother, Lela Arnett, on a trip to Germany and heard her make loud snorts during the night.

It got so noisy that Donna Arnett ended up sleeping in the hotel room's bathroom with the door closed. It turns out her mother had sleep apnea and severe hypertension. Her mother knew she sometimes awoke when she took big breaths, but she didn't realize the severity of what was happening.

Getting Proper Treatment

Through treatment known as continuous positive airway pressure, or CPAP, her mother's blood pressure stabilized. The CPAP device involves wearing a mask while sleeping.

It keeps air pressure in the breathing passages so they don't close down. Some patients have bad reactions to the masks, Dr. Arnett said, but their design has evolved significantly, making it easier to find a suitable one.

In a sleep study, doctors count pauses in breathing to determine whether the patient has mild sleep apnea, characterized by five to fifteen episodes per hour; moderate sleep apnea, defined by fifteen to thirty per hour; or severe sleep apnea, meaning more than thirty each hour.

It's certainly possible to have simple, loud snoring without sleep apnea. But with regular snoring, the person continues to inhale and exhale.

With sleep apnea, the sleeping person tends to have periods when he or she stops breathing and nothing can be heard. The good news is treatment that keeps the breathing passages open and oxygen flowing can yield fast results, Dr. Arnett said. "Blood pressure comes down really quite quickly."

Section 3.7

Stress and Cardiovascular Disease

The stresses of life have long been thought to increase a person's risk of cardiovascular disease or a serious coronary or cerebral event. But it is not universally agreed which stress causes heart disease.

In Australia, an expert group concluded that there is strong and consistent link between depression, social isolation and lack of quality social support, and heart disease. These factors were as risky to heart health as abnormal blood lipid levels, smoking, and high blood pressure.

But the same group did not find a link between heart disease and chronic life events, job stress, Type A behavior patterns, hostility, anxiety disorders, or panic disorders.

Elsewhere, other researchers have found a strong link between anxiety and heart disease.

One study found a linear progression between self-reported psychological stress and damage to the carotid artery. The extensive Whitehall Study in the United Kingdom among government employees found that those with the least control over their work had the highest rates of heart disease.

Research is continuing in this area to define more clearly which kinds of stress are more likely to trigger cardiovascular disease. Whatever the outcome may be, we already know that different types of stress tend to cluster together. When they do, the resultant risk for cardiac events is often substantially elevated.

How Stress Causes Cardiovascular Disease

Living a stressful life can cause people to adopt poor habits like smoking and eating badly, which in turn are risk factors for cardiovascular disease.

But being stressed itself can alter the way the body behaves and this can bring about changes to the blood and nervous system, which can have negative effects on your heart health.

Studies show that acute stress triggers reduced blood flow to the heart, promotes your heart beating irregularly and increases the likelihood of your blood clotting. All of these can trigger the development of cardiovascular disease.

If you already have atherosclerosis and become acutely stressed you may experience chest pains caused by the arteries to your heart contracting and reducing the blood flow.

When experienced over an extended period of time, all these effects can cause damage to the lining of the blood vessels. This makes the blood vessels more susceptible to atherosclerosis.

Can You Protect Yourself?

Changing your behavior and your circumstances, where possible, may help you reduce your risk of developing cardiovascular disease.

Section 3.8

Thyroid Disease and Heart Disease

"Thyroid Condition Linked to Heart Problems: Study" by Randy Dotinga, April 23, 2012. Copyright © 2012 HealthDay (www.healthday.com). All rights reserved. Reprinted with permission.

New evidence suggests that a type of overactive thyroid condition appears to boost the risk of heart problems, especially atrial fibrillation (a form of irregular heartbeat) and premature death.

Patients sometimes are reluctant to do anything about the condition, known as subclinical hyperthyroidism, because it often doesn't cause any symptoms. The findings show, however, that "physicians and patients should take it seriously and consider the appropriate way to treat it to prevent increases in heart disease, bone problems, and death," said Dr. Kenneth Burman, chief of the endocrine section at Washington Hospital Center, in Washington, D.C.

Patients with subclinical hyperthyroidism have too much of the hormone created by the thyroid gland, which helps control people's metabolism. An estimated 10 percent of the population has the condition, which is considered to be less serious than overt hyperthyroidism.

Researchers have wondered for years whether subclinical hyperthyroidism puts people at risk of a variety of health problems. Previous research has suggested it does, and a new study takes a closer look and finds more reasons to suspect the condition is dangerous.

The report authors examined the results of ten studies, which included nearly fifty-three thousand participants. After adjusting their statistics so they wouldn't be skewed by high or low numbers of participants of certain ages or genders, the researchers found that those with subclinical hyperthyroidism were 24 percent more likely to die during the study periods, 29 percent more likely to die of heart-related problems, and 68 percent more likely to have atrial fibrillation.

Burman, who wrote a commentary accompanying the study, said the risk of early death and heart problems were still low even with the increased risk. The risk of death during the study period, for example, rose overall from 16 percent in those with normal thyroid levels to 18 percent in those with subclinical hyperthyroidism. But the heightened risk of atrial fibrillation was a significant jump, he said. Atrial fibrillation causes the heart to fail to beat properly, putting patients at higher risk of stroke.

What to do? Physicians often turn to medication first, then surgery or treatment with radioactive iodine, Burman said. But medication raises questions, he said: "Do you keep them on medication indefinitely when they feel fine and the medications have side effects?"

Study co-author Dr. Nicolas Rodondi, head of ambulatory care at the University of Bern, in Switzerland, said treatment should be considered if patients are in certain risk groups and only if their thyroid levels remain abnormal after they're rechecked in three to six months.

The next step in research is to confirm the analysis findings and explore how treatment may help patients lower their risks of problems, he said.

The study appears online April 23, 2012, in the journal *Archives of Internal Medicine*. A second study, also published in the journal, examined whether the drug levothyroxine sodium—a man-made form of the thyroid hormone—would help reduce the risk of cardiovascular problems in patients with subclinical hypothyroidism.

The study of about 4,800 patients, led by researchers at Newcastle University in England, found that the drug (brand names include Synthroid), appeared to reduce the risk of heart problems in relatively younger patients (aged forty to seventy) but not in older patients (over seventy).

In younger patients, about 4 percent of those treated with the drug had heart disease, compared with nearly 7 percent of those who weren't treated with it. After adjusting their statistics so they wouldn't be skewed by various factors, the researchers found that those who took the drug had a 39 percent lower risk of heart disease.

The drug can, however, cause a variety of side effects. Researchers could not definitively explain why older patients didn't receive the same health benefit.

A co-author for this study has received a speaking fee from drug manufacturer Merck Serono.

Chapter 4

Aging and Cardiovascular Risk Factors

Chapter Contents

Section 4.1

Changes in the Heart and Blood Vessels during Aging

Some changes in the heart and blood vessels normally occur with age, but many other changes that are common with aging are due to modifiable factors that, if not treated, can lead to heart disease.

Background

The heart has two sides. The right side pumps blood to the lungs to receive oxygen and get rid of carbon dioxide. The left side pumps oxygen-rich blood to the body.

Blood flows out of the heart through arteries, which branch out and get smaller and smaller as they go into the tissues. In the tissues, they become tiny capillaries.

Capillaries are where the blood gives up oxygen and nutrients to the tissues, and receives carbon dioxide and wastes back from the tissues. Then, the vessels begin to collect together into larger and larger veins, which return blood to the heart.

Aging Changes

Heart

- The heart has a natural pacemaker system that controls the heartbeat. Some of the pathways of this system may develop fibrous tissue and fat deposits. The natural pacemaker (the sinoatrial [SA] node) loses some of its cells. These changes may result in a slightly slower heart rate.

- A slight increase in the size of the heart, especially the left ventricle, is not uncommon. The heart wall thickens, so the amount of blood that the chamber can hold may actually decrease despite the increased overall heart size. The heart may fill more slowly.

- Heart changes cause the electrocardiogram (ECG) of a normal, healthy older person to be slightly different than the ECG of a healthy younger adult. Abnormal rhythms (arrhythmias) such as atrial fibrillation are more common in older people. They may be caused by heart disease.

- Normal changes in the heart include deposits of the "aging pigment," lipofuscin. The heart muscle cells degenerate slightly. The valves inside the heart, which control the direction of blood flow, thicken and become stiffer. A heart murmur caused by valve stiffness is fairly common in the elderly.

Blood Vessels

- Receptors called baroreceptors monitor the blood pressure and make changes to help maintain a fairly constant blood pressure when a person changes positions or activities. The baroreceptors become less sensitive with aging. This may explain why many older people have orthostatic hypotension, a condition in which the blood pressure falls when a person goes from lying or sitting to standing. This causes dizziness because there is less blood flow to the brain.

- The capillary walls thicken slightly. This may cause a slightly slower rate of exchange of nutrients and wastes.

- The main artery from the heart (aorta) becomes thicker, stiffer, and less flexible. This is probably related to changes in the connective tissue of the blood vessel wall. This makes the blood pressure higher and makes the heart work harder, which may lead to thickening of the heart muscle (hypertrophy). The other arteries also thicken and stiffen. In general, most elderly people have a moderate increase in blood pressure.

Blood

- The blood itself changes slightly with age. Normal aging causes a reduction in total body water. As part of this, there is less fluid in the bloodstream, so blood volume decreases.

- The speed with which red blood cells are produced in response to stress or illness is reduced. This creates a slower response to blood loss and anemia.

- Most of the white blood cells stay at the same levels, although certain white blood cells important to immunity (neutrophils) decrease in their number and ability to fight off bacteria. This reduces the ability to resist infection.

Effect of Changes

Normally, the heart continues to pump enough blood to supply all parts of the body. However, an older heart may not be able to pump blood as well when you make it work harder.

Some of the things that make your heart work harder are:

- certain medications;

- emotional stress;

- extreme physical exertion;

- illness;

- infections;

- injuries.

Common Problems

- Angina (chest pain caused by temporarily reduced blood flow to the heart muscle), shortness of breath with exertion, and heart attack can result from coronary artery disease.

- Abnormal heart rhythms (arrhythmias) of various types can occur.

- Anemia may occur, possibly related to malnutrition, chronic infections, blood loss from the gastrointestinal tract, or as a complication of other diseases or medications.

- Arteriosclerosis (hardening of the arteries) is very common. Fatty plaque deposits inside the blood vessels cause them to narrow and can totally block blood vessels.

- Congestive heart failure is also very common in the elderly. In people older than seventy-five, congestive heart failure occurs ten times more often than in younger adults.

- Coronary artery disease is fairly common. It is often a result of arteriosclerosis.

- High blood pressure and orthostatic hypotension are more common with older age.

- Heart valve diseases are fairly common. Aortic stenosis, or narrowing of the aortic valve, is the most common valve disease in the elderly.

- Transient ischemic attacks (TIA) or strokes can occur if blood flow to the brain is disrupted.

Other problems with the heart and blood vessels include the following:

- Blood clots:
  - Deep vein thrombosis
  - Thrombophlebitis
- Peripheral vascular disease, resulting in intermittent pain in the legs when walking (claudication)
- Varicose veins

Prevention

You can help your circulatory system (heart and blood vessels). Heart disease risk factors that you have some control over include high blood pressure, cholesterol levels, diabetes, obesity, and smoking:

- Eat a heart-healthy diet with reduced amounts of saturated fat and cholesterol, and control your weight. Follow your health care provider's recommendations for treating high blood pressure, high cholesterol, or diabetes. Reduce or stop smoking.

- Exercise may help prevent obesity, and it helps people with diabetes control their blood sugar.

- Exercise may help you maintain your abilities as much as possible and it reduces stress.

- Have regular check-ups for your heart:
  - Have your blood pressure checked every year. If you have diabetes, heart disease, kidney problems, or certain other conditions, your blood pressure may need to be monitored more closely.
  - If your cholesterol level is normal, have it rechecked every five years. If you have diabetes, heart disease, kidney problems, or certain other conditions, your cholesterol may need to be monitored more closely.

- Moderate exercise is one of the best things you can do to keep your heart, and the rest of your body, healthy. Consult with your health care provider before beginning a new exercise program. Exercise moderately and within your capabilities, but do it regularly.

- People who exercise usually have less body fat and smoke less than people who do not exercise. They also tend to have fewer blood pressure problems and less heart disease.

Alternative Names

Heart disease—aging; Atherosclerosis—aging

References

Minaker KL. Common clinical sequelae of aging. In Goldman L, Schafer AI, eds. *Cecil Medicine. 24th ed*. Philadelphia, Pa: Saunders Elsevier;2011:chap 24.

Schwartz JB, Zipes DP. Cardiovascular disease in the elderly. In: Bonow RO, Mann DL, Zipes DP, Libby P, eds. *Braunwald's Heart Disease: A Textbook of Cardiovascular Medicine. 9th ed*. Philadelphia, Pa: Saunders; 2011:chap 80.

Section 4.2

Visible Signs of Aging May Predict Heart Disease

If you look old, your heart may feel old, according to research presented at the American Heart Association's Scientific Sessions 2012.

In a new study, those who had three to four aging signs—receding hairline at the temples, baldness at the head's crown, earlobe crease, or yellow fatty deposits around the eyelid (xanthelasmata)—had a 57 percent increased risk for heart attack and a 39 percent increased risk for heart disease.

"The visible signs of aging reflect physiologic or biological age, not chronological age, and are independent of chronological age," said Anne Tybjaerg-Hansen, M.D., the study's senior author and professor of clinical biochemistry at the University of Copenhagen in Denmark.

Researchers analyzed 10,885 participants forty years and older (45 percent women) in the Copenhagen Heart Study. Of these, 7,537 had frontoparietal baldness (receding hairline at the temples), 3,938 had crown top baldness, 3,405 had earlobe crease, and 678 had fatty deposits around the eye.

In thirty-five years of follow-up, 3,401 participants developed heart disease and 1,708 had a heart attack.

Individually and combined, these signs predicted heart attack and heart disease independent of traditional risk factors. Fatty deposits around the eye were the strongest individual predictor of both heart attack and heart disease.

Heart attack and heart disease risk increased with each additional sign of aging in all age groups and among men and women. The highest risk was for those in their seventies and those with multiple signs of aging.

In the study, nurses and laboratory technicians noted the quantity of gray hair, the prominence of wrinkles, the type and extent of baldness, the presence of earlobe crease and eyelid deposits.

"Checking these visible aging signs should be a routine part of every doctor's physical examination," Tybjaerg-Hansen said.

Chapter 5

Recent Research Regarding Cardiovascular Disease Risks

Chapter Contents

Section 5.1

Berries May Cut Heart Attack Risk

Eating three or more servings of blueberries and strawberries per week may help women reduce their risk of a heart attack by as much as one-third, researchers reported in *Circulation: Journal of the American Heart Association*.

Blueberries and strawberries contain high levels of naturally occurring compounds called dietary flavonoids, also found in grapes and wine, blackberries, eggplant, and other fruits and vegetables. A specific subclass of flavonoids, called anthocyanins, may help dilate arteries, counter the buildup of plaque, and provide other cardiovascular benefits, according to the study.

"Blueberries and strawberries can easily be incorporated into what women eat every week," said Eric Rimm D.Sc., senior author and associate professor of nutrition and epidemiology at the Harvard School of Public Health in Boston, Massachusetts. "This simple dietary change could have a significant impact on prevention efforts."

Blueberries and strawberries were part of this analysis simply because they are the most-eaten berries in the United States. Thus, it's possible that other foods could produce the same results, researchers said.

Scientists from the Harvard School of Public Health in the United States and the University of East Anglia, United Kingdom, conducted a prospective study among 93,600 women ages twenty-five to forty-two who were registered with the Nurses' Health Study II. The women completed questionnaires about their diet every four years for eighteen years.

During the study, 405 heart attacks occurred. Women who ate the most blueberries and strawberries had a 32 percent reduction in their risk of heart attack compared to women who ate the berries once a month or less—even in women who otherwise ate a diet rich in other fruits and vegetables.

"We have shown that even at an early age, eating more of these fruits may reduce risk of a heart attack later in life," said Aedín Cassidy, Ph.D., lead author and head of the Department of Nutrition at Norwich Medical School of the University of East Anglia in Norwich, United Kingdom.

The findings were independent of other risk factors, such as age, high blood pressure, family history of heart attack, body mass, exercise, smoking, and caffeine or alcohol intake.

The American Heart Association supports eating berries as part of an overall balanced diet that also includes other fruits, vegetables, and whole-grain products. Eating a variety of foods is the best way to get the right amounts of nutrients.

Section 5.2

Calcium Supplements May Increase Cardiovascular Risk

Calcium Supplements May Increase Cardiovascular Risk in Men

Many of us know that calcium is important for bone health, especially as we age. And since we may not always get enough calcium through our diet, many Americans take dietary supplements to help ensure that they get enough calcium. In fact, as many as 50 percent of older men and 70 percent of older women in the United States take supplemental calcium, like through pills or chewable tablets. Although it was once believed that calcium may decrease cardiovascular risk by reducing cholesterol and blood pressure, many experts are now concerned about the negative impact calcium supplements may have on our hearts. Could calcium supplements be hurting our hearts, and increasing risk for heart disease, heart attack, and stroke?

According to a study published in the *Journal of the American Medical Association*, the answer is: maybe. This study included more than 388,000 middle-aged men and women, all of whom completed dietary questionnaires in the mid-1990s and were followed for an average of twelve years. What researchers found was that calcium supplements increased risk of death from heart disease in men, but not in women. But the good news? Dietary calcium intake, like through milk and foods, was unrelated to death from heart disease in men and women.

So what should we take away from this study? There is more research needed to fully understand the impact of calcium supplements on heart health. Some studies have shown that getting too much calcium through supplements can increase risk for heart disease, heart attack, stroke, and even death in both men and women. Other studies have shown that calcium supplements actually lower risk for heart disease. While experts try to figure out exactly how calcium supplementation impacts heart health, a safe alternative to calcium supplements is to get calcium from food. Low-fat dairy foods, beans, and green leafy vegetables are a great way to get your calcium and other minerals and vitamins that promote good health. And if you are taking supplements, stick to the recommended daily amounts. Most adults over nineteen years of age need 1,000 mg a day of calcium (except for women fifty-one to seventy years old who need 1,200 mg a day), and older adults (over seventy-one) need 1,200 mg of calcium a day.

Calcium Supplements May Raise Odds of Heart Death in Women

Women eating a high-calcium diet and taking calcium supplements adding up to more than 1,400 milligrams a day may be running nearly twice the risk of dying from heart disease, a large Swedish study suggests.

Both men and women take calcium supplements to prevent bone loss. The new findings come on the heels of another recent study that found a similar increased risk of death related to calcium intake among men.

"Many older adults increase dietary intake of calcium or take calcium supplements to prevent bone loss, and there had been speculation that increased calcium intake with or without vitamin D could improve cardiovascular health," said Dr. Gregg Fonarow, an American Heart Association spokesman who wasn't involved in the study.

However, a number of recent studies have suggested that higher dietary intake or calcium supplementation may not only not improve cardiovascular health—they may be associated with increased risk for cardiovascular events and mortality, said Fonarow, a professor of cardiology at University of California, Los Angeles.

The new report was published in the February 12, 2013, online edition of the *BMJ*.

To see if calcium supplements raised the risk of dying from heart disease, a team led by Dr. Karl Michaelsson, a clinical professor in the department of orthopedic surgical sciences at Uppsala University in Sweden, analyzed data collected on more than 61,000 women enrolled in a study on mammograms.

Over nineteen years of follow-up, nearly 12,000 women died— almost 4,000 dying from cardiovascular disease, about 1,900 from heart disease and 1,100 from stroke, the researchers found.

The highest rates of death were seen among women whose calcium intake was higher than 1,400 milligrams a day, the researchers noted. On the other hand, women who took less than 600 milligrams of calcium a day were also at an increased risk of death.

Moreover, women taking 1,400 milligrams of calcium a day and also using a supplement had even a higher risk of dying than women not using supplements, Michaelsson's group found.

All in all, women getting more than 1,400 milligrams of calcium a day were more than twice as likely to die than women getting 600 to 999 milligrams a day, the researchers said.

The U.S. Office of Dietary Supplements recommends 1,000 to 1,200 milligrams of calcium a day for most adults.

According to the study authors, diets very low or very high in calcium can override normal control by the body, causing changes in blood levels of calcium.

Rather than worry about increasing calcium intake of those getting enough through their diet, emphasis should be placed on people with a low intake of calcium, the authors suggest.

Taylor Wallace, a representative of the supplement industry, faults this study because, he said, it was not specifically meant to address calcium supplements and heart disease.

"We are comparing apples and oranges," said Wallace, who is senior director for Scientific and Regulatory Affairs at the Council for Responsible Nutrition. He noted that in the new study, the data that researchers used to draw their conclusions looked at diet and cancer, not whether calcium supplements were bad for the heart.

"Still, there is not a single human cause-and-effect study that demonstrates a hazard for calcium either from the diet or supplements and cardiovascular disease," he said.

Although the new study tied total calcium intake to increased risk of death from heart disease in women, it didn't establish a cause-and-effect relationship.

Wallace did say it's important to know how much calcium a person is getting from diet and supplements. "It is important to talk with your doctor to make sure you are getting the right amount for you," he said.

For his part, heart association spokesman Fonarow said: "While further studies are needed, calcium supplements should be used only after careful consideration of whether the potential benefits in terms of bone health outweigh the potential cardiovascular risks."

Section 5.3

Migraine with Aura May Raise Risk of Heart Trouble

Women who suffer from migraines with visual effects called aura may face an increased risk for heart attacks, strokes, and blood clots, new studies find.

Only high blood pressure was a more powerful predictor of cardiovascular trouble, the researchers said.

There are things women with this type of migraine can do to reduce that risk, they added: lower blood pressure and cholesterol levels, avoid smoking, eat healthfully, and exercise.

"Other studies have found that this form of migraine has been associated with the risk of stroke, and may be associated with any cardiovascular disease," said lead author Dr. Tobias Kurth, from the French National Institute of Health and Medical Research in Bordeaux and Brigham and Women's Hospital in Boston. "We find migraine with aura is a quite strong contributor to major cardiovascular disease. It is one of the top two risk factors."

Other studies have found the risk for cardiovascular disease for people who suffer from migraines with aura is roughly double that of people without the condition, Kurth noted.

People who suffer from migraines with aura see flickering lights or other visual effects just before the headache kicks in, he explained.

The findings were presented in March 2013 at the American Academy of Neurology annual meeting in San Diego.

For the study, Kurth's team collected data on nearly 28,000 women who took part in the Women's Health Study. Among these women, more than 1,400 suffered from migraines with aura.

During fifteen years of follow-up, more than 1,000 women had a heart attack, had a stroke, or died from cardiovascular causes, the researchers found.

After high blood pressure, migraine with aura was the strongest predictor for having a heart attack or stroke among these women. The risk was even more pronounced than that associated with diabetes, smoking, obesity, and a family history of heart disease, the investigators noted.

Whether controlling migraines reduces the risk for heart disease isn't known, Kurth said.

The study found a link between migraines with aura and cardiovascular trouble, but it didn't prove cause and effect.

Although women who have migraine with aura seem to have this increased risk, it doesn't doom everyone who has migraines with aura to have a heart attack or stroke, Kurth noted.

One expert was worried by the finding.

"What is concerning about this is that migraine with aura is more of a risk than diabetes," said Dr. Noah Rosen, director of the Headache Center at Cushing Neuroscience Institute at North Shore-LIJ Health System in Manhasset, New York. "Maybe this will change the way we stratify risk based on a history of migraine."

Rosen doesn't think that controlling migraine will reduce the cardiovascular risks. "Migraine, in all likelihood, is a genetic phenomena, so it is not a modifiable risk factor," he said. That makes it even more important to control other risk factors for cardiovascular disease, he added.

Results of another study scheduled to be presented at the neurology meeting show that women who have migraines with aura who take hormonal contraceptives have a higher risk of blood clots than women with migraine without aura.

The study found that 7.6 percent of women with migraine with aura who used a newer generation contraceptive that combines the hormones estrogen and progestin had deep vein thrombosis (a clot in a leg vein), compared with 6.3 percent of women with migraine without aura.

This risk for clots, such as deep vein thrombosis, has been associated with all women taking hormonal contraceptives, but it is even more elevated in women with migraine, the researchers noted.

In addition, the complications from these clots is greater among women with migraine with aura. The danger of these clots is they can travel to the heart, lungs, or brain and cause heart attacks, strokes, or severe breathing problems.

For this study, researchers from Brigham and Women's Falkner Hospital collected data on more than 145,000 women who used hormonal contraceptives. Among these women, nearly 2,700 had migraine with aura and more than 3,400 had migraine without aura.

The reasons why migraine is linked to clotting and cardiovascular disease aren't known, Rosen said.

"Women making the decision to be on a hormonal contraceptive should discuss their headache history with their doctor," he added.

The data and conclusions of research presented at medical meetings should be considered preliminary until published in a peer-reviewed journal.

Section 5.4

Even Moderate Smoking Is Associated with Sudden Cardiac Death

Women who are even light-to-moderate cigarette smokers may be significantly more likely than nonsmokers to suffer sudden cardiac death, according to new research in *Circulation: Arrhythmia & Electrophysiology*, an American Heart Association journal.

The findings indicate long-term smokers may be at even greater risk. But quitting smoking can reduce and eliminate the risk over time.

"Cigarette smoking is a known risk factor for sudden cardiac death, but until now, we didn't know how the quantity and duration of smoking affected the risk among apparently healthy women, nor did we have long-term follow-up," said Roopinder K. Sandhu, M.D., M.P.H., the study's lead author and a cardiac electrophysiologist at the University of Alberta's Mazankowski Heart Institute in Edmonton, Alberta, Canada.

Researchers examined the incidence of sudden cardiac death among more than 101,000 healthy women in the Nurses' Health Study, which has collected biannual health questionnaires from female nurses nationwide since 1976. They included records dating back to 1980 with thirty years of follow-up. Most of the participants were white, and all were between thirty to fifty-five years old at the study's start. On average, those who smoked reported that they started in their late teens.

During the study, 351 participants died of sudden cardiac death. Other findings include:

- Light-to-moderate smokers, defined in this study as those who smoked one to fourteen cigarettes daily, had nearly two times the risk of sudden cardiac death as their nonsmoking counterparts.

- Women with no history of heart disease, cancer, or stroke who smoked had almost two and a half times the risk of sudden cardiac death compared with healthy women who never smoked.

- For every five years of continued smoking, the risk climbed by 8 percent.

- Among women with heart disease, the risk of sudden cardiac death dropped to that of a nonsmoker within fifteen to twenty years after smoking cessation. In the absence of heart disease, there was an immediate reduction in sudden cardiac death risk, occurring in fewer than five years.

Sudden cardiac death results from the abrupt loss of heart function, usually within minutes after the heart stops. It's a primary cause of heart-related deaths, accounting for between three hundred thousand and four hundred thousand deaths in the United States each year.

"Sudden cardiac death is often the first sign of heart disease among women, so lifestyle changes that reduce that risk are particularly important," said Sandhu, who is also a visiting scientist at Brigham and Women's Hospital in Boston, Massachusetts. "Our study shows that cigarette smoking is an important modifiable risk factor for sudden cardiac death among all women. Quitting smoking before heart disease develops is critical."

Section 5.5

Sugar-Sweetened Drinks Linked to Increased Risk of Heart Disease

Excerpted from "Sugar-Sweetened Drinks Linked to Increased Risk of Heart Disease in Men," reprinted with permission from www.heart.org. © 2013 American Heart Association, Inc. All rights reserved.

Men who drank a twelve-ounce sugar-sweetened beverage a day had a 20 percent higher risk of heart disease compared to men who didn't drink any sugar-sweetened drinks, according to research published in *Circulation*, an American Heart Association journal.

"This study adds to the growing evidence that sugary beverages are detrimental to cardiovascular health," said Frank B. Hu, M.D., Ph.D., study lead author and professor of nutrition and epidemiology in the Harvard School of Public Health in Boston, Massachusetts. "Certainly, it provides strong justification for reducing sugary beverage consumption among patients, and more importantly, in the general population."

Heart disease is the leading cause of death in the United States. Risk factors include obesity, smoking, physical inactivity, diabetes, and poor diet.

Researchers, who studied 42,883 men in the Health Professionals Follow-Up Study, found that the increase persisted even after controlling for other risk factors, including smoking, physical inactivity, alcohol use, and family history of heart disease. Less frequent consumption—twice weekly and twice monthly—didn't increase risk.

Researchers also measured different lipids and proteins in the blood, which are indicators, or biomarkers, for heart disease. These included the inflammation marker C-reactive protein (CRP), harmful lipids called triglycerides, and good lipids called high-density lipoproteins (HDL). Compared to nondrinkers, those who consumed sugary beverages daily had higher triglyceride and CRP and lower HDL levels.

Artificially sweetened beverages were not linked to increased risk or biomarkers for heart disease in this study.

Beginning in January 1986 and every two years until December 2008, participants answered questionnaires about diet and other health habits. They also provided a blood sample midway through the survey. Follow-up was twenty-two years.

Participants were primarily Caucasian men forty to seventy-five years old. All were employed in a health-related profession.

Health habits of the men in the study may differ from those of the general public, but findings in women from the 2009 Nurses' Health Study were comparable, Hu said.

The American Heart Association recommends no more than half of discretionary calories come from added sugars. For most American men, that's no more than 150 calories per day, and 100 for most American women. Discretionary calories are those left in your "energy allowance" after consuming the recommended types and amounts of foods to meet all daily nutrient requirements.

Section 5.6

Yo-Yo Dieting Can Hurt the Heart

"Yo-Yo Dieting Can Hurt the Heart, Study Finds" by Steven Reinberg, December 13, 2012. Copyright © 2012 HealthDay (www.healthday.com). All rights reserved. Reprinted with permission.

Older women who lose weight and gain it back again may be increasing their risk for heart disease, Wake Forest University researchers report.

Although cholesterol, blood pressure, triglycerides, and blood sugar all improve with weight loss, with weight regain they all return to pre-diet levels and, in some cases, to even higher levels, the researchers found.

"For postmenopausal women considering weight loss, maintaining weight loss is just as important as losing weight," said lead researcher Daniel Beavers, an assistant professor in the department of biostatistics and public health sciences at Wake Forest University School of Medicine in Winston-Salem, North Carolina. "Even partial weight regain is associated with worsened diabetes and cardiovascular risk factors."

In an earlier study of these same women, the researchers found that those who regained weight during the year following weight loss regained fat mass to a greater degree than lean mass, Beavers said.

The report was published in the December 13, 2012, online edition of the *Journal of Gerontology: Medical Sciences*.

For the study, the researchers studied more than one hundred post-menopausal obese women while they took part in a five-month weight-loss program. They continued to monitor the women for a year. During the weight-loss program the women lost an average of twenty-five pounds.

After a year, two-thirds of the women had regained at least four pounds, on average regaining about 70 percent of the weight they had lost, the researchers found.

"Women who regained 4.4 pounds or more in the year following the weight-loss intervention had several worsened cardiovascular and diabetes risk factors," Beavers said.

"What was striking about the women who regained weight was that although they did not return to their full baseline weight on average—women only regained about 70 percent of lost weight—several chronic disease risk factors were right back at baseline values and in some cases, particularly for the diabetic risk factors, slightly worse than baseline values," he added. "Meanwhile, women who maintained their weight loss a year later managed to preserve most of the benefits."

Dr. Gregg Fonarow, professor of cardiology at the University of California, Los Angeles, said that "this study highlights the importance of not just losing weight, but the need to develop effective and enduring strategies so that this weight loss can be successfully maintained long term."

Another expert advises taking a lifestyle approach to dieting.

"This small study is a great example of why we need to avoid fad diets and diet programs, potions, and pills that promise quick weight loss," said Samantha Heller, an exercise physiologist and clinical nutrition coordinator at the Center for Cancer Care at Griffin Hospital in Derby, Connecticut.

Most people regain the weight within five years, she said. "This study indicates that regaining as little as five pounds can spell cardio-metabolic trouble, especially for postmenopausal women," Heller said.

People should be focusing on being healthy, not skinny, she said, and they should create strategies for reaching and maintaining a healthy weight throughout their lifetime.

"The roller coaster of weight loss and regain is deleterious both physically and psychologically," Heller said.

"While it can be frustrating to take the slower, healthier route to weight loss, the long-term results are ultimately more satisfying and healthier," she said. "Start with simple changes such as swapping seltzer for soda, keeping a daily food record, adding a salad to lunch, and substituting a second vegetable for half the starch at dinner."

Chapter 6

Research Regarding Genetics and Heart Disease

Chapter Contents

Section 6.1

Scientists Identify Mechanism Behind Genetic Link to Heart Disease

Scientists from Queen Mary, University of London, have discovered that carriers of a specific genetic variant linked to heart disease are at increased risk of developing a more severe form of the condition.

The research, which has furthered understanding of how this gene variant increases the risk of coronary artery disease (CAD), opens up possibilities for the development of new treatments.

Coronary artery disease (also known as coronary heart disease) happens when the blood supply to the heart is blocked by a buildup of fatty deposits within the walls of one or more of the coronary arteries, causing chest pain. CAD can lead to a heart attack if these buildups of plaque break down, suddenly blocking the flow of blood to the heart.

Lifestyle factors—including smoking, a bad diet, and lack of exercise—contribute to an individual's risk of heart disease, but a number of genes have also been found to play a role. In this study the scientists focused on the gene region known as 9p21. This region has been strongly associated with heart disease, but it has been unclear whether it contributes to risk by increasing the buildup of plaque or by making it more likely that the plaque may break down, leading to a heart attack.

The team analyzed genetic data from more than thirty thousand individuals drawn from multiple international studies focused on the 9p21 gene region. They found that individuals carrying two versions (homozygous) of the risk variant of the 9p21 gene were 23 percent more likely to develop a more serious form of the disease, with blockages in more than one of the three coronary arteries carrying blood to the heart.

The study also showed that individuals carrying the genetic risk variant were no more likely to have a heart attack than individuals with CAD who do not carry the genetic risk variant.

Shu Ye, professor of molecular medicine and genetics at Queen Mary, led the study. Professor Ye said: "This finding is important as it suggests this genetic variant, carried by around 75 percent of the population, increases the risk of heart disease by promoting the buildup of deposits within the walls of the arteries.

"Understanding the mechanisms involved means it is now possible to look at developing new therapies and treatments which can potentially reduce this buildup. Genetic tests which can identify this variant already exist and so it's vital that we are able to more accurately interpret these risks."

Kenneth Chan is joint first author of the study and a current medical student at Barts and the London School of Medicine and Dentistry, part of Queen Mary. He got involved with Professor Ye's work through the school's summer research studentship scheme.

Kenneth said: "It has been a privilege working in Professor Ye's lab and being involved in this international collaboration in the voyage to understand the human genome, which propels us closer to delivering the promised novel treatments in the near future."

The findings are published in the *Journal of the American College of Cardiology*.

Section 6.2

Studies Double the Known Genetic Links to Coronary Heart Disease

"Studies Double the Known Genetic Links to Coronary Heart Disease," March 2011. Reprinted with permission. © 2011 Wellcome Trust Centre for Human Genetics (http://www.well.ox.ac.uk). All rights reserved.

Researchers in two major international studies have discovered seventeen new genetic variants linked with increased heart disease risk. The research more than doubles the known firm genetic links to coronary heart disease.

The studies, published online in *Nature Genetics*, were funded by several leading research institutions, including the Wellcome Trust, the British Heart Foundation, and the Medical Research Council, and used data generated by the Wellcome Trust Case Control Consortium.

The studies—one from the CARDIoGRAM consortium and one from the Coronary Artery Disease (C4D) Genetics Consortium—compared the deoxyribonucleic acid (DNA) of thousands of people with coronary heart disease against the DNA of people unaffected by the disease in search of genetic variations that are more likely to be found in people with the disease.

The CARDIoGRAM research involved in-depth analyses of the DNA of more than 140,000 people, more than 50,000 of whom had coronary heart disease. The C4D scientists looked at the DNA of more than 70,000 people, more than half of whom had the disease.

Some genes were associated with pathways known to be involved in the development of coronary heart disease, but the researchers also identified many other relevant genetic variants.

Professor Hugh Watkins from the Wellcome Trust Centre for Human Genetics (WTCHG), who co-led the C4D research, says: "Our research strengthens the argument that lots of genes have a small effect on your heart disease risk, rather than a few genes having a large effect. Knowing about them will be important for directing research to find new treatments.

"We also show that our five new genetic culprits are found equally in European and South Asian populations, indicating that large international studies may be the best way forward in the hunt for the genetic causes of heart disease."

"The most exciting thing about our study—the largest ever of its type—is that we have discovered several new genes not previously known to be involved in the development of coronary heart disease," says Professor Nilesh Samani from the University of Leicester, who co-led the CARDIoGRAM research.

"Understanding how these genes work, which is the next step, will vastly improve our knowledge of how the disease develops, and could ultimately help to develop new treatments."

Section 6.3

Researchers Find New Genetic Variants Associated with Lipid Levels and Risk for Coronary Artery Disease

Excerpted from "International Effort Finds New Genetic Variants Associated with Lipid Levels, Risk for Coronary Artery Disease," National Institutes of Health, January 13, 2008. Reviewed by David A. Cooke, M.D., FACP, October 2013.

Environmental and genetic factors influence a person's blood fat, or lipid levels, important risk factors for coronary artery disease (CAD). While there is some understanding of the environmental contribution, the role of genetics has been less defined. Now, in an international collaboration supported primarily by the National Institutes of Health (NIH), scientists have discovered more than twenty-five genetic variants in eighteen genes connected to cholesterol and lipid levels. Seven of the eighteen genes previously had not been connected to these levels, while the eleven others confirm previous discoveries. In the investigation, published online January 13, 2008, and in the February 2008 print issue of *Nature Genetics*, the associated genes were found through studies of more than twenty thousand individuals and more than two million genetic variants, spanning the entire genome. These variants potentially open the door to strategies for the treatment and prevention of CAD.

"Heart disease is a leading cause of illness, disability, and death in industrialized countries, particularly for older people," says National Institute on Aging (NIA) Director Richard J. Hodes, M.D. "We know that certain lifestyle factors like smoking, diet, and physical activity greatly affect a person's lipid profiles. This study is an important, basic step in finding the genes that influence lipid levels and heart disease so that we can better understand the genetic contribution to cardiovascular risk."

Cristen Willer, Ph.D., at the University of Michigan's School of Public Health, Ann Arbor, and Serena Sanna, Ph.D., at the C.N.R. Institute of Neurogenetics and Neuropharmacology, Monserrato, Italy, and other members of the SardiNIA Study of Aging, including investigators at NIA, conducted the study, along with members of the Finland-United States Investigation of Non-Insulin-Dependent Diabetes Mellitus Genetics (FUSION) study, which included investigators in North Carolina, Michigan, Finland, Los Angeles, and from the National Human Genome Research Institute (NHGRI). SardiNIA and FUSION investigators also coordinated the efforts of other groups in France, the United Kingdom, and across the United States.

The purpose of the study was to identify comprehensively genetic variants that influence lipid levels and to examine the relationships between these genetic variants and risk of CAD. High levels of low-density lipoprotein (LDL; "bad" cholesterol) appear to increase the risk of CAD by narrowing or blocking arteries that carry blood to the heart. High levels of high-density lipoprotein (HDL; "good" cholesterol) appear to lower the risk. High levels of triglycerides, which make up a large part of the body's fat and are also found in the bloodstream, are also associated with increased risk of CAD.

To identify genetic variants that play a role in lipid levels, researchers turned to a relatively new approach, known as a genome-wide association study (GWAS). The GWAS strategy enables researchers to survey the entire human genetic blueprint, or genome, not just the genetic variants in a few genes. The human genome contains approximately three billion base pairs, or letters, of deoxyribonucleic acid (DNA). Small, single-letter variations naturally occur about once in every one thousand letters of the DNA code. Most of these genetic variants have not yet been associated with particular traits or disease risks. However, in some instances, people with a certain trait, such as higher levels of LDL cholesterol, tend to have one version of the variant, while those with lower levels are more likely to have the other version. In such instances, researchers may infer that there is an association between the values of the trait and the variants in the gene.

Typically, GWAS studies have been carried out in samples where all individuals are examined with the same gene chip, an experimental device that allows investigators to measure more than one hundred thousand genetic variants in a single experiment. But in this study, investigators developed and employed new statistical methods that allowed them to combine data across different gene chips and thus examine much larger numbers of participants.

With the statistical power gained by new programs that facilitated pooling of the large SardiNIA, FUSION, and Diabetes Genetic Initiative (DGI) datasets, researchers were able to identify variations in eighteen genes that influence HDL, LDL and/or triglyceride levels. This list of lipid-associated genes is substantially longer than what was generated by analyses of individual datasets, which had only pointed to one to three genes each. Of the seven newly implicated genes, two were associated with HDL levels, one with LDL levels, three with triglyceride levels, and one with both triglycerides and LDL levels.

"These results are yet another example of how genome-wide association studies are opening exciting new avenues for biomedical research," says NHGRI Director Francis S. Collins, M.D., Ph.D., who is a coauthor of the study and an investigator in NHGRI's Genome Technology Branch. "While some of the genetic variants we identified are known to play a well-established role in lipid metabolism, others have no obvious connection. Further studies to identify the precise genes and biological pathways involved could shed new light on lipid metabolism."

Scientists estimate that the genetic contribution to lipid levels is about 30 to 40 percent; the genetic variants uncovered in the new study are responsible for about 5 to 8 percent of that contribution, the scientists note, which means there is more work to be done. "In this study we carried out a comprehensive search for common variants of large effect. The genetic factors still to be discovered might turn out to be common variants with smaller effects or rare variants with a large effect," says Karen L. Mohlke, Ph.D., of the University of North Carolina, Chapel Hill, who co-directed the study with Gonçalo R. Abecasis, Ph.D., of the University of Michigan's School of Public Health.

To determine if the genetic variants associated with lipid levels also influence risk of heart disease, the researchers compared their results with results from the Wellcome Trust Case Control Consortium's recent genome-wide association study of CAD involving fifteen thousand British individuals. They found that all gene variants associated with increased LDL levels also were more prevalent among people with CAD. People with the gene variant for high triglyceride levels also had an increased risk for CAD, although the relationship was not as strong. No relationship was found between HDL and CAD.

"It was surprising that while it was clear that genetic variants that increase your 'bad' cholesterol are also associated with increased risk of heart disease, we did not find that variants influencing your 'good' cholesterol were associated with decreased risk of coronary artery disease. Perhaps that result will lead us to reexamine the roles of good and bad cholesterol in susceptibility to heart disease," remarks Abecasis.

Identifying a correlation among genes influencing lipid levels and risk for coronary heart disease is a first step in a long path to potentially important clinical implications. "What we're looking for, ultimately, are novel therapeutics and/or lifestyle modifications that can be recommended to individuals to help manage blood lipid levels and reduce risk of heart disease," says David Schlessinger, Ph.D., chief of the NIA's Laboratory of Genetics and NIA project officer for SardiNIA.

Chapter 7

Warning Signs of Cardiovascular Emergencies

Chapter Contents

Section 7.1

Signs and Symptoms of a Heart Attack

"Know the Signs and Symptoms of a Heart Attack," Centers
for Disease Control and Prevention, March 19, 2013.

Heart Attack

- A heart attack happens when the blood supply to the heart is cut off. Cells in the heart muscle that do not receive enough oxygen-carrying blood begin to die. The more time that passes without treatment to restore blood flow, the greater the damage to the heart.

- Every year about 715,000 Americans have a heart attack. Of these, 525,000 are a first heart attack and 190,000 happen in people who have already had a heart attack.[1]

- About 15 percent of people who have a heart attack will die from it.[1]

- Almost half of sudden cardiac deaths happen outside a hospital.[2]

- Having high blood pressure or high blood cholesterol, smoking, having had a previous heart attack or stroke, or having diabetes can increase your chance of developing heart disease and having a heart attack.

- It is important to recognize the signs of a heart attack and to act immediately by calling 9-1-1. A person's chance of surviving a heart attack increases if emergency treatment is administered as soon as possible.

Symptoms of a Heart Attack

The National Heart Attack Alert Program notes these major signs of a heart attack:

- Chest pain or discomfort. Most heart attacks involve discomfort in the center or left side of the chest that lasts for more than a few minutes, or that goes away and comes back. The discomfort can feel like uncomfortable pressure, squeezing, fullness, or pain.

- Discomfort in other areas of the upper body. Can include pain or discomfort in one or both arms, the back, neck, jaw, or stomach.

- Shortness of breath. Often comes along with chest discomfort. But it also can occur before chest discomfort.

- Other symptoms. May include breaking out in a cold sweat, nausea, or light-headedness.

If you think that you or someone you know is having a heart attack, you should call 9-1-1 immediately.

References

1. Roger VL, Go AS, Lloyd-Jones DM, et al. Heart disease and stroke statistics—2012 update: a report from the American Heart Association. *Circulation*. 2012;125(1):e2–220.

2. Zheng ZJ, Croft JB, Giles WH, Ayala CI, Greenlund KJ, Keenan NL, Neff L, Wattigney WA, Mensah GA. State Specific Mortality from Sudden Cardiac Death: United States, 1999. *MMWR* 2002;51(6):123–26.

Section 7.2

Heart Attack or Sudden Cardiac Arrest: How Are They Different?

People often use these terms interchangeably, but they are not synonyms. A heart attack is when blood flow to the heart is blocked, and sudden cardiac arrest is when the heart malfunctions and suddenly stops beating unexpectedly. A heart attack is a "circulation" problem and sudden cardiac arrest is an "electrical" problem.

What Is a Heart Attack?

A heart attack occurs when a blocked artery prevents oxygen-rich blood from reaching a section of the heart. If the blocked artery is not reopened quickly, the part of the heart normally nourished by that artery begins to die. The longer a person goes without treatment, the greater the damage. Symptoms of a heart attack may be immediate and intense. More often, though, symptoms start slowly and persist for hours, days, or weeks before a heart attack. Unlike with sudden cardiac arrest, the heart usually does not stop beating during a heart attack. The heart attack symptoms in women can be different than men.

What Is Cardiac Arrest?

Sudden cardiac arrest occurs suddenly and often without warning. It is triggered by an electrical malfunction in the heart that causes an irregular heartbeat (arrhythmia). With its pumping action disrupted, the heart cannot pump blood to the brain, lungs, and other organs. Seconds later, a person loses consciousness and has no pulse. Death occurs within minutes if the victim does not receive treatment.

What Is the Link?

These two distinct heart conditions are linked. Sudden cardiac arrest can occur after a heart attack, or during recovery. Heart attacks increase the risk for sudden cardiac arrest. Most heart attacks do not lead to sudden cardiac arrest. But when sudden cardiac arrest occurs, heart attack is a common cause. Other heart conditions may also disrupt the heart's rhythm and lead to sudden cardiac arrest. These include a thickened heart muscle (cardiomyopathy), heart failure, arrhythmias, particularly ventricular fibrillation, and long Q-T syndrome.

What to Do: Heart Attack

Even if you're not sure it's a heart attack, don't wait more than five minutes to call 9-1-1 or your emergency response number. Every minute matters! It's best to call emergency medical services (EMS) to get to the emergency room right away. Emergency medical services staff can begin treatment when they arrive—up to an hour sooner than if someone gets to the hospital by car. EMS staff are also trained to revive someone whose heart has stopped. Patients with chest pain who arrive by ambulance usually receive faster treatment at the hospital, too.

What to Do: Sudden Cardiac Arrest

Cardiac arrest is reversible in most victims if it's treated within a few minutes. First, call 9-1-1 for emergency medical services. Then get an automated external defibrillator (AED) if one is available and use it as soon as it arrives. Begin cardiopulmonary resuscitation (CPR) immediately and continue until professional emergency medical services arrive. If two people are available to help, one should begin CPR immediately while the other calls 9-1-1 and finds an AED.

Sudden cardiac arrest is a leading cause of death—nearly four hundred thousand out-of-hospital cardiac arrests occur annually in the United States. By performing hands-only CPR to the beat of the classic disco song "Stayin' Alive," you can double or even triple a victim's chance of survival.

Section 7.3

Warning Signs of a Stroke

Learn the many warning signs of a stroke. Act FAST and CALL 9-1-1 IMMEDIATELY at any sign of a stroke.

Use FAST to remember the warning signs:

- **Face:** Ask the person to smile. Does one side of the face droop?

- **Arms:** Ask the person to raise both arms. Does one arm drift downward?

- **Speech:** Ask the person to repeat a simple phrase. Is their speech slurred or strange?

- **Time:** If you observe any of these signs, call 9-1-1 immediately.

Note the time when any symptoms first appear. If given within three hours of the first symptom, there is a U.S. Food and Drug Association (FDA)–approved clot-buster medication that may reduce long-term disability for the most common type of stroke. There are also two other types of stroke treatment available that might help reduce the effects of stroke.

Learn as many stroke symptoms as possible so you can recognize stroke as FAST as possible.

Stroke symptoms include:

- Sudden numbness or weakness of face, arm or leg—especially on one side of the body

- Sudden confusion, trouble speaking or understanding

- Sudden trouble seeing in one or both eyes

- Sudden trouble walking, dizziness, loss of balance or coordination

- Sudden severe headache with no known cause

Call 9-1-1 immediately if you have any of these symptoms.

Note the time you experienced your first symptom. This information is important to your health care provider and can affect treatment decisions.

Chapter 8

What to Do in a Cardiac Emergency

Chapter Contents

Section 8.1

What to Do During a Heart Attack

"What to Do During a Heart Attack: Heart Attack Action Plan," U.S. Department of Health and Human Services, Office on Women's Health, 2011.

Call 9-1-1 for Emergency Medical Care

Calling 9-1-1 is the best and fastest way to get to the hospital. When you notice heart attack symptoms, call 9-1-1 immediately (within five minutes at most). If you call 9-1-1, emergency medical personnel can begin life-saving treatment right away, even before you get to the hospital. Don't drive yourself or have someone drive you unless you have no other choice.

Talk to the 9-1-1 Operator and Follow His or Her Instructions

Try not to panic. Take long, deep breaths, stay calm, and speak slowly and clearly. The dispatcher will ask for your name, where you are, and what is wrong. Say: "I think I am having a heart attack." Stay on the line until you are sure the operator has all the information he or she needs.

The 9-1-1 operator may tell you to chew and swallow an aspirin if you are not allergic and don't have any other medical reason not to take it. Never delay calling 9-1-1 to take an aspirin.

Follow Your Heart Attack Action Plan

If you have heart disease, or have had a heart attack before, ask your doctor ahead of time what you should do in case of emergency. Your heart attack action plan should tell you when to call 9-1-1, and may also include the following:

- Chewing an aspirin (one normal aspirin or two baby aspirin)
- Putting a nitroglycerin pill under your tongue
- Keeping a copy of your resting electrocardiogram (ECG) and a list of medications you are allergic to close by at all times

Wait For Help to Arrive

If you feel faint or dizzy after you hang up the phone, unlock the door and lie down on the floor where emergency responders can see you as soon as they come in. Try to stay calm and take slow, deep breaths.

Section 8.2

Symptoms and Emergency Treatment of Cardiac Arrest

"Symptoms and Emergency Treatment of Cardiac Arrest," reprinted with permission from www.heart.org. © 2013 American Heart Association, Inc. All rights reserved.

Signs of Cardiac Arrest

It strikes suddenly and without warning:

- Sudden loss of responsiveness:
    - No response to tapping on shoulders
    - Does nothing when you ask if he is okay
- No normal breathing:
    - The victim does not take a normal breath when you tilt the head up
    - Check for at least five seconds

If these signs of cardiac arrest are present:

- Call 9-1-1 for emergency medical services.
- Get an automated external defibrillator (AED) if one is available.
- Begin cardiopulmonary resuscitation (CPR) immediately. Continue until professional emergency medical services arrive.
- Use the AED as soon as it arrives.

If two people are available to help, one should begin CPR immediately while the other calls 9-1-1 and finds an AED.

Cardiac arrest is reversible in most victims if it's treated within a few minutes. This first became clear in the early 1960s with the development of coronary care units. Electrical devices that shocked the heart were discovered to turn an abnormally rapid rhythm into a normal one. Before then, heart attack victims had a 30 percent chance of dying if they got to the hospital alive; 50 percent of these deaths were due to cardiac arrest. In-hospital survival after cardiac arrest in heart attack patients improved dramatically when the DC defibrillator and bedside monitoring were developed. Later, it also became clear that cardiac arrest could be reversed outside a hospital by properly staffed emergency rescue teams trained to give CPR and defibrillate.

Immediate treatment is essential to survival of cardiac arrest. The problem isn't whether cardiac arrest can be reversed but reaching the victim in time to do so. The American Heart Association supports implementing a "chain of survival" to rescue people who suffer cardiac arrest. The chain consists of:

- early recognition of the emergency and activation of the emergency medical services (EMS);
- early defibrillation when indicated;
- early bystander CPR (cardiopulmonary resuscitation);
- early advanced life support followed by postresuscitation care delivered by health care providers.

Care for Children

Not as much is known about care for children who experience cardiac arrest, but critical elements include managing temperature, glucose, blood pressure, ventilation, and cardiac output. Survival is higher in hospitals with specialized pediatric staff.

Section 8.3

What to Do During a Stroke

"Know Stroke. Know the Signs. Act in Time," National Institute
of Neurological Disorders and Stroke, National Institutes of Health,
June 19, 2013.

Know Stroke

Stroke is the third leading cause of death in the United States and a leading cause of serious, long-term disability in adults. About six hundred thousand new strokes are reported in the United States each year. The good news is that treatments are available that can greatly reduce the damage caused by a stroke. However, you need to recognize the symptoms of a stroke and get to a hospital quickly. Getting treatment within sixty minutes can prevent disability.

What Is a Stroke?

A stroke, sometimes called a "brain attack," occurs when blood flow to the brain is interrupted. When a stroke occurs, brain cells in the immediate area begin to die because they stop getting the oxygen and nutrients they need to function.

What Causes a Stroke?

There are two major kinds of stroke.

The first, called an ischemic stroke, is caused by a blood clot that blocks or plugs a blood vessel or artery in the brain. About 80 percent of all strokes are ischemic. The second, known as a hemorrhagic stroke, is caused by a blood vessel in the brain that breaks and bleeds into the brain. About 20 percent of strokes are hemorrhagic.

What Disabilities Can Result from a Stroke?

Although stroke is a disease of the brain, it can affect the entire body. The effects of a stroke range from mild to severe and can include paralysis, problems with thinking, problems with speaking, and emotional problems. Patients may also experience pain or numbness after a stroke.

Know the Signs

Because stroke injures the brain, you may not realize that you are having a stroke. To a bystander, someone having a stroke may just look unaware or confused. Stroke victims have the best chance if someone around them recognizes the symptoms and acts quickly.

What Are the Symptoms of a Stroke?

The symptoms of stroke are distinct because they happen quickly:

- Sudden numbness or weakness of the face, arm, or leg (especially on one side of the body)

- Sudden confusion, trouble speaking or understanding speech

- Sudden trouble seeing in one or both eyes

- Sudden trouble walking, dizziness, loss of balance or coordination

- Sudden severe headache with no known cause

What Should a Bystander Do?

If you believe someone is having a stroke—if he or she suddenly loses the ability to speak or move an arm or leg on one side or experiences facial paralysis on one side—call 9-1-1 immediately.

Act in Time

Stroke is a medical emergency. Every minute counts when someone is having a stroke. The longer blood flow is cut off to the brain, the greater the damage. Immediate treatment can save people's lives and enhance their chances for successful recovery.

Why Is There a Need to Act Fast?

Ischemic strokes, the most common type of strokes, can be treated with a drug called t-PA that dissolves blood clots obstructing blood flow to the brain. The window of opportunity to start treating stroke patients is three hours, but to be evaluated and receive treatment, patients need to get to the hospital within sixty minutes.

What Is the Benefit of Treatment?

A five-year study by the National Institute of Neurological Disorders and Stroke (NINDS) found that some stroke patients who received t-PA within three hours of the start of stroke symptoms were at least 30 percent more likely to recover with little or no disability after three months.

What Can I Do to Prevent a Stroke?

The best treatment for stroke is prevention. There are several risk factors that increase your chances of having a stroke:

- High blood pressure
- Heart disease
- Smoking
- Diabetes
- High cholesterol

If you smoke—quit. If you have high blood pressure, heart disease, diabetes, or high cholesterol, getting them under control—and keeping them under control—will greatly reduce your chances of having a stroke.

Chapter 9

Cardiopulmonary Resuscitation (CPR)

Chapter Contents

Section 9.1

How to Perform Cardiopulmonary Resuscitation

Reprinted from "CPR in Three Simple Steps," "Complications of CPR," and "Checking the Pulse," © 2013 Learn CPR (learncpr.org). All rights reserved. Reprinted with permission.

CPR in Three Simple Steps

1. **Call:** Check the victim for unresponsiveness. If the person is not responsive and not breathing or not breathing normally, call 9-1-1 and return to the victim. In most locations the emergency dispatcher can assist you with CPR instructions.

2. **Pump:** If the victim is still not breathing normally, coughing, or moving, begin chest compressions. Push down in the center of the chest two inches thirty times. Pump hard and fast at the rate of at least one hundred per minute, faster than once per second.

3. **Blow:** Tilt the head back and lift the chin. Pinch nose and cover the mouth with yours and blow until you see the chest rise. Give two breaths. Each breath should take one second.

Continue with thirty pumps and two breaths until help arrives.

Note: This ratio is the same for one-person and two-person CPR. In two-person CPR the person pumping the chest stops while the other gives mouth-to-mouth breathing.

Complications of CPR

Vomiting is the most frequently encountered complication of CPR. If the victim starts to vomit, turn the head to the side and try to sweep out or wipe off the vomit. Continue with CPR.

The spread of infection from the victim to the rescuer is exceedingly rare. Most cardiac arrests occur in people's homes—relatives or friends will be the ones needing to do CPR. Even CPR performed on strangers has an exceedingly rare risk of infection. There is *no* documentation of human immunodeficiency virus (HIV) or acquired immunodeficiency syndrome (AIDS) ever being transmitted via CPR.

Checking the Pulse

The pulse check is no longer taught or expected of laypersons. Instead, if there is no response after two mouth-to-mouth breaths, begin to pump on the chest. Please note that the pulse check is still expected of health care providers.

Section 9.2

Hands-Only Cardiopulmonary Resuscitation

"CPR in Two Simple Steps: Hands-Only CPR," © 2013 Learn CPR
(learncpr.org). All rights reserved. Reprinted with permission.

This method of cardiopulmonary resuscitation (CPR) was recommended by the American Heart Association in 2010. It is intended for bystanders untrained in CPR. It is also recommended for situations when the rescuer is unable or unwilling to provide mouth-to-mouth ventilations.

1. **Call:** Check the victim for unresponsiveness. If the person is not responsive and not breathing or not breathing normally, call 9-1-1 and return to the victim. In most locations the emergency dispatcher can assist you with CPR instructions.

2. **Pump:** Begin chest compressions. Push down in the center of the chest two inches and keep doing it. Pump hard and fast at the rate of at least one hundred per minute, faster than once per second.

Continue until help arrives.

Chapter 10

Automated External Defibrillators

What Is an Automated External Defibrillator?

An automated external defibrillator (AED) is a portable device that checks the heart rhythm. If needed, it can send an electric shock to the heart to try to restore a normal rhythm. AEDs are used to treat sudden cardiac arrest (SCA).

SCA is a condition in which the heart suddenly and unexpectedly stops beating. When this happens, blood stops flowing to the brain and other vital organs.

SCA usually causes death if it's not treated within minutes. In fact, each minute of SCA leads to a 10 percent reduction in survival. Using an AED on a person who is having SCA may save the person's life.

When Should an Automated External Defibrillator Be Used?

Using an automated external defibrillator (AED) on a person who is having sudden cardiac arrest (SCA) can save the person's life.

The most common cause of SCA is an arrhythmia called ventricular fibrillation (v-fib). In v-fib, the ventricles (the heart's lower chambers) don't beat normally. Instead, they quiver very rapidly and irregularly.

Excerpted from "Automated External Defibrillator," National Heart, Lung, and Blood Institute, National Institutes of Health, December 2, 2011.

Another arrhythmia that can lead to SCA is ventricular tachycardia. This is a fast, regular beating of the ventricles that may last for a few seconds or much longer.

In people who have either of these arrhythmias, an electric shock from an AED can restore the heart's normal rhythm (if done within minutes of the onset of SCA).

What Are the Signs of Sudden Cardiac Arrest?

If someone is having SCA, you may see him or her suddenly collapse and pass out. Or, you may find the person unconscious and unable to respond when you call or shake him or her.

The person may not be breathing, or he or she may have an abnormal breathing pattern. If you check, you usually can't find a pulse. The person's skin may become dark or blue from lack of oxygen. Also, the person may not move, or his or her movements may look like a seizure (spasms).

An AED can check the person's heart rhythm and determine whether an electric shock is needed to try to restore a normal rhythm.

How Does an Automated External Defibrillator Work?

Automated external defibrillators (AEDs) are lightweight, battery-operated, portable devices that are easy to use. Sticky pads with sensors (called electrodes) are attached to the chest of the person who is having sudden cardiac arrest (SCA).

The electrodes send information about the person's heart rhythm to a computer in the AED. The computer analyzes the heart rhythm to find out whether an electric shock is needed. If a shock is needed, the AED uses voice prompts to tell you when to give the shock, and the electrodes deliver it.

Using an AED to shock the heart within minutes of the start of SCA may restore a normal heart rhythm. Every minute counts. Each minute of SCA leads to a 10 percent reduction in survival.

Training to Use an Automated External Defibrillator

Learning how to use an AED and taking a CPR (cardiopulmonary resuscitation) course are helpful. However, if trained personnel aren't available, untrained people also can use an AED to help save someone's life.

How to Use an Automated External Defibrillator

Before using an automated external defibrillator (AED) on someone who you think is having sudden cardiac arrest (SCA), check him or her.

If you see a person suddenly collapse and pass out, or if you find a person already unconscious, confirm that the person can't respond. Shout at and shake the person to make sure he or she isn't sleeping.

Never shake an infant or young child. Instead, you can pinch the child to try to wake him or her up.

Call 9-1-1 or have someone else call 9-1-1. If two rescuers are present, one can provide cardiopulmonary resuscitation (CPR) while the other calls 9-1-1 and gets the AED.

Check the person's breathing and pulse. If breathing and pulse are absent or irregular, prepare to use the AED as soon as possible. (SCA causes death if it's not treated within minutes.)

If no one knows how long the person has been unconscious, or if an AED isn't readily available, do two minutes of CPR. Then use the AED (if you have one) to check the person.

After you use the AED, or if you don't have an AED, give CPR until emergency medical help arrives or until the person begins to move. Try to limit pauses in CPR.

After two minutes of CPR, you can use the AED again to check the person's heart rhythm and give another shock, if needed. If a shock isn't needed, continue CPR.

Using an Automated External Defibrillator

AEDs are user-friendly devices that untrained bystanders can use to save the life of someone having SCA.

Before using an AED, check for puddles or water near the person who is unconscious. Move him or her to a dry area, and stay away from wetness when delivering shocks (water conducts electricity).

Turn on the AED's power. The device will give you step-by-step instructions. You'll hear voice prompts and see prompts on a screen.

Expose the person's chest. If the person's chest is wet, dry it. AEDs have sticky pads with sensors called electrodes. Apply the pads to the person's chest as pictured on the AED's instructions.

Place one pad on the right center of the person's chest above the nipple. Place the other pad slightly below the other nipple and to the left of the ribcage.

Make sure the sticky pads have good connection with the skin. If the connection isn't good, the machine may repeat the phrase "check electrodes."

If the person has a lot of chest hair, you may have to trim it. (AEDs usually come with a kit that includes scissors and/or a razor.) If the person is wearing a medication patch that's in the way, remove it and clean the medicine from the skin before applying the sticky pads.

Remove metal necklaces and underwire bras. The metal may conduct electricity and cause burns. You can cut the center of the bra and pull it away from the skin.

Check the person for implanted medical devices, such as a pacemaker or implantable cardioverter defibrillator. (The outline of these devices is visible under the skin on the chest or abdomen, and the person may be wearing a medical alert bracelet.) Also check for body piercings.

Move the defibrillator pads at least one inch away from implanted devices or piercings so the electric current can flow freely between the pads.

Check that the wires from the electrodes are connected to the AED. Make sure no one is touching the person, and then press the AED's "analyze" button. Stay clear while the machine checks the person's heart rhythm.

If a shock is needed, the AED will let you know when to deliver it. Stand clear of the person and make sure others are clear before you push the AED's "shock" button.

Start or resume CPR until emergency medical help arrives or until the person begins to move. Stay with the person until medical help arrives, and report all of the information you know about what has happened.

What Are the Risks of Using an Automated External Defibrillator?

Automated external defibrillators (AEDs) are safe to use. There are no reports of AEDs harming bystanders or users. Also, there are no reports of AEDs delivering inappropriate shocks.

If someone is having sudden cardiac arrest, using an AED and giving cardiopulmonary resuscitation (CPR) can improve the person's chance of survival.

Part Two

Heart Disorders

Chapter 11

Problems with the Heart's Blood Supply

Chapter Contents

Section 11.1

Coronary Artery Disease

Coronary Artery Disease: Overview

Your heart is a muscle—a very important muscle that your entire body depends on. As with all muscles, the heart is dependent on blood supply to provide necessary nutrients, fuel, and oxygen. The heart gets its blood supply from the coronary arteries. When the coronary arteries become blocked, narrowed, or completely obstructed, the heart cannot get the nutrients, fuel, and oxygen it needs. This can cause the heart to become weak or stop altogether or cause a heart attack. This blockage, narrowing, or obstruction is known as coronary artery disease (CAD).

Who Gets Coronary Artery Disease?

CAD is the number one killer in the United States. For persons aged forty years, the lifetime risk of developing CAD is 49 percent in men and 32 percent in women. For those reaching age seventy years, the lifetime risk is 35 percent in men and 24 percent in women. For total coronary events, the incidence rises steeply with age, with women lagging behind men by ten years.

A variety of other factors can increase risk, including:

• smoking;

• excess fats and cholesterol in the blood;

• high blood pressure;

• excess sugar in the blood (often due to diabetes).

Coronary Artery Disease: Symptoms

Coronary artery disease (CAD) makes it more difficult for oxygen-rich blood to move through arteries. Common symptoms of CAD include:

- **Angina:** Upper body pain or pressure. It's usually felt in the chest, but can also be experienced in the back, belly, and even the jaw.

- **Shortness of breath:** Shortness of breath (dyspnea) with exertion, or chest tightness, squeezing, or burning.

Sometimes CAD has no symptoms, called silent CAD. It can go undiagnosed up until someone has a heart attack, irregular heartbeat, or other heart condition.

Coronary Artery Disease: Diagnosis

Often, symptoms bring a patient in to see a cardiologist. The cardiologist will take into account several factors in diagnosing coronary artery disease (CAD), such as family history, symptoms, and risk factors. In addition, there are several diagnostic tests that are helpful when used together to diagnose the condition:

- **Stress testing:** In a stress test, you perform a physical activity, such as jogging on a treadmill, to increase the speed of your heartbeat. This helps determine how well your heart performs. Usually, the stress test is accompanied by either nuclear or echocardiographic imaging.

- **Echocardiography:** An echocardiogram uses sound waves to produce an image of the heart, showing how well it's working. It can help determine which areas of the heart are having problems and help identify any damage to the heart.

- **Coronary computed tomography (CT):** During a coronary CT angiogram pictures are taken of cross-sections or slices of the heart. A coronary artery calcium scoring CT can detect and measure the extent of the calcium deposits in the coronary arteries.

- **Cardiac catheterization:** This is a minimally invasive test which not only allows visualization of your coronary arteries, but also will allow for possible opening of blockages using a piece of metal scaffolding called a stent.

Coronary Artery Disease: Treatment

The key to treating coronary artery disease (CAD) is to prevent it, or at least reduce the risk of serious cardiac events (such as heart attacks). This is usually done through diet, moderate exercise, and a healthy, nonsmoking, active lifestyle. In addition to several lifestyle changes, your health care provider may recommend various medications, medical procedures, or rehabilitation to treat coronary artery disease (CAD).

Medication

Medicines can be important to:

- relieve the stress on your heart and lessen CAD symptoms;
- decrease the risk of heart attack;
- lower cholesterol levels and decrease blood pressure;
- prevent harmful blood clots.

Medicines used to treat CAD include anticoagulants, aspirin, angiotensin-converting enzyme (ACE) inhibitors, beta blockers, calcium channel blockers, nitroglycerin, glycoprotein IIb-IIIa, statins, and fish oil and other supplements high in omega-3 fatty acids.

Believe it or not, intensive lifestyle medication is the most important of all "medicine" to improve your heart health. Besides being free, regular physical activity (after speaking with your doctor) and eating a more plant-based diet can markedly improve symptoms and reduce co-morbid conditions.

Medical Procedures

Severe cases of CAD may warrant medical procedures, such as:

- **Angioplasty:** This procedure opens blocked or narrowed coronary arteries. A thin tube with a balloon or other device is threaded through a blood vessel until it reaches the blocked artery. The balloon is then inflated, pushing the plaque against the artery wall, which widens the artery. The procedure helps to restore blood flow to the heart, alleviate chest pain, and decrease the chance of a heart attack.

- **Coronary artery bypass graft (CABG):** This procedure creates new routes for arteries and veins so they can bypass the clogged coronary arteries and reach the heart.

Rehabilitation

Cardiac rehabilitation is another treatment option, usually combined with medicine and surgical methods. Cardiac rehab usually consists of:

- **Exercise training:** Learning how to exercise safely, building muscle strength, and improving stamina can be very important in strengthening your heart and making it healthier.

- **Education, counseling, and training:** Patient education seeks to inform you of anything you may want to know about your condition, helping you make the best decisions possible to maintain good health. Counseling is available to help you cope with the stress of the condition and managing lifestyle changes.

Section 11.2

Coronary Microvascular Disease

Excerpted from "Coronary Microvascular Disease,"
National Heart, Lung, and Blood Institute, National Institutes of Health,
November 2, 2011.

What Is Coronary Microvascular Disease?

Coronary microvascular disease (MVD) is heart disease that affects the tiny coronary (heart) arteries. In coronary MVD, the walls of the heart's tiny arteries are damaged or diseased.

Coronary MVD is different from traditional coronary heart disease (CHD), also called coronary artery disease. In CHD, a waxy substance called plaque builds up in the large coronary arteries.

Plaque narrows the heart's large arteries and reduces the flow of oxygen-rich blood to your heart muscle. The buildup of plaque also makes it more likely that blood clots will form in your arteries. Blood clots can mostly or completely block blood flow through a coronary artery.

In coronary MVD, however, the heart's tiny arteries are affected. Plaque doesn't create blockages in these vessels as it does in the heart's large arteries.

What Causes Coronary Microvascular Disease?

The same risk factors that cause atherosclerosis may cause coronary microvascular disease (MVD). Atherosclerosis is a disease in which plaque builds up inside the arteries.

Risk factors for atherosclerosis include the following:

- Unhealthy blood cholesterol levels
- High blood pressure
- Smoking
- Insulin resistance
- Diabetes
- Overweight and obesity
- Lack of physical activity
- Unhealthy diet
- Older age
- Family history of early heart disease

In women, coronary MVD also may be linked to low estrogen levels occurring before or after menopause. Also, the disease may be linked to anemia or conditions that affect blood clotting. Anemia is thought to slow the growth of cells needed to repair damaged blood vessels.

Researchers continue to explore other possible causes of coronary MVD.

Who Is at Risk for Coronary Microvascular Disease?

Studies have shown that women are more likely than men to have coronary microvascular disease (MVD). Women at high risk for the disease often have multiple risk factors for atherosclerosis.

Women may be at risk for coronary MVD if they have lower than normal levels of estrogen at any point in their adult lives. (This refers to the estrogen that the ovaries produce, not the estrogen used in hormone therapy.)

Low estrogen levels before menopause can raise younger women's risk for coronary MVD. One cause of low estrogen levels in younger women is mental stress. Another cause is a problem with the function of the ovaries.

Women who have high blood pressure before menopause, especially high systolic blood pressure, are at increased risk for coronary MVD.

(Systolic blood pressure is the top or first number of a blood pressure measurement.)

After menopause, women tend to have more of the traditional risk factors for atherosclerosis, which also puts them at higher risk for coronary MVD.

Women who have heart disease are more likely to have a worse outcome, such as a heart attack, if they also have anemia. Anemia is thought to slow the growth of cells needed to repair damaged blood vessels.

What Are the Signs and Symptoms of Coronary Microvascular Disease?

The signs and symptoms of coronary microvascular disease (MVD) often differ from the signs and symptoms of traditional coronary heart disease (CHD).

Many women with coronary MVD have angina. Angina is chest pain or discomfort that occurs when your heart muscle doesn't get enough oxygen-rich blood.

Angina may feel like pressure or squeezing in your chest. You also may feel it in your shoulders, arms, neck, jaw, or back. Angina pain may even feel like indigestion.

Angina also is a common symptom of CHD. However, the angina that occurs in coronary MVD may differ from the typical angina that occurs in CHD. In coronary MVD, the chest pain usually lasts longer than ten minutes, and it can last longer than thirty minutes. Typical angina is more common in women older than sixty-five.

Other signs and symptoms of coronary MVD are shortness of breath, sleep problems, fatigue (tiredness), and lack of energy.

Coronary MVD symptoms often are first noticed during routine daily activities (such as shopping, cooking, cleaning, and going to work) and times of mental stress. It's less likely that women will notice these symptoms during physical activity (such as jogging or walking fast).

This differs from CHD, in which symptoms often first appear while a person is being physically active—such as while jogging, walking on a treadmill, or going up stairs.

How Is Coronary Microvascular Disease Diagnosed?

Your doctor will diagnose coronary microvascular disease (MVD) based on your medical history, a physical exam, and test results. He or she will check to see whether you have any risk factors for heart disease.

The risk factors for coronary MVD and traditional coronary heart disease (CHD) often are the same. Thus, your doctor may recommend tests for CHD, such as the following:

- **Coronary angiography:** This test uses dye and special x-rays to show the insides of your coronary arteries. Coronary angiography can show plaque buildup in the large coronary arteries. This test often is done during a heart attack to help find blockages in the coronary arteries.

- **Stress testing:** This test shows how blood flows through your heart during physical stress, such as exercise. Even if coronary angiography doesn't show plaque buildup in the large coronary arteries, a stress test may still show abnormal blood flow. This may be a sign of coronary MVD.

- **Cardiac magnetic resonance imaging (MRI) stress test:** Doctors may use this test to evaluate people who have chest pain.

Unfortunately, standard tests for CHD aren't designed to detect coronary MVD. These tests look for blockages in the large coronary arteries. Coronary MVD affects the tiny coronary arteries.

If test results show that you don't have CHD, your doctor might still diagnose you with coronary MVD. This could happen if signs are present that not enough oxygen is reaching your heart's tiny arteries.

Coronary MVD symptoms often first occur during routine daily tasks. Thus, your doctor may ask you to fill out a questionnaire called the Duke Activity Status Index (DASI). The questionnaire will ask you how well you're able to do daily activities, such as shopping, cooking, and going to work.

The DASI results will help your doctor decide which kind of stress test you should have. The results also give your doctor information about how well blood is flowing through your coronary arteries.

Your doctor also may recommend blood tests, including a test for anemia. Anemia is thought to slow the growth of cells needed to repair damaged blood vessels.

Research is ongoing for better ways to detect and diagnose coronary MVD. Currently, researchers have not agreed on the best way to diagnose the disease.

How Is Coronary Microvascular Disease Treated?

Relieving pain is one of the main goals of treating coronary microvascular disease (MVD). Treatments also are used to control risk factors and other symptoms.

Treatments may include medicines such as the following:

- Statins to improve cholesterol levels

- Angiotensin-converting enzyme (ACE) inhibitors and beta blockers to lower blood pressure and decrease the heart's workload

- Aspirin to help prevent blood clots or control inflammation

- Nitroglycerin to relax blood vessels, improve blood flow to the heart muscle, and treat chest pain

If you're diagnosed with coronary MVD and also have anemia, you may benefit from treatment for that condition. Anemia is thought to slow the growth of cells needed to repair damaged blood vessels.

If you're diagnosed with and treated for coronary MVD, you should get ongoing care from your doctor.

Research is under way to find the best treatments for coronary MVD.

Chapter 12

Angina

What Is Angina?

Angina is chest pain or discomfort that occurs if an area of your heart muscle doesn't get enough oxygen-rich blood.

Angina may feel like pressure or squeezing in your chest. The pain also can occur in your shoulders, arms, neck, jaw, or back. Angina pain may even feel like indigestion.

Angina isn't a disease; it's a symptom of an underlying heart problem. Angina usually is a symptom of coronary heart disease (CHD).

CHD is the most common type of heart disease in adults. It occurs if a waxy substance called plaque builds up on the inner walls of your coronary arteries. These arteries carry oxygen-rich blood to your heart.

Plaque narrows and stiffens the coronary arteries. This reduces the flow of oxygen-rich blood to the heart muscle, causing chest pain. Plaque buildup also makes it more likely that blood clots will form in your arteries. Blood clots can partially or completely block blood flow, which can cause a heart attack.

Angina also can be a symptom of coronary microvascular disease (MVD). This is heart disease that affects the heart's smallest coronary arteries. In coronary MVD, plaque doesn't create blockages in the arteries like it does in CHD.

Excerpted from "Angina," National Heart, Lung, and Blood Institute, National Institutes of Health, June 1, 2011.

Studies have shown that coronary MVD is more likely to affect women than men. Coronary MVD also is called cardiac syndrome X and nonobstructive CHD.

Types of Angina

The major types of angina are stable, unstable, variant (Prinzmetal), and microvascular. Knowing how the types differ is important. This is because they have different symptoms and require different treatments.

Stable angina: Stable angina is the most common type of angina. It occurs when the heart is working harder than usual. Stable angina has a regular pattern. ("Pattern" refers to how often the angina occurs, how severe it is, and what factors trigger it.)

If you have stable angina, you can learn its pattern and predict when the pain will occur. The pain usually goes away a few minutes after you rest or take your angina medicine.

Stable angina isn't a heart attack, but it suggests that a heart attack is more likely to happen in the future.

Unstable angina: Unstable angina doesn't follow a pattern. It may occur more often and be more severe than stable angina. Unstable angina also can occur with or without physical exertion, and rest or medicine may not relieve the pain.

Unstable angina is very dangerous and requires emergency treatment. This type of angina is a sign that a heart attack may happen soon.

Variant (Prinzmetal) angina: Variant angina is rare. A spasm in a coronary artery causes this type of angina. Variant angina usually occurs while you're at rest, and the pain can be severe. It usually happens between midnight and early morning. Medicine can relieve this type of angina.

Microvascular angina: Microvascular angina can be more severe and last longer than other types of angina. Medicine may not relieve this type of angina.

Overview

Experts believe that nearly seven million people in the United States suffer from angina. The condition occurs equally among men and women.

Angina can be a sign of CHD, even if initial tests don't point to the disease. However, not all chest pain or discomfort is a sign of CHD.

Other conditions also can cause chest pain, including the following:

- Pulmonary embolism (a blockage in a lung artery)
- A lung infection
- Aortic dissection (tearing of a major artery)
- Aortic stenosis (narrowing of the heart's aortic valve)
- Hypertrophic cardiomyopathy (heart muscle disease)
- Pericarditis (inflammation in the tissues that surround the heart)
- A panic attack

All chest pain should be checked by a doctor.

What Causes Angina?

Underlying Causes

Angina usually is a symptom of coronary heart disease (CHD). This means that the underlying causes of angina generally are the same as the underlying causes of CHD.

Research suggests that CHD starts when certain factors damage the inner layers of the coronary arteries. These factors include the following:

- Smoking
- High amounts of certain fats and cholesterol in the blood
- High blood pressure
- High amounts of sugar in the blood due to insulin resistance or diabetes

Plaque may begin to build up where the arteries are damaged. When plaque builds up in the arteries, the condition is called atherosclerosis.

Plaque narrows or blocks the arteries, reducing blood flow to the heart muscle. Some plaque is hard and stable and causes the arteries to become narrow and stiff. This can greatly reduce blood flow to the heart and cause angina.

Other plaque is soft and more likely to rupture (break open) and cause blood clots. Blood clots can partially or totally block the coronary arteries and cause angina or a heart attack.

Immediate Causes

Many factors can trigger angina pain, depending on the type of angina you have.

Stable angina: Physical exertion is the most common trigger of stable angina. Severely narrowed arteries may allow enough blood to reach the heart when the demand for oxygen is low, such as when you're sitting.

However, with physical exertion—like walking up a hill or climbing stairs—the heart works harder and needs more oxygen.

Other triggers of stable angina include the following:

- Emotional stress

- Exposure to very hot or cold temperatures

- Heavy meals

- Smoking

Unstable angina: Blood clots that partially or totally block an artery cause unstable angina.

If plaque in an artery ruptures, blood clots may form. This creates a blockage. A clot may grow large enough to completely block the artery and cause a heart attack.

Blood clots may form, partially dissolve, and later form again. Angina can occur each time a clot blocks an artery.

Variant angina: A spasm in a coronary artery causes variant angina. The spasm causes the walls of the artery to tighten and narrow. Blood flow to the heart slows or stops. Variant angina can occur in people who have CHD and in those who don't.

The coronary arteries can spasm as a result of the following things:

- Exposure to cold

- Emotional stress

- Medicines that tighten or narrow blood vessels

- Smoking

- Cocaine use

Microvascular angina: This type of angina may be a symptom of coronary microvascular disease (MVD). Coronary MVD is heart disease that affects the heart's smallest coronary arteries.

Reduced blood flow in the small coronary arteries may cause microvascular angina. Plaque in the arteries, artery spasms, or damaged or diseased artery walls can reduce blood flow through the small coronary arteries.

Who Is at Risk for Angina?

Angina is a symptom of an underlying heart problem. It's usually a symptom of coronary heart disease (CHD), but it also can be a symptom of coronary microvascular disease (MVD). So, if you're at risk for CHD or coronary MVD, you're also at risk for angina.

The major risk factors for CHD and coronary MVD include the following:

- Unhealthy cholesterol levels.
- High blood pressure.
- Smoking.
- Insulin resistance or diabetes.
- Overweight or obesity.
- Metabolic syndrome.
- Lack of physical activity.
- Unhealthy diet.
- Older age. (The risk increases for men after forty-five years of age and for women after fifty-five years of age.)
- Family history of early heart disease.

People sometimes think that because men have more heart attacks than women, men also suffer from angina more often. In fact, overall, angina occurs equally among men and women.

Microvascular angina, however, occurs more often in women. About 70 percent of the cases of microvascular angina occur in women around the time of menopause.

Unstable angina occurs more often in older adults. Variant angina is rare; it accounts for only about two out of one hundred cases of angina. People who have variant angina often are younger than those who have other forms of angina.

What Are the Signs and Symptoms of Angina?

Pain and discomfort are the main symptoms of angina. Angina often is described as pressure, squeezing, burning, or tightness in the chest. The pain or discomfort usually starts behind the breastbone.

Pain from angina also can occur in the arms, shoulders, neck, jaw, throat, or back. The pain may feel like indigestion. Some people say that angina pain is hard to describe or that they can't tell exactly where the pain is coming from.

Signs and symptoms such as nausea (feeling sick to your stomach), fatigue (tiredness), shortness of breath, sweating, light-headedness, and weakness also may occur.

Women are more likely to feel discomfort in the neck, jaw, throat, abdomen, or back. Shortness of breath is more common in older people and those who have diabetes. Weakness, dizziness, and confusion can mask the signs and symptoms of angina in elderly people.

Symptoms also vary based on the type of angina you have.

Because angina has so many possible symptoms and causes, all chest pain should be checked by a doctor. Chest pain that lasts longer than a few minutes and isn't relieved by rest or angina medicine may be a sign of a heart attack. Call 9-1-1 right away.

Stable Angina

The pain or discomfort has the following characteristics:

- Occurs when the heart must work harder, usually during physical exertion

- Doesn't come as a surprise, and episodes of pain tend to be alike

- Usually lasts a short time (five minutes or less)

- Is relieved by rest or medicine

- May feel like gas or indigestion

- May feel like chest pain that spreads to the arms, back, or other areas

Unstable Angina

The pain or discomfort has the following characteristics:

- Often occurs at rest, while sleeping at night, or with little physical exertion

- Comes as a surprise

- Is more severe and lasts longer than stable angina (as long as thirty minutes)

- Usually isn't relieved by rest or medicine

- May get worse over time
- May mean that a heart attack will happen soon

Variant Angina

The pain or discomfort has the following characteristics:

- Usually occurs at rest and during the night or early morning hours
- Tends to be severe
- Is relieved by medicine

Microvascular Angina

The pain or discomfort has the following characteristics:

- May be more severe and last longer than other types of angina pain
- May occur with shortness of breath, sleep problems, fatigue, and lack of energy
- Often is first noticed during routine daily activities and times of mental stress

How Is Angina Diagnosed?

The most important issues to address when you go to the doctor with chest pain are the following:

- What's causing the chest pain
- Whether you're having or are about to have a heart attack

Angina is a symptom of an underlying heart problem, usually coronary heart disease (CHD). The type of angina pain you have can be a sign of how severe the CHD is and whether it's likely to cause a heart attack.

If you have chest pain, your doctor will want to find out whether it's angina. He or she also will want to know whether the angina is stable or unstable. If it's unstable, you may need emergency medical treatment to try to prevent a heart attack.

To diagnose chest pain as stable or unstable angina, your doctor will do a physical exam, ask about your symptoms, and ask about your risk factors for and your family history of CHD or other heart diseases.

Diagnostic Tests and Procedures

If your doctor thinks that you have unstable angina or that your angina is related to a serious heart condition, he or she may recommend one or more tests.

Electrocardiogram (EKG): An EKG is a simple, painless test that detects and records the heart's electrical activity. The test shows how fast the heart is beating and its rhythm (steady or irregular). An EKG also records the strength and timing of electrical signals as they pass through the heart.

An EKG can show signs of heart damage due to CHD and signs of a previous or current heart attack. However, some people who have angina have normal EKGs.

Stress testing: During stress testing, you exercise to make your heart work hard and beat fast while heart tests are done. If you can't exercise, you may be given medicine to make your heart work hard and beat fast.

When your heart is working hard and beating fast, it needs more blood and oxygen. Plaque-narrowed arteries can't supply enough oxygen-rich blood to meet your heart's needs.

A stress test can show possible signs and symptoms of CHD, such as the following:

• Abnormal changes in your heart rate or blood pressure

• Shortness of breath or chest pain

• Abnormal changes in your heart rhythm or your heart's electrical activity

As part of some stress tests, pictures are taken of your heart while you exercise and while you rest. These imaging stress tests can show how well blood is flowing in various parts of your heart. They also can show how well your heart pumps blood when it beats.

Chest x-ray: A chest x-ray takes pictures of the organs and structures inside your chest, such as your heart, lungs, and blood vessels.

A chest x-ray can reveal signs of heart failure. It also can show signs of lung disorders and other causes of symptoms not related to CHD. However, a chest x-ray alone is not enough to diagnose angina or CHD.

Coronary angiography and cardiac catheterization: Your doctor may recommend coronary angiography if he or she suspects you have CHD. This test uses dye and special x-rays to show the inside of your coronary arteries.

To get the dye into your coronary arteries, your doctor will use a procedure called cardiac catheterization.

A thin, flexible tube called a catheter is put into a blood vessel in your arm, groin (upper thigh), or neck. The tube is threaded into your coronary arteries, and the dye is released into your bloodstream.

Special x-rays are taken while the dye is flowing through your coronary arteries. The dye lets your doctor study the flow of blood through your heart and blood vessels.

Cardiac catheterization usually is done in a hospital. You're awake during the procedure. It usually causes little or no pain, although you may feel some soreness in the blood vessel where your doctor inserts the catheter.

Computed tomography angiography: Computed tomography angiography (CTA) uses dye and special x-rays to show blood flow through the coronary arteries. This test is less invasive than coronary angiography with cardiac catheterization.

For CTA, a needle connected to an intravenous (IV) line is put into a vein in your hand or arm. Dye is injected through the IV line during the scan. You may have a warm feeling when this happens. The dye highlights your blood vessels on the computed tomography (CT) scan pictures.

Sticky patches called electrodes are put on your chest. The patches are attached to an EKG machine to record your heart's electrical activity during the scan.

The CT scanner is a large machine that has a hollow, circular tube in the middle. You lie on your back on a sliding table. The table slowly slides into the opening of the machine.

Inside the scanner, an x-ray tube moves around your body to take pictures of different parts of your heart. A computer puts the pictures together to make a three-dimensional (3D) picture of the whole heart.

Blood tests: Blood tests check the levels of certain fats, cholesterol, sugar, and proteins in your blood. Abnormal levels may show that you have risk factors for CHD.

Your doctor may recommend a blood test to check the level of a protein called C-reactive protein (CRP) in your blood. Some studies suggest that high levels of CRP in the blood may increase the risk for CHD and heart attack.

Your doctor also may recommend a blood test to check for low levels of hemoglobin in your blood. Hemoglobin is an iron-rich protein in red blood cells. It helps the blood cells carry oxygen from the lungs to all parts of your body. If your hemoglobin level is low, you may have a condition called anemia.

How Is Angina Treated?

Treatments for angina include lifestyle changes, medicines, medical procedures, cardiac rehabilitation (rehab), and other therapies. The main goals of treatment are as follows:

- To reduce pain and discomfort and how often it occurs
- To prevent or lower your risk for heart attack and death by treating your underlying heart condition

Lifestyle changes and medicines may be the only treatments needed if your symptoms are mild and aren't getting worse. If lifestyle changes and medicines don't control angina, you may need medical procedures or cardiac rehab.

Unstable angina is an emergency condition that requires treatment in a hospital.

Chapter 13

Heart Attack (Myocardial Infarction)

What Is a Heart Attack?

A heart attack occurs if the flow of oxygen-rich blood to a section of heart muscle suddenly becomes blocked. If blood flow isn't restored quickly, the section of heart muscle begins to die.

Heart attacks are a leading killer of both men and women in the United States. The good news is that excellent treatments are available for heart attacks. These treatments can save lives and prevent disabilities.

Heart attack treatment works best when it's given right after symptoms occur. If you think you or someone else is having a heart attack, call 9-1-1 right away.

What Causes a Heart Attack?

Coronary Heart Disease

A heart attack happens if the flow of oxygen-rich blood to a section of heart muscle suddenly becomes blocked. Most heart attacks occur as a result of coronary heart disease (CHD).

CHD is a condition in which a waxy substance called plaque builds up inside of the coronary arteries. These arteries supply oxygen-rich blood to your heart.

Excerpted from "Heart Attack," National Heart, Lung, and Blood Institute, National Institutes of Health, March 1, 2011.

When plaque builds up in the arteries, the condition is called atherosclerosis. The buildup of plaque occurs over many years.

Eventually, an area of plaque can rupture (break open) inside of an artery. This causes a blood clot to form on the plaque's surface. If the clot becomes large enough, it can mostly or completely block blood flow through a coronary artery.

If the blockage isn't treated quickly, the portion of heart muscle fed by the artery begins to die. Healthy heart tissue is replaced with scar tissue. This heart damage may not be obvious, or it may cause severe or long-lasting problems.

Coronary Artery Spasm

A less common cause of heart attack is a severe spasm (tightening) of a coronary artery. The spasm cuts off blood flow through the artery. Spasms can occur in coronary arteries that aren't affected by atherosclerosis.

What causes a coronary artery to spasm isn't always clear. A spasm may be related to the following:

- Taking certain drugs, such as cocaine

- Emotional stress or pain

- Exposure to extreme cold

- Cigarette smoking

Who Is at Risk for a Heart Attack?

Certain risk factors make it more likely that you'll develop coronary heart disease (CHD) and have a heart attack. You can control many of these risk factors.

Risk Factors You Can Control

The major risk factors for a heart attack that you can control include the following:

- Smoking

- High blood pressure

- High blood cholesterol

- Overweight and obesity

- An unhealthy diet (for example, a diet high in saturated fat, trans fat, cholesterol, and sodium)

- Lack of routine physical activity

- High blood sugar due to insulin resistance or diabetes

Risk Factors You Can't Control

Risk factors that you can't control include the following:

- **Age:** The risk of heart disease increases for men after age forty-five and for women after age fifty-five (or after menopause).

- **Family history of early heart disease:** Your risk increases if your father or a brother was diagnosed with heart disease before fifty-five years of age, or if your mother or a sister was diagnosed with heart disease before sixty-five years of age.

- **Preeclampsia:** This condition can develop during pregnancy. The two main signs of preeclampsia are a rise in blood pressure and excess protein in the urine. Preeclampsia is linked to an increased lifetime risk of heart disease, including CHD, heart attack, heart failure, and high blood pressure.

What Are the Signs and Symptoms of a Heart Attack?

Not all heart attacks begin with the sudden, crushing chest pain that often is shown on TV or in the movies. In one study, for example, one-third of the patients who have heart attacks have no chest pain. These patients are more likely to be older, female, or diabetic.

The warning signs and symptoms of a heart attack aren't the same for everyone. Many heart attacks start slowly as mild pain or discomfort. Some people don't have symptoms at all. Heart attacks that occur without any symptoms or very mild symptoms are called silent heart attacks.

Chest Pain or Discomfort

The most common heart attack symptom is chest pain or discomfort. This includes new chest pain or discomfort or a change in the pattern of existing chest pain or discomfort.

Most heart attacks involve discomfort in the center or left side of the chest that often lasts for more than a few minutes or goes away and comes back. The discomfort can feel like uncomfortable pressure, squeezing, fullness, or pain. The feeling can be mild or severe.

Heart attack pain sometimes feels like indigestion or heartburn.

The symptoms of angina can be similar to the symptoms of a heart attack. Angina is chest pain that occurs in people who have coronary heart disease, usually when they're active. Angina pain usually lasts for only a few minutes and goes away with rest.

Chest pain or discomfort that doesn't go away or changes from its usual pattern (for example, occurs more often or while you're resting) can be a sign of a heart attack.

All chest pain should be checked by a doctor.

Other Common Signs and Symptoms

Other common signs and symptoms of a heart attack include new onset of the following:

- Upper body discomfort in one or both arms, the back, neck, jaw, or upper part of the stomach

- Shortness of breath, which may occur with or before chest discomfort

- Nausea (feeling sick to your stomach), vomiting, light-headedness or sudden dizziness, or breaking out in a cold sweat

- Sleep problems, fatigue (tiredness), or lack of energy

Not everyone having a heart attack has typical symptoms. If you've already had a heart attack, your symptoms may not be the same for another one. However, some people may have a pattern of symptoms that recur.

The more signs and symptoms you have, the more likely it is that you're having a heart attack.

Act Fast

The signs and symptoms of a heart attack can develop suddenly. However, they also can develop slowly—sometimes within hours, days, or weeks of a heart attack.

Know the warning signs of a heart attack so you can act fast to get treatment for yourself or someone else. The sooner you get emergency help, the less damage your heart will sustain.

Call 9-1-1 for help right away if you think you or someone else may be having a heart attack. You also should call for help if your chest pain doesn't go away as it usually does when you take medicine prescribed for angina.

Do not drive to the hospital or let someone else drive you. Call an ambulance so that medical personnel can begin life-saving treatment on the way to the emergency room.

How Is a Heart Attack Diagnosed?

Your doctor will diagnose a heart attack based on your signs and symptoms, your medical and family histories, and test results.

Diagnostic Tests

Electrocardiogram (EKG): An EKG is a simple, painless test that detects and records the heart's electrical activity. The test shows how fast the heart is beating and its rhythm (steady or irregular). An EKG also records the strength and timing of electrical signals as they pass through each part of the heart.

An EKG can show signs of heart damage due to coronary heart disease (CHD) and signs of a previous or current heart attack.

Blood tests: During a heart attack, heart muscle cells die and release proteins into the bloodstream. Blood tests can measure the amount of these proteins in the bloodstream. Higher than normal levels of these proteins suggest a heart attack.

Coronary angiography: Coronary angiography is a test that uses dye and special x-rays to show the insides of your coronary arteries. This test often is done during a heart attack to help find blockages in the coronary arteries.

How Is a Heart Attack Treated?

Early treatment for a heart attack can prevent or limit damage to the heart muscle. Acting fast, at the first symptoms of a heart attack, can save your life. Medical personnel can begin diagnosis and treatment even before you get to the hospital.

Certain treatments usually are started right away if a heart attack is suspected, even before the diagnosis is confirmed. These include the following:

- Oxygen therapy

- Aspirin to thin your blood and prevent further blood clotting

- Nitroglycerin to reduce your heart's workload and improve blood flow through the coronary arteries

- Treatment for chest pain

Once the diagnosis of a heart attack is confirmed or strongly suspected, doctors start treatments to try to promptly restore blood flow to the heart. The two main treatments are "clot-busting" medicines and angioplasty, a procedure used to open blocked coronary arteries.

Clot-Busting Medicines

Thrombolytic medicines, also called "clot busters," are used to dissolve blood clots that are blocking the coronary arteries. To work best, these medicines must be given within several hours of the start of heart attack symptoms. Ideally, the medicine should be given as soon as possible.

Angioplasty

Angioplasty is a nonsurgical procedure that opens blocked or narrowed coronary arteries. This procedure also is called percutaneous coronary intervention, or PCI.

A thin, flexible tube with a balloon or other device on the end is threaded through a blood vessel to the narrowed or blocked coronary artery.

Once in place, the balloon is inflated to compress the plaque against the wall of the artery. This restores blood flow through the artery.

During the procedure, the doctor may put a small mesh tube called a stent in the artery. The stent helps prevent blockages in the artery in the months or years after angioplasty.

Other Treatments for Heart Attack

Medicines: A number of different types of medicines are used to treat heart attacks. They include the following:

- *Beta blockers:* Beta blockers decrease your heart's workload. These medicines also are used to relieve chest pain and discomfort and to help prevent repeat heart attacks. Beta blockers also are used to treat arrhythmias (irregular heartbeats).

- *Angiotensin-converting enzyme (ACE) inhibitors:* ACE inhibitors lower blood pressure and reduce strain on your heart. They also help slow down further weakening of the heart muscle.

- *Anticoagulants:* Anticoagulants, or "blood thinners," prevent blood clots from forming in your arteries. These medicines also keep existing clots from getting larger.

- *Anticlotting medicines:* Anticlotting medicines stop platelets from clumping together and forming unwanted blood clots. Examples of anticlotting medicines include aspirin and clopidogrel.

You also may be given medicines to relieve pain and anxiety, treat arrhythmias (which often occur during a heart attack), or lower your cholesterol (these medicines are called statins).

Medical procedures: Coronary artery bypass grafting (CABG) also may be used to treat a heart attack. During CABG, a surgeon removes a healthy artery or vein from your body. The artery or vein is then connected, or grafted, to the blocked coronary artery.

The grafted artery or vein bypasses (that is, goes around) the blocked portion of the coronary artery. This provides a new route for blood to flow to the heart muscle.

Treatment After You Leave the Hospital

Most people spend several days in the hospital after a heart attack. When you leave the hospital, treatment doesn't stop. At home, your treatment may include daily medicines and cardiac rehabilitation (rehab). Your doctor may want you to have a flu shot and pneumococcal vaccine each year.

Your doctor also may recommend lifestyle changes, including following a heart healthy diet, being physically active, maintaining a healthy weight, and quitting smoking. Taking these steps can lower your chances of having another heart attack.

Cardiac rehabilitation: Your doctor may recommend cardiac rehab to help you recover from a heart attack and to help prevent another heart attack. Almost everyone who has had a heart attack can benefit from rehab.

Cardiac rehab is a medically supervised program that may help improve the health and well-being of people who have heart problems. Rehab has two parts:

- *Exercise training:* This part helps you learn how to exercise safely, strengthen your muscles, and improve your stamina. Your exercise plan will be based on your personal abilities, needs, and interests.

- *Education, counseling, and training:* This part of rehab helps you understand your heart condition and find ways to reduce your risk of future heart problems. The rehab team will help you learn

119

how to cope with the stress of adjusting to a new lifestyle and deal with your fears about the future.

How Can a Heart Attack Be Prevented?

Lowering your risk factors for coronary heart disease (CHD) can help you prevent a heart attack.

Even if you already have CHD, you can still take steps to lower your risk for a heart attack. These steps involve following a heart healthy lifestyle and getting ongoing care.

Heart Healthy Lifestyle

Following a healthy diet is an important part of a heart healthy lifestyle. A healthy diet includes a variety of fruits, vegetables, and whole grains. It also includes lean meats, poultry, fish, beans, and fat-free or low-fat milk or milk products. A healthy diet is low in saturated fat, trans fat, cholesterol, sodium (salt), and added sugars.

If you're overweight or obese, work with your doctor to create a reasonable weight-loss plan that involves diet and physical activity. Controlling your weight helps you control risk factors for CHD and heart attack.

Be as physically active as you can. Physical activity can improve your fitness level and your health. Talk with your doctor about what types of activity are safe for you.

If you smoke, quit. Smoking can raise your risk of CHD and heart attack. Talk with your doctor about programs and products that can help you quit. Also, try to avoid secondhand smoke.

Ongoing Care

Treat related conditions: Treating conditions that make a heart attack more likely also can help lower your risk for a heart attack. These conditions may include the following:

- *High blood cholesterol:* Your doctor may prescribe medicine to lower your cholesterol if diet and exercise aren't enough.

- *High blood pressure:* You doctor may prescribe medicine to keep your blood pressure under control.

- *Diabetes (high blood sugar):* If you have diabetes, try to control your blood sugar level through diet and physical activity (as your doctor recommends). If needed, take medicine as prescribed.

Have an emergency action plan: Make sure that you have an emergency action plan in case you or someone in your family has a heart attack. This is very important if you're at high risk for a heart attack or have already had a heart attack.

Talk with your doctor about the signs and symptoms of a heart attack, when you should call 9-1-1, and steps you can take while waiting for medical help to arrive.

Life After a Heart Attack

Many people survive heart attacks and live active, full lives. If you get help quickly, treatment can limit damage to your heart muscle. Less heart damage improves your chances for a better quality of life after a heart attack.

Medical Follow-up

After a heart attack, you'll need treatment for coronary heart disease (CHD). This will help prevent another heart attack. Your doctor may recommend the following things:

- Lifestyle changes, such as following a healthy diet, being physically active, maintaining a healthy weight, and quitting smoking

- Medicines to control chest pain or discomfort, high blood cholesterol, high blood pressure, and your heart's workload

- A cardiac rehabilitation program

If you find it hard to get your medicines or take them, talk with your doctor. Don't stop taking medicines that can help you prevent another heart attack.

Returning to Normal Activities

After a heart attack, most people who don't have chest pain or discomfort or other problems can safely return to most of their normal activities within a few weeks.

Sexual activity also can begin within a few weeks for most patients. Talk with your doctor about a safe schedule for returning to your normal routine.

If allowed by state law, driving usually can begin within a week for most patients who don't have chest pain or discomfort or other problems. Each state has rules about driving a motor vehicle following a serious illness. People who have complications shouldn't drive until their symptoms have been stable for a few weeks.

Anxiety and Depression After a Heart Attack

After a heart attack, many people worry about having another heart attack. Sometimes they feel depressed and have trouble adjusting to new lifestyle changes.

Talk about how you feel with your health care team. Talking to a professional counselor also can help. If you're very depressed, your doctor may recommend medicines or other treatments that can improve your quality of life.

Joining a patient support group may help you adjust to life after a heart attack. You can see how other people who have the same symptoms have coped with them. Talk with your doctor about local support groups or check with an area medical center.

Support from family and friends also can help relieve stress and anxiety. Let your loved ones know how you feel and what they can do to help you.

Risk of a Repeat Heart Attack

Once you've had a heart attack, you're at higher risk for another one. Knowing the difference between angina and a heart attack is important. Angina is chest pain that occurs in people who have CHD.

The pain from angina usually occurs after physical exertion and goes away in a few minutes when you rest or take medicine as directed.

The pain from a heart attack usually is more severe than the pain from angina. Heart attack pain doesn't go away when you rest or take medicine.

If you don't know whether your chest pain is angina or a heart attack, call 9-1-1.

The symptoms of a second heart attack may not be the same as those of a first heart attack. Don't take a chance if you're in doubt. Always call 9-1-1 right away if you or someone else has heart attack symptoms.

Chapter 14

Sudden Cardiac Arrest

What is sudden cardiac arrest?

Sudden cardiac arrest (SCA) is a condition in which the heartbeat stops abruptly and unexpectedly. This usually is caused by ventricular fibrillation (VF), an abnormality in the heart's electrical system. When this happens, blood stops flowing to the brain, the heart, and the rest of the body, and the person collapses. In fact, the victim is clinically dead and will remain so unless someone helps immediately. A quick combination of cardiopulmonary resuscitation (CPR) and defibrillation can restore life.

Is SCA the same as a heart attack?

No. A heart attack is a condition in which a blood clot suddenly blocks a coronary artery, resulting in the death of the heart muscle supplied by that artery unless the clot is opened within a few hours. Heart attack victims usually experience symptoms such as chest discomfort or pain and remain conscious. Most people who have a heart attack survive the event. Some will develop an SCA. Other people have an SCA independently from a heart attack and without warning signs. SCA results in death if it is not treated immediately.

"Sudden Cardiac Arrest FAQs," by Mary M. Newman, MS. Reprinted by permission of the author and the Sudden Cardiac Arrest Foundation, © 2013. All rights reserved. For additional information, visit http://www.sca-aware.org.

Who is at risk for SCA?

SCA often occurs in active people who seem to be healthy and have no known medical conditions. In these patients, SCA is the first indication of a heart condition. However, some people can be identified in advance as being at risk for SCA. Risk factors include:

- previous heart attack;
- coronary artery disease (and risk factors for coronary artery disease, including smoking, high blood pressure, diabetes, elevated low-density lipoprotein [LDL] cholesterol, family history of heart disease, sedentary lifestyle);
- heart failure from other causes;
- abnormal heart rate or rhythm (arrhythmia) of unknown cause;
- episodes of fainting of unknown cause;
- low ejection fraction (EF) (less than 35 percent).

What is an ejection fraction?

The ejection fraction (EF) is a measurement of how much blood is pumped by the ventricles with each heartbeat. A healthy heart pumps 55 percent or more of its blood with each beat.

What causes SCA in young people?

There are three common causes. Long QT syndrome is an often unrecognized congenital condition that predisposes the child to an abnormality in the heart's electrical system, which can lead to SCA. This is a genetic disease that affects one in seven thousand young people. Episodes are most commonly triggered by physical exertion or emotional stress. Commotio cordis is an electrical disturbance caused by a blow to the chest. It occurs most often in baseball, but has been reported in other sports and situations in which there is a blow to the chest. Researchers at the U.S. Commotio Cordis Registry studied 124 cases and found the average age is fourteen. Only 18 victims (14 percent) survived; most who survived received prompt CPR and defibrillation. Hypertrophic cardiomyopathy is a congenital heart muscle disease. The walls of the heart's left ventricle become abnormally thickened (hypertrophy). The structural abnormality can lead to obstruction of blood flow from the heart, causing loss of consciousness and irregular heartbeat, leading to SCA. About one in five hundred to one thousand young people have this condition.

How can SCA be prevented?

Living a healthy lifestyle—exercising regularly, eating healthy foods, maintaining a reasonable weight, and avoiding smoking—can help prevent SCA. Monitoring and controlling blood pressure, cholesterol levels, and diabetes is also important. If abnormal heart rhythms or arrhythmias are detected, they can be treated through implantable cardioverter defibrillator (ICD) therapy; use of medications such as angiotensin-converting enzyme (ACE) inhibitors, beta blockers, and calcium channel blockers; and catheter ablation.

How should SCA be treated?

SCA is treatable most of the time, especially when it is due to an electrical abnormality called ventricular fibrillation (VF). Immediate treatment includes cardiopulmonary resuscitation (CPR) and use of defibrillators. This treatment must be provided within moments of collapse to be effective, preferably within three to five minutes. Even the fastest emergency medical services may not be able to reach a victim this quickly. That is why prompt action by bystanders is so critical and why it is so important that more laypersons learn CPR and how to use an automated external defibrillator (AED).

Subsequent care includes administration of medications and other advanced cardiac life support (ACLS) techniques by emergency medical personnel. In patients who have been successfully resuscitated but remain in a coma after cardiac arrest due to VF, mild hypothermia can improve the chances of survival with good brain function. SCA survivors should see heart specialists (cardiologists and electrophysiologists) for follow-up care.

What is an AED?

An AED, or automated external defibrillator, is a device that automatically analyzes heart rhythms and advises the operator to deliver a shock if the heart is in a fatal heart rhythm. AEDs are safe and will not shock anyone who is not in a fatal heart rhythm. Nonmedical personnel can use AEDs safely and effectively with minimal training.

How does an AED work?

A computer inside the defibrillator analyzes the victim's heart rhythm. The device decides whether a shock is needed. Some devices shock the victim automatically if a shock is needed. Other devices require that the operator press a button to deliver the shock. The shock is delivered through pads stuck to the victim's bare chest. The shock stuns the heart, stopping abnormal heart activity, and allowing a normal heart rhythm to resume.

Who can use an AED?

Modern AEDs are designed to be used by any motivated bystander, regardless of training. The devices are designed to advise the user about how to apply the device and whether or not to administer a shock. Some devices shock automatically if the victim has a fatal heart rhythm. Training is important, however, particularly since almost all victims also need CPR. Most of the time, the AED will advise the user to administer CPR, depending on the needs of the victim, and in these cases it is quite helpful to have CPR training. AEDs have been used successfully by police, firefighters, flight attendants, security guards, and lay rescuers.

Can I accidentally hurt the victim with an AED?

No. Most SCA victims will die if they are not treated immediately. Your actions can only help. AEDs are designed in such a way that they will only shock victims who need to be shocked.

Can I hurt myself or others with an AED?

No, not if you use it properly. The electric shock is programmed to go from one pad to the other through the victim's chest. Basic precautions, such as not touching the victim during the shock, ensure the safety of rescuers and bystanders.

Can the AED be used safely if the victim is on a metal surface such as a bleacher or stretcher?

Yes. AEDs can be used safely as long as the electrode pads do not come into contact with the metal surface.

Are there special considerations when placing electrodes on a female victim?

If the victim is wearing a bra, remove it before placing electrodes.

What if the victim has a medication patch, such as nitroglycerin?

Never place electrodes directly on top of medication patches. If the patch is in the way of the AED pads, remove it and wipe off the area with the victim's shirt. Then apply the pads to the clean, bare skin.

What if the victim has an implantable pacemaker or defibrillator?

If the victim has a pacemaker or internal defibrillator with a battery pack (visible as a lump under the skin about two inches long), avoid placing pad directly on top of the implanted medical device.

Do AEDs always help SCA victims?

No. AEDs are designed to treat victims in SCA with an irregular heart rhythm called ventricular fibrillation (VF). AEDs work best in these victims if they are used quickly and if the victim has received cardiopulmonary resuscitation (CPR). SCA victims who suffer from other irregular heart rhythms benefit from CPR, drug therapy, and advanced treatments such as hypothermia.

What is the difference between AEDs and defibrillators commonly used on ambulances and in hospitals?

Defibrillators sometimes used on ambulances and in hospitals, and often seen on TV, are manual defibrillators. They are larger than AEDs and are designed to be used by qualified medical personnel with special training. In contrast, AEDs are smaller and computerized so that virtually any operator can use the device and simply follow the audio and visual prompts. The decision to shock or not to shock is determined by the device, not the operator.

Where should AEDs be deployed?

Logical locations for AED placement include police cars, airports, train and bus stations, highway rest stops, sports arenas, doctor and dentist offices, health clinics, fitness clubs, shopping malls, large grocery stores, theatres, workplaces, schools, churches, and retirement communities. Increasingly, consumers are choosing to purchase AEDs for their homes and vehicles.

Do I have to have a prescription to acquire an AED?

A prescription from a physician is required for purchasing most AED models. However, at least one model has been cleared by the Food and Drug Administration for use without a prescription and is available over the counter.

Do AEDs replace the use of CPR?

No. CPR is still very important, and high-quality CPR can greatly improve the chances of survival.

After resuscitation, will the victim be able to resume a normal life?

More than 80 percent of SCA victims who are discharged home from the hospital live at least one year. More than half live another five years after resuscitation. Most people who survive SCA can return to their previous level of functioning. All survivors need follow-up care with physicians who specialize in heart conditions (cardiologists and electrophysiologists.)

Chapter 15

Cardiogenic Shock

What Is Cardiogenic Shock?

Cardiogenic shock is a condition in which a suddenly weakened heart isn't able to pump enough blood to meet the body's needs. The condition is a medical emergency and is fatal if not treated right away.

The most common cause of cardiogenic shock is damage to the heart muscle from a severe heart attack. However, not everyone who has a heart attack has cardiogenic shock. In fact, on average, only about 7 percent of people who have heart attacks develop the condition.

If cardiogenic shock does occur, it's very dangerous. When people die from heart attacks in hospitals, cardiogenic shock is the most common cause of death.

Outlook

In the past, almost no one survived cardiogenic shock. Now, about half of the people who go into cardiogenic shock survive. This is because of prompt recognition of symptoms and improved treatments, such as medicines and devices. These treatments can restore blood flow to the heart and help the heart pump better.

In some cases, devices that take over the pumping function of the heart are used. Implanting these devices requires major surgery.

Excerpted from "Cardiogenic Shock," National Heart, Lung, and Blood Institute, National Institutes of Health, July 1, 2011.

What Causes Cardiogenic Shock?

Immediate Causes

Cardiogenic shock occurs if the heart suddenly can't pump enough oxygen-rich blood to the body. The most common cause of cardiogenic shock is damage to the heart muscle from a severe heart attack.

This damage prevents the heart's main pumping chamber, the left ventricle, from working well. As a result, the heart can't pump enough oxygen-rich blood to the rest of the body.

In about 3 percent of cardiogenic shock cases, the heart's lower right chamber, the right ventricle, doesn't work well. This means the heart can't properly pump blood to the lungs, where it picks up oxygen to bring back to the heart and the rest of the body.

Without enough oxygen-rich blood reaching the body's major organs, many problems can occur:

- Cardiogenic shock can cause death if the flow of oxygen-rich blood to the organs isn't restored quickly. This is why emergency medical treatment is required.

- If organs don't get enough oxygen-rich blood, they won't work well. Cells in the organs die, and the organs may never work well again.

- As some organs stop working, they may cause problems with other bodily functions. This, in turn, can worsen shock. For example, if the kidneys aren't working well, the levels of important chemicals in the body change. This may cause the heart and other muscles to become even weaker, limiting blood flow even more. If the liver isn't working well, the body stops making proteins that help the blood clot. This can lead to more bleeding if the shock is due to blood loss.

How well the brain, kidneys, and other organs recover will depend on how long a person is in shock. The less time a person is in shock, the less damage will occur to the organs. This is another reason why emergency treatment is so important.

Underlying Causes

The underlying causes of cardiogenic shock are conditions that weaken the heart and prevent it from pumping enough oxygen-rich blood to the body.

Heart attack: Most heart attacks occur as a result of coronary heart disease (CHD). CHD is a condition in which a waxy substance called plaque narrows or blocks the coronary (heart) arteries.

Plaque reduces blood flow to your heart muscle. It also makes it more likely that blood clots will form in your arteries. Blood clots can partially or completely block blood flow.

Conditions caused by heart attack: Heart attacks can cause some serious heart conditions that can lead to cardiogenic shock. One example is ventricular septal rupture. This condition occurs if the wall that separates the ventricles (the heart's two lower chambers) breaks down.

The breakdown happens because cells in the wall have died due to a heart attack. Without the wall to separate them, the ventricles can't pump properly.

Heart attacks also can cause papillary muscle infarction or rupture. This condition occurs if the muscles that help anchor the heart valves stop working or break because a heart attack cuts off their blood supply. If this happens, blood doesn't flow correctly between the heart's chambers. This prevents the heart from pumping properly.

Other heart conditions: Serious heart conditions that may occur with or without a heart attack can cause cardiogenic shock. Examples include the following:

- *Myocarditis:* This is inflammation of the heart muscle.

- *Endocarditis:* This is an infection of the inner lining of the heart chambers and valves.

- *Life-threatening arrhythmias:* These are problems with the rate or rhythm of the heartbeat.

- *Pericardial tamponade:* This is too much fluid or blood around the heart. The fluid squeezes the heart muscle so it can't pump properly.

Pulmonary embolism: Pulmonary embolism (PE) is a sudden blockage in a lung artery. This condition usually is caused by a blood clot that travels to the lung from a vein in the leg. PE can damage your heart and other organs in your body.

Who Is at Risk for Cardiogenic Shock?

The most common risk factor for cardiogenic shock is having a heart attack. If you've had a heart attack, the following factors can further increase your risk for cardiogenic shock:

- Older age
- A history of heart attacks or heart failure
- Coronary heart disease that affects all of the heart's major blood vessels
- High blood pressure
- Diabetes

Women who have heart attacks are at higher risk for cardiogenic shock than men who have heart attacks.

What Are the Signs and Symptoms of Cardiogenic Shock?

A lack of oxygen-rich blood reaching the brain, kidneys, skin, and other parts of the body causes the signs and symptoms of cardiogenic shock.

Some of the typical signs and symptoms of shock usually include at least two or more of the following:

- Confusion or lack of alertness
- Loss of consciousness
- A sudden and ongoing rapid heartbeat
- Sweating
- Pale skin
- A weak pulse
- Rapid breathing
- Decreased or no urine output
- Cool hands and feet

Any of these alone is unlikely to be a sign or symptom of shock.

If you or someone else is having these signs and symptoms, call 9-1-1 right away for emergency treatment. Prompt medical care can save your life and prevent or limit organ damage.

How Is Cardiogenic Shock Diagnosed?

The first step in diagnosing cardiogenic shock is to identify that a person is in shock. At that point, emergency treatment should begin.

Once emergency treatment starts, doctors can look for the specific cause of the shock. If the reason for the shock is that the heart isn't pumping strongly enough, then the diagnosis is cardiogenic shock.

Tests and Procedures to Diagnose Shock and Its Underlying Causes

Blood pressure test: Medical personnel can use a simple blood pressure cuff and stethoscope to check whether a person has very low blood pressure. This is the most common sign of shock. A blood pressure test can be done before the person goes to a hospital.

Electrocardiogram (EKG): An EKG is a simple test that detects and records the heart's electrical activity. The test shows how fast the heart is beating and its rhythm (steady or irregular).

An EKG also records the strength and timing of electrical signals as they pass through each part of the heart. Doctors use EKGs to diagnose severe heart attacks and monitor the heart's condition.

Echocardiography: Echocardiography (echo) uses sound waves to create a moving picture of the heart. The test provides information about the size and shape of the heart and how well the heart chambers and valves are working.

Echo also can identify areas of poor blood flow to the heart, areas of heart muscle that aren't contracting normally, and previous injury to the heart muscle caused by poor blood flow.

Chest x-ray: A chest x-ray takes pictures of organs and structures in the chest, including the heart, lungs, and blood vessels. This test shows whether the heart is enlarged or whether fluid is present in the lungs. These can be signs of cardiogenic shock.

Cardiac enzyme test: When cells in the heart die, they release enzymes into the blood. These enzymes are called markers or biomarkers. Measuring these markers can show whether the heart is damaged and the extent of the damage.

Coronary angiography: Coronary angiography is an x-ray exam of the heart and blood vessels. The doctor passes a catheter (a thin, flexible tube) through an artery in the leg or arm to the heart. The catheter can measure the pressure inside the heart chambers.

Dye that can be seen on an x-ray image is injected into the bloodstream through the tip of the catheter. The dye lets the doctor study the flow of blood through the heart and blood vessels and see any blockages.

Pulmonary artery catheterization: For this procedure, a catheter is inserted into a vein in the arm or neck or near the collarbone. Then, the catheter is moved into the pulmonary artery. This artery connects the right side of the heart to the lungs.

The catheter is used to check blood pressure in the pulmonary artery. If the blood pressure is too high or too low, treatment may be needed.

Blood tests: Some blood tests also are used to help diagnose cardiogenic shock. These include the following:

- *Arterial blood gas measurement:* For this test, a blood sample is taken from an artery. The sample is used to measure oxygen, carbon dioxide, and pH (acidity) levels in the blood. Certain levels of these substances are associated with shock.

- *Tests that measure the function of various organs, such as the kidneys and liver:* If these organs aren't working well, they may not be getting enough oxygen-rich blood. This could be a sign of cardiogenic shock.

How Is Cardiogenic Shock Treated?

Cardiogenic shock is life threatening and requires emergency medical treatment. The condition usually is diagnosed after a person has been admitted to a hospital for a heart attack. If the person isn't already in a hospital, emergency treatment can start as soon as medical personnel arrive.

The first goal of emergency treatment for cardiogenic shock is to improve the flow of blood and oxygen to the body's organs.

Sometimes both the shock and its cause are treated at the same time. For example, doctors may quickly open a blocked blood vessel that's damaging the heart. Often, this can get the patient out of shock with little or no additional treatment.

Emergency Life Support

Emergency life support treatment is needed for any type of shock. This treatment helps get oxygen-rich blood flowing to the brain, kidneys, and other organs.

Restoring blood flow to the organs keeps the patient alive and may prevent long-term damage to the organs. Emergency life support treatment includes the following:

- Giving the patient extra oxygen to breathe so that more oxygen reaches the lungs, the heart, and the rest of the body.

- Providing breathing support if needed. A ventilator might be used to protect the airway and provide the patient with extra oxygen. A ventilator is a machine that supports breathing.

- Giving the patient fluids, including blood and blood products, through a needle inserted in a vein (when the shock is due to blood loss). This can help get more blood to major organs and the rest of the body. This treatment usually isn't used for cardiogenic shock because the heart can't pump the blood that's already in the body. Also, too much fluid is in the lungs, making it hard to breathe.

Medicines

Treatment for cardiogenic shock will depend on its cause. Doctors may prescribe medicines to do the following things:

- Prevent blood clots from forming

- Increase the force with which the heart muscle contracts

- Treat a heart attack

Medical Devices

Medical devices can help the heart pump and improve blood flow. Devices used to treat cardiogenic shock may include the following:

- *An intra-aortic balloon pump:* This device is placed in the aorta, the main blood vessel that carries blood from the heart to the body. A balloon at the tip of the device is inflated and deflated in a rhythm that matches the heart's pumping rhythm. This allows the weakened heart muscle to pump as much blood as it can, which helps get more blood to vital organs, such as the brain and kidneys.

- *A left ventricular assist device (LVAD):* This device is a battery-operated pump that takes over part of the heart's pumping action. An LVAD helps the heart pump blood to the body. This device may be used if damage to the left ventricle, the heart's main pumping chamber, is causing shock.

Medical Procedures and Surgery

Medical procedures and surgery can restore blood flow to the heart and the rest of the body, repair heart damage, and help keep a patient alive while he or she recovers from shock.

Surgery also can improve the chances of long-term survival. Surgery done within six hours of the onset of shock symptoms has the greatest chance of improving survival.

The types of procedures and surgery used to treat underlying causes of cardiogenic shock include the following:

- Angioplasty

- Coronary artery bypass grafting

- Surgery to repair damaged heart valves

- Surgery to repair a break in the wall that separates the heart's chambers

- Heart transplant

Chapter 16

Cardiomyopathy

What Is Cardiomyopathy?

Cardiomyopathy refers to diseases of the heart muscle. These diseases have many causes, signs and symptoms, and treatments.

In cardiomyopathy, the heart muscle becomes enlarged, thick, or rigid. In rare cases, the muscle tissue in the heart is replaced with scar tissue.

As cardiomyopathy worsens, the heart becomes weaker. It's less able to pump blood through the body and maintain a normal electrical rhythm. This can lead to heart failure or irregular heartbeats called arrhythmias. In turn, heart failure can cause fluid to build up in the lungs, ankles, feet, legs, or abdomen.

The weakening of the heart also can cause other complications, such as heart valve problems.

Overview

The main types of cardiomyopathy are as follows:

- Dilated cardiomyopathy
- Hypertrophic cardiomyopathy
- Restrictive cardiomyopathy

Excerpted from "Cardiomyopathy," National Heart, Lung, and Blood Institute, National Institutes of Health, January 1, 2011.

• Arrhythmogenic right ventricular dysplasia

Other types of cardiomyopathy sometimes are referred to as "unclassified cardiomyopathy."

Cardiomyopathy can be acquired or inherited. "Acquired" means you aren't born with the disease, but you develop it due to another disease, condition, or factor. "Inherited" means your parents passed the gene for the disease on to you. Many times, the cause of cardiomyopathy isn't known.

Cardiomyopathy can affect people of all ages. However, people in certain age groups are more likely to have certain types of cardiomyopathy. This chapter focuses on cardiomyopathy in adults.

Outlook

Some people who have cardiomyopathy have no signs or symptoms and need no treatment. For other people, the disease develops quickly, symptoms are severe, and serious complications occur.

Treatments for cardiomyopathy include lifestyle changes, medicines, surgery, implanted devices to correct arrhythmias, and a nonsurgical procedure. These treatments can control symptoms, reduce complications, and stop the disease from getting worse.

Types of Cardiomyopathy

Dilated Cardiomyopathy

Dilated cardiomyopathy is the most common type of the disease. It mostly occurs in adults aged twenty to sixty. Men are more likely than women to have this type of cardiomyopathy.

Dilated cardiomyopathy affects the heart's ventricles and atria. These are the lower and upper chambers of the heart, respectively.

The disease often starts in the left ventricle, the heart's main pumping chamber. The heart muscle begins to dilate (stretch and become thinner). This causes the inside of the chamber to enlarge. The problem often spreads to the right ventricle and then to the atria as the disease gets worse.

When the heart chambers dilate, the heart muscle doesn't contract normally. Also, the heart can't pump blood very well. Over time, the heart becomes weaker and heart failure can occur.

Common symptoms of heart failure include shortness of breath, fatigue (tiredness), and swelling of the ankles, feet, legs, abdomen, and veins in the neck.

Dilated cardiomyopathy also can lead to heart valve problems, arrhythmias (irregular heartbeats), and blood clots in the heart.

Hypertrophic Cardiomyopathy

Hypertrophic cardiomyopathy (HCM) is very common and can affect people of any age. About one out of every five hundred people has HCM. It affects men and women equally.

HCM is a common cause of sudden cardiac arrest (SCA) in young people, including young athletes.

HCM occurs if heart muscle cells enlarge and cause the walls of the ventricles (usually the left ventricle) to thicken. Despite this thickening, the ventricle size often remains normal. However, the thickening may block blood flow out of the ventricle. If this happens, the condition is called obstructive hypertrophic cardiomyopathy.

Sometimes, the septum thickens and bulges into the left ventricle. This also can block blood flow out of the left ventricle. (The septum is the wall that divides the left and right sides of the heart.)

If a blockage occurs, the ventricle must work hard to pump blood to the body. Symptoms can include chest pain, dizziness, shortness of breath, or fainting.

HCM also can affect the heart's mitral valve, causing blood to leak backward through the valve.

Sometimes the thickened heart muscle doesn't block blood flow out of the left ventricle. This is called nonobstructive hypertrophic cardiomyopathy. The entire ventricle may thicken, or the thickening may happen only at the bottom of the heart. The right ventricle also may be affected.

In both types of HCM (obstructive and nonobstructive), the thickened muscle makes the inside of the left ventricle smaller, so it holds less blood. The walls of the ventricle also may stiffen. As a result, the ventricle is less able to relax and fill with blood.

These changes can raise blood pressure in the ventricles and the blood vessels of the lungs. Changes also occur to the cells in the damaged heart muscle. This may disrupt the heart's electrical signals and lead to arrhythmias.

Some people who have HCM have no signs or symptoms. The disease doesn't affect their lives. Others have severe symptoms and complications. For example, they may have shortness of breath, serious arrhythmias, or an inability to exercise.

Rarely, people who have HCM can have SCA during very vigorous physical activity. The physical activity can trigger dangerous arrhythmias. If you have HCM, ask your doctor what types and amounts of physical activity are safe for you.

Restrictive Cardiomyopathy

Restrictive cardiomyopathy tends to mostly affect older adults. With this disease, the ventricles become stiff and rigid. This happens because abnormal tissue, such as scar tissue, replaces the normal heart muscle.

As a result, the ventricles can't relax normally and fill with blood, and the atria become enlarged. Over time, blood flow in the heart is reduced. This can lead to problems such as heart failure or arrhythmias.

Arrhythmogenic Right Ventricular Dysplasia

Arrhythmogenic right ventricular dysplasia (ARVD) is a rare type of cardiomyopathy. ARVD occurs if the muscle tissue in the right ventricle dies and is replaced with scar tissue.

This process disrupts the heart's electrical signals and causes arrhythmias. Symptoms include palpitations and fainting after physical activity. (Palpitations are feelings that your heart is skipping a beat, fluttering, or beating too hard or too fast.)

ARVD usually affects teens or young adults. It can cause SCA in young athletes.

What Causes Cardiomyopathy?

Cardiomyopathy can be acquired or inherited. "Acquired" means you aren't born with the disease, but you develop it due to another disease, condition, or factor.

"Inherited" means your parents passed the gene for the disease on to you. Researchers continue to look for the genetic links to cardiomyopathy. They also continue to explore how these links cause or contribute to the various types of the disease.

Many times, the cause of cardiomyopathy isn't known. This often is the case when the disease occurs in children.

Dilated Cardiomyopathy

The cause of dilated cardiomyopathy often isn't known. As many as one-third of the people who have dilated cardiomyopathy inherit it from their parents.

Certain diseases, conditions, and substances also can cause the disease, such as the following:

- Coronary heart disease, heart attack, high blood pressure, diabetes, thyroid disease, viral hepatitis, and human immunodeficiency virus (HIV)

- Infections, especially viral infections that inflame the heart muscle
- Alcohol, especially if you also have a poor diet
- Complications during the last month of pregnancy or within five months of birth
- Certain toxins, such as cobalt
- Certain drugs (such as cocaine and amphetamines) and two medicines used to treat cancer (doxorubicin and daunorubicin)

Hypertrophic Cardiomyopathy

Hypertrophic cardiomyopathy (HCM) usually is inherited. It's caused by a mutation (change) in some of the genes in heart muscle proteins. HCM also can develop over time because of high blood pressure or aging.

Other diseases, such as diabetes or thyroid disease, also can cause HCM. Sometimes the cause of the disease isn't known.

Restrictive Cardiomyopathy

Certain diseases, conditions, and factors can cause restrictive cardiomyopathy, including the following:

- **Hemochromatosis:** This is a disease in which too much iron builds up in your body. The extra iron is toxic to the body and can damage the organs, including the heart.
- **Sarcoidosis:** This disease causes inflammation and can affect various organs in the body. Researchers believe that an abnormal immune response may cause sarcoidosis. This abnormal response causes tiny lumps of cells to form in the body's organs, including the heart.
- **Amyloidosis:** This is a disease in which abnormal proteins build up in the body's organs, including the heart.
- **Connective tissue disorders.**
- **Some cancer treatments, such as radiation and chemotherapy.**

Arrhythmogenic Right Ventricular Dysplasia

Researchers think that arrhythmogenic right ventricular dysplasia is an inherited disease.

Who Is at Risk for Cardiomyopathy?

People of all ages and races can have cardiomyopathy. However, certain types of the disease are more common in certain groups.

Dilated cardiomyopathy is more common in African Americans than whites. This type of the disease also is more common in men than women.

Teens and young adults are more likely than older people to have arrhythmogenic right ventricular dysplasia, although it's rare in both groups.

Major Risk Factors

Certain diseases, conditions, or factors can raise your risk for cardiomyopathy. Major risk factors include the following:

- A family history of cardiomyopathy, heart failure, or sudden cardiac arrest (SCA)

- A disease or condition that can lead to cardiomyopathy, such as coronary heart disease, heart attack, or a viral infection that inflames the heart muscle

- Diabetes or other metabolic diseases, or severe obesity

- Diseases that can damage the heart, such as hemochromatosis, sarcoidosis, or amyloidosis

- Long-term alcoholism

- Long-term high blood pressure

Some people who have cardiomyopathy never have signs or symptoms. Thus, it's important to identify people who may be at high risk for the disease. This can help prevent future problems, such as serious arrhythmias (irregular heartbeats) or SCA.

What Are the Signs and Symptoms of Cardiomyopathy?

Some people who have cardiomyopathy never have signs or symptoms. Others don't have signs or symptoms in the early stages of the disease.

As cardiomyopathy worsens and the heart weakens, signs and symptoms of heart failure usually occur. These signs and symptoms include the following:

- Shortness of breath or trouble breathing, especially with physical exertion

- Fatigue (tiredness)
- Swelling in the ankles, feet, legs, abdomen, and veins in the neck

Other signs and symptoms may include dizziness; light-headedness; fainting during physical activity; arrhythmias (irregular heartbeats); chest pain, especially after physical exertion or heavy meals; and heart murmurs. (Heart murmurs are extra or unusual sounds heard during a heartbeat.)

How Is Cardiomyopathy Diagnosed?

Your doctor will diagnose cardiomyopathy based on your medical and family histories, a physical exam, and the results from tests and procedures.

Medical and Family Histories

Your doctor will want to learn about your medical history. He or she will want to know what signs and symptoms you have and how long you've had them.

Your doctor also will want to know whether anyone in your family has had cardiomyopathy, heart failure, or sudden cardiac arrest.

Physical Exam

Your doctor will use a stethoscope to listen to your heart and lungs for sounds that may suggest cardiomyopathy. These sounds may even suggest a certain type of the disease.

For example, the loudness, timing, and location of a heart murmur may suggest obstructive hypertrophic cardiomyopathy. A "crackling" sound in the lungs may be a sign of heart failure. (Heart failure often develops in the later stages of cardiomyopathy.)

Physical signs also help your doctor diagnose cardiomyopathy. Swelling of the ankles, feet, legs, abdomen, or veins in your neck suggests fluid buildup, a sign of heart failure.

Your doctor may notice signs and symptoms of cardiomyopathy during a routine exam. For example, he or she may hear a heart murmur, or you may have abnormal test results.

Diagnostic Tests

Your doctor may recommend one or more of the following tests to diagnose cardiomyopathy:

- Blood tests
- Chest x-ray
- Electrocardiogram (EKG)
- Echocardiography
- Stress Test

Diagnostic Procedures

You may have one or more medical procedures to confirm a diagnosis or to prepare for surgery (if surgery is planned). These procedures may include cardiac catheterization, coronary angiography, or myocardial biopsy.

Genetic Testing

Some types of cardiomyopathy run in families. Thus, your doctor may suggest genetic testing to look for the disease in your parents, brothers and sisters, or other family members.

Genetic testing can show how the disease runs in families. It also can find out the chances of parents passing the genes for the disease on to their children.

Genetic testing also may be useful if your doctor thinks you have cardiomyopathy, but you don't yet have signs or symptoms. If the test shows you have the disease, your doctor can start treatment early, when it may work best.

How Is Cardiomyopathy Treated?

People who have cardiomyopathy but no signs or symptoms may not need treatment. Sometimes, dilated cardiomyopathy that comes on suddenly may even go away on its own.

For other people who have cardiomyopathy, treatment is needed. Treatment depends on the type of cardiomyopathy you have, the severity of your symptoms and complications, and your age and overall health.

Treatments may include lifestyle changes, medicines, surgery, implanted devices to correct arrhythmias (irregular heartbeats), and/or a nonsurgical procedure.

Lifestyle Changes

Your doctor may suggest lifestyle changes to manage a condition that's causing your cardiomyopathy. These changes can help reduce symptoms. They include the following:

- Eating a healthy diet
- Being physically active
- Quitting smoking
- Losing excess weight
- Avoiding the use of alcohol and illegal drugs
- Getting enough sleep and rest
- Reducing stress
- Treating underlying conditions, such as diabetes and high blood pressure

Medicines

Many medicines are used to treat cardiomyopathy. Your doctor may prescribe medicines to do the following things:

- **Lower your blood pressure**: angiotensin-converting enzyme (ACE) inhibitors, angiotensin II receptor blockers, beta blockers, and calcium channel blockers are examples of medicines that lower blood pressure.

- **Slow your heart rate:** Beta blockers, calcium channel blockers, and digoxin are examples of medicines that slow the heart rate. Beta blockers and calcium channel blockers also are used to lower blood pressure.

- **Keep your heart beating with a normal rhythm:** These medicines, called antiarrhythmics, help prevent arrhythmias.

- **Balance electrolytes in your body:** Electrolytes are minerals that help maintain fluid levels and acid-base balance in the body. They also help muscle and nerve tissues work properly. Abnormal electrolyte levels may be a sign of dehydration (lack of fluid in your body), heart failure, high blood pressure, or other disorders. Aldosterone blockers are an example of a medicine used to balance electrolytes.

- **Remove excess fluid and sodium from your body:** Diuretics, or "water pills," are an example of a medicine that helps remove excess fluid and sodium from the body.

- **Prevent blood clots from forming:** Anticoagulants, or "blood thinners," are an example of a medicine that prevents blood clots. Blood thinners often are used to prevent blood clots from forming in people who have dilated cardiomyopathy.

- **Reduce inflammation:** Corticosteroids are an example of a medicine used to reduce inflammation.

Surgery

Doctors use several types of surgery to treat cardiomyopathy. They include septal myectomy, implanted devices to help the heart work better, and heart transplant.

Septal myectomy: Septal myectomy is open-heart surgery. It's used for people who have obstructive hypertrophic cardiomyopathy and severe symptoms. This surgery generally is used for younger patients and for people whose medicines aren't working well.

During the surgery, a surgeon removes part of the thickened septum that's bulging into the left ventricle. This improves blood flow through the heart and out to the body. The removed tissue doesn't grow back.

The surgeon also can repair or replace the mitral valve at the same time (if needed). Septal myectomy often is successful and allows you to return to a normal life with no symptoms.

Surgically implanted devices: Surgeons can place several types of devices in the heart to help it work better. One example is a pacemaker. This is a small device that's placed under the skin of your chest or abdomen to help control arrhythmias. The device uses electrical pulses to prompt the heart to beat at a normal rate.

Sometimes doctors choose to use a cardiac resynchronization therapy (CRT) device. A CRT device coordinates contractions between the heart's left and right ventricles.

A left ventricular assist device (LVAD) helps the heart pump blood to the body. An LVAD can be used as a long-term therapy or as a short-term treatment for people who are waiting for a heart transplant.

An implantable cardioverter defibrillator (ICD) helps control life-threatening arrhythmias that may lead to SCA. This small device is implanted in the chest or abdomen and connected to the heart with wires.

If an ICD senses a dangerous change in heart rhythm, it will send an electric shock to the heart to restore a normal heartbeat.

Heart transplant: For this surgery, a surgeon replaces a person's diseased heart with a healthy heart from a deceased donor. A heart transplant is a last resort treatment for people who have end-stage heart failure. "End-stage" means the condition has become so severe that all treatments, other than heart transplant, have failed.

Nonsurgical Procedure

Doctors may use a nonsurgical procedure called alcohol septal ablation to treat cardiomyopathy.

For this procedure, your doctor injects ethanol (a type of alcohol) through a tube into the small artery that supplies blood to the thickened area of heart muscle. The alcohol kills cells, and the thickened tissue shrinks to a more normal size.

This procedure allows blood to flow freely through the ventricle, which improves symptoms.

Chapter 17

Heart Failure

What Is Heart Failure?

Heart failure is a condition in which the heart can't pump enough blood to meet the body's needs. In some cases, the heart can't fill with enough blood. In other cases, the heart can't pump blood to the rest of the body with enough force. Some people have both problems.

The term "heart failure" doesn't mean that your heart has stopped or is about to stop working. However, heart failure is a serious condition that requires medical care.

What Causes Heart Failure?

Conditions that damage or overwork the heart muscle can cause heart failure. Over time, the heart weakens. It isn't able to fill with and/or pump blood as well as it should.

As the heart weakens, certain proteins and substances might be released into the blood. These substances have a toxic effect on the heart and blood flow, and they worsen heart failure.

Common Causes of Heart Failure

The most common causes of heart failure are coronary heart disease (CHD), high blood pressure, and diabetes. Treating these problems can prevent or improve heart failure.

Excerpted from "Heart Failure," National Heart, Lung, and Blood Institute, National Institutes of Health, January 9, 2012.

Other Causes

Other diseases and conditions also can lead to heart failure, including the following:

- **Cardiomyopathy, or heart muscle disease:** Cardiomyopathy may be present at birth or caused by injury or infection.

- **Heart valve disease:** Problems with the heart valves may be present at birth or caused by infection, heart attack, or damage from heart disease.

- **Arrhythmias, or irregular heartbeats:** These heart problems may be present at birth or caused by heart disease or heart defects.

- **Congenital heart defects:** These problems with the heart's structure are present at birth.

Other factors also can injure the heart muscle and lead to heart failure. Examples include the following:

- Treatments for cancer, such as radiation and chemotherapy

- Thyroid disorders (having either too much or too little thyroid hormone in the body)

- Alcohol abuse or cocaine and other illegal drug use

- Human immunodeficiency virus (HIV)/acquired immune deficiency syndrome (AIDS)

- Too much vitamin E

Heart damage from obstructive sleep apnea may worsen heart failure. Sleep apnea is a common disorder in which you have one or more pauses in breathing or shallow breaths while you sleep.

Sleep apnea can deprive your heart of oxygen and increase its workload. Treating this sleep disorder might improve heart failure.

Who Is at Risk for Heart Failure?

About 5.8 million people in the United States have heart failure. The number of people who have this condition is growing.

Heart failure is more common in the following groups:

- **People who are sixty-five years old or older:** Aging can weaken the heart muscle. Older people also may have had diseases for many years that led to heart failure. Heart failure is a leading cause of hospital stays among people on Medicare.

- **African Americans:** African Americans are more likely to have heart failure than people of other races. They're also more likely to have symptoms at a younger age, have more hospital visits due to heart failure, and die from heart failure.
- **People who are overweight:** Excess weight puts strain on the heart. Being overweight also increases your risk of heart disease and type 2 diabetes. These diseases can lead to heart failure.
- **People who have had a heart attack.**
- **Men:** Men have a higher rate of heart failure than women.

Children who have congenital heart defects also can develop heart failure. These defects occur if the heart, heart valves, or blood vessels near the heart don't form correctly while a baby is in the womb.

Congenital heart defects can make the heart work harder. This weakens the heart muscle, which can lead to heart failure.

Children don't have the same symptoms of heart failure or get the same treatments as adults. This chapter focuses on heart failure in adults.

What Are the Signs and Symptoms of Heart Failure?

The most common signs and symptoms of heart failure are as follows:

- Shortness of breath or trouble breathing
- Fatigue (tiredness)
- Swelling in the ankles, feet, legs, abdomen, and veins in the neck

All of these symptoms are the result of fluid buildup in your body. When symptoms start, you may feel tired and short of breath after routine physical effort, like climbing stairs.

As your heart grows weaker, symptoms get worse. You may begin to feel tired and short of breath after getting dressed or walking across the room. Some people have shortness of breath while lying flat.

Fluid buildup from heart failure also causes weight gain, frequent urination, and a cough that's worse at night and when you're lying down. This cough may be a sign of acute pulmonary edema. This is a condition in which too much fluid builds up in your lungs. The condition requires emergency treatment.

How Is Heart Failure Diagnosed?

Your doctor will diagnose heart failure based on your medical and family histories, a physical exam, and test results.

Medical and Family Histories

Your doctor will ask whether you or others in your family have or have had a disease or condition that can cause heart failure.

Your doctor also will ask about your symptoms. He or she will want to know which symptoms you have, when they occur, how long you've had them, and how severe they are. Your answers will help show whether and how much your symptoms limit your daily routine.

Physical Exam

During the physical exam, your doctor will do the following things:

* Listen to your heart for sounds that aren't normal

* Listen to your lungs for the sounds of extra fluid buildup

* Look for swelling in your ankles, feet, legs, abdomen, and the veins in your neck

Diagnostic Tests

No single test can diagnose heart failure. If you have signs and symptoms of heart failure, your doctor may recommend one or more tests.

Electrocardiogram (EKG): An EKG is a simple, painless test that detects and records the heart's electrical activity. The test shows how fast your heart is beating and its rhythm (steady or irregular). An EKG also records the strength and timing of electrical signals as they pass through your heart.

An EKG may show whether the walls in your heart's pumping chambers are thicker than normal. Thicker walls can make it harder for your heart to pump blood. An EKG also can show signs of a previous or current heart attack.

Chest x-ray: A chest x-ray takes pictures of the structures inside your chest, such as your heart, lungs, and blood vessels. This test can show whether your heart is enlarged, you have fluid in your lungs, or you have lung disease.

Brain natriuretic peptide (BNP) blood test: This test checks the level of a hormone in your blood called BNP. The level of this hormone rises during heart failure.

Echocardiography: Echocardiography (echo) uses sound waves to create a moving picture of your heart. The test shows the size and shape of your heart and how well your heart chambers and valves work.

Echo also can identify areas of poor blood flow to the heart, areas of heart muscle that aren't contracting normally, and heart muscle damage caused by lack of blood flow.

Echo might be done before and after a stress test. A stress echo can show how well blood is flowing through your heart. The test also can show how well your heart pumps blood when it beats.

Doppler ultrasound: A Doppler ultrasound uses sound waves to measure the speed and direction of blood flow. This test often is done with echo to give a more complete picture of blood flow to the heart and lungs.

Doctors often use Doppler ultrasound to help diagnose right-side heart failure.

Holter monitor: A Holter monitor records your heart's electrical activity for a full twenty-four- or forty-eight-hour period, while you go about your normal daily routine.

You wear small patches called electrodes on your chest. Wires connect the patches to a small, portable recorder. The recorder can be clipped to a belt, kept in a pocket, or hung around your neck.

Nuclear heart scan: A nuclear heart scan shows how well blood is flowing through your heart and how much blood is reaching your heart muscle.

During a nuclear heart scan, a safe, radioactive substance called a tracer is injected into your bloodstream through a vein. The tracer travels to your heart and releases energy. Special cameras outside of your body detect the energy and use it to create pictures of your heart.

A nuclear heart scan can show where the heart muscle is healthy and where it's damaged.

A positron emission tomography (PET) scan is a type of nuclear heart scan. It shows the level of chemical activity in areas of your heart. This test can help your doctor see whether enough blood is flowing to these areas. A PET scan can show blood flow problems that other tests might not detect.

Cardiac catheterization: During cardiac catheterization, a long, thin, flexible tube called a catheter is put into a blood vessel in your arm, groin (upper thigh), or neck and threaded to your heart. This allows your doctor to look inside your coronary (heart) arteries.

During this procedure, your doctor can check the pressure and blood flow in your heart chambers, collect blood samples, and use x-rays to look at your coronary arteries.

Coronary angiography: Coronary angiography usually is done with cardiac catheterization. A dye that can be seen on x-ray is injected into your bloodstream through the tip of the catheter.

The dye allows your doctor to see the flow of blood to your heart muscle. Angiography also shows how well your heart is pumping.

Stress test: Some heart problems are easier to diagnose when your heart is working hard and beating fast. During stress testing, you exercise to make your heart work hard and beat fast.

You may walk or run on a treadmill or pedal a bicycle. If you can't exercise, you may be given medicine to raise your heart rate.

Heart tests, such as nuclear heart scanning and echo, often are done during stress testing.

Cardiac magnetic resonance imaging (MRI): Cardiac MRI (magnetic resonance imaging) uses radio waves, magnets, and a computer to create pictures of your heart as it's beating. The test produces both still and moving pictures of your heart and major blood vessels.

A cardiac MRI can show whether parts of your heart are damaged. Doctors also have used MRI in research studies to find early signs of heart failure, even before symptoms appear.

Thyroid function tests: Thyroid function tests show how well your thyroid gland is working. These tests include blood tests, imaging tests, and tests to stimulate the thyroid. Having too much or too little thyroid hormone in the blood can lead to heart failure.

How Is Heart Failure Treated?

Early diagnosis and treatment can help people who have heart failure live longer, more active lives. Treatment for heart failure will depend on the type and stage of heart failure (the severity of the condition).

The goals of treatment for all stages of heart failure include the following:

- Treating the condition's underlying cause, such as coronary heart disease (CHD), high blood pressure, or diabetes
- Reducing symptoms
- Stopping the heart failure from getting worse
- Increasing your lifespan and improving your quality of life

Treatments usually include lifestyle changes, medicines, and ongoing care. If you have severe heart failure, you also may need medical procedures or surgery.

Lifestyle Changes

Simple changes can help you feel better and control heart failure. The sooner you make these changes, the better off you'll likely be.

A heart healthy diet: Following a heart healthy diet is an important part of managing heart failure. In fact, not having a proper diet can make heart failure worse. Ask your doctor and health care team to create an eating plan that works for you.

A balanced, nutrient-rich diet can help your heart work better. Getting enough potassium is important for people who have heart failure. Some heart failure medicines deplete the potassium in your body. Lack of potassium can cause very rapid heart rhythms that can lead to sudden death.

Talk with your health care team about getting the correct amount of potassium. Too much potassium also can be harmful.

Fluid intake: It's important for people who have heart failure to drink the correct amounts and types of fluid. Drinking too much fluid can worsen heart failure. Also, if you have heart failure, you shouldn't drink alcohol.

Talk with your doctor about what amounts and types of fluid you should have each day.

Other lifestyle changes: Taking steps to control risk factors for CHD, high blood pressure, and diabetes will help control heart failure. Here are some steps you can take:

- Lose weight if you're overweight or obese. Work with your health care team to lose weight safely.

- Be physically active (as your doctor advises) to become more fit and stay as active as possible.

- Quit smoking and avoid using illegal drugs. Talk with your doctor about programs and products that can help you quit smoking. Also, try to avoid secondhand smoke. Smoking and drugs can worsen heart failure and harm your health.

- Get enough rest.

Medicines

Your doctor will prescribe medicines based on the type of heart failure you have, how severe it is, and your response to certain medicines. The following medicines are commonly used to treat heart failure:

- Diuretics (water or fluid pills) help reduce fluid buildup in your lungs and swelling in your feet and ankles.

- Angiotensin-converting enzyme (ACE) inhibitors lower blood pressure and reduce strain on your heart. They also may reduce the risk of a future heart attack.

- Aldosterone antagonists trigger the body to get rid of salt and water through urine. This lowers the volume of blood that the heart must pump.

- Angiotensin receptor blockers relax your blood vessels and lower blood pressure to decrease your heart's workload.

- Beta blockers slow your heart rate and lower your blood pressure to decrease your heart's workload.

- Isosorbide dinitrate/hydralazine hydrochloride helps relax your blood vessels so your heart doesn't work as hard to pump blood. Studies have shown that this medicine can reduce the risk of death in African Americans. More studies are needed to find out whether this medicine will benefit other racial groups.

- Digoxin makes the heart beat stronger and pump more blood.

Ongoing Care

You should watch for signs that heart failure is getting worse. For example, weight gain may mean that fluids are building up in your body. Ask your doctor how often you should check your weight and when to report weight changes.

Getting medical care for other related conditions is important. If you have diabetes or high blood pressure, work with your health care team to control these conditions. Have your blood sugar level and blood pressure checked. Talk with your doctor about when you should have tests and how often to take measurements at home.

Try to avoid respiratory infections like the flu and pneumonia. Talk with your doctor or nurse about getting flu and pneumonia vaccines.

Many people who have severe heart failure may need treatment in a hospital from time to time. Your doctor may recommend oxygen therapy (oxygen given through nasal prongs or a mask). Oxygen therapy can be given in a hospital or at home.

Medical Procedures and Surgery

As heart failure worsens, lifestyle changes and medicines may no longer control your symptoms. You may need a medical procedure or surgery.

If you have heart damage and severe heart failure symptoms, your doctor might recommend a cardiac resynchronization therapy (CRT) device or an implantable cardioverter defibrillator (ICD).

In heart failure, the right and left sides of the heart may no longer contract at the same time. This disrupts the heart's pumping. To correct this problem, your doctor might implant a CRT device (a type of pacemaker) near your heart.

This device helps both sides of your heart contract at the same time, which can decrease heart failure symptoms.

Some people who have heart failure have very rapid, irregular heartbeats. Without treatment, these heartbeats can cause sudden cardiac arrest. Your doctor might implant an ICD near your heart to solve this problem. An ICD checks your heart rate and uses electrical pulses to correct irregular heart rhythms.

People who have severe heart failure symptoms at rest, despite other treatments, may need the following:

- **A mechanical heart pump, such as a left ventricular assist device:** This device helps pump blood from the heart to the rest of the body. You may use a heart pump until you have surgery or as a long-term treatment.

- **Heart transplant:** A heart transplant is an operation in which a person's diseased heart is replaced with a healthy heart from a deceased donor. Heart transplants are done as a life-saving measure for end-stage heart failure when medical treatment and less drastic surgery have failed.

- **Experimental treatments:** Studies are under way to find new and better ways to treat heart failure.

Chapter 18

Arrhythmias

Chapter Contents

Section 18.1

Atrial Fibrillation

Excerpted from "Atrial Fibrillation," National Heart, Lung, and
Blood Institute, National Institutes of Health, July 1, 2011.

What Is Atrial Fibrillation?

Atrial fibrillation, or AF, is the most common type of arrhythmia.
An arrhythmia is a problem with the rate or rhythm of the heartbeat.
During an arrhythmia, the heart can beat too fast, too slow, or with
an irregular rhythm.

AF occurs if rapid, disorganized electrical signals cause the heart's
two upper chambers—called the atria—to fibrillate. The term "fibrillate" means to contract very fast and irregularly.

In AF, blood pools in the atria. It isn't pumped completely into
the heart's two lower chambers, called the ventricles. As a result, the
heart's upper and lower chambers don't work together as they should.

People who have AF may not feel symptoms. However, even when
AF isn't noticed, it can increase the risk of stroke. In some people, AF
can cause chest pain or heart failure, especially if the heart rhythm
is very rapid.

AF may happen rarely or every now and then, or it may become an
ongoing or long-term heart problem that lasts for years.

Types of Atrial Fibrillation

Paroxysmal atrial fibrillation: In paroxysmal atrial fibrillation
(AF), the faulty electrical signals and rapid heart rate begin suddenly
and then stop on their own. Symptoms can be mild or severe. They
stop within about a week, but usually in less than twenty-four hours.

Persistent atrial fibrillation: Persistent AF is a condition in
which the abnormal heart rhythm continues for more than a week. It
may stop on its own, or it can be stopped with treatment.

Permanent atrial fibrillation: Permanent AF is a condition in
which a normal heart rhythm can't be restored with treatment. Both

paroxysmal and persistent AF may become more frequent and, over time, result in permanent AF.

What Causes Atrial Fibrillation?

Atrial fibrillation (AF) occurs if the heart's electrical signals don't travel through the heart in a normal way. Instead, they become very rapid and disorganized.

Damage to the heart's electrical system causes AF. The damage most often is the result of other conditions that affect the health of the heart, such as high blood pressure and coronary heart disease.

The risk of AF increases as you age. Inflammation also is thought to play a role in causing AF.

Sometimes, the cause of AF is unknown.

Who Is at Risk for Atrial Fibrillation?

Atrial fibrillation (AF) affects millions of people, and the number is rising. Men are more likely than women to have the condition. In the United States, AF is more common among whites than African Americans or Hispanic Americans.

The risk of AF increases as you age. This is mostly because your risk for heart disease and other conditions that can cause AF also increases as you age. However, about half of the people who have AF are younger than seventy-five.

AF is uncommon in children.

What Are the Signs and Symptoms of Atrial Fibrillation?

Atrial fibrillation (AF) usually causes the heart's lower chambers, the ventricles, to contract faster than normal.

When this happens, the ventricles can't completely fill with blood. Thus, they may not be able to pump enough blood to the lungs and body. This can lead to signs and symptoms, such as the following:

- Palpitations (feelings that your heart is skipping a beat, fluttering, or beating too hard or fast)

- Shortness of breath

- Weakness or problems exercising

- Chest pain

- Dizziness or fainting

- Fatigue (tiredness)

- Confusion

Atrial Fibrillation Complications

AF has two major complications—stroke and heart failure.

Stroke: During AF, the heart's upper chambers, the atria, don't pump all of their blood to the ventricles. Some blood pools in the atria. When this happens, a blood clot (also called a thrombus) can form.

If the clot breaks off and travels to the brain, it can cause a stroke. (A clot that forms in one part of the body and travels in the bloodstream to another part of the body is called an embolus.)

Blood-thinning medicines that reduce the risk of stroke are an important part of treatment for people who have AF.

Heart failure: Heart failure occurs if the heart can't pump enough blood to meet the body's needs. AF can lead to heart failure because the ventricles are beating very fast and can't completely fill with blood. Thus, they may not be able to pump enough blood to the lungs and body.

Fatigue and shortness of breath are common symptoms of heart failure. A buildup of fluid in the lungs causes these symptoms. Fluid also can build up in the feet, ankles, and legs, causing weight gain.

Lifestyle changes, medicines, and procedures or surgery (rarely, a mechanical heart pump or heart transplant) are the main treatments for heart failure.

How Is Atrial Fibrillation Diagnosed?

Atrial fibrillation (AF) is diagnosed based on your medical and family histories, a physical exam, and the results from tests and procedures.

Sometimes AF doesn't cause signs or symptoms. Thus, it may be found during a physical exam or electrocardiogram (EKG) test done for another purpose.

If you have AF, your doctor will want to find out what is causing it. This will help him or her plan the best way to treat the condition.

Physical Exam

Your doctor will do a complete cardiac exam. He or she will listen to the rate and rhythm of your heartbeat and take your pulse and blood pressure reading. Your doctor will likely check for any signs of heart muscle or heart valve problems. He or she will listen to your lungs to check for signs of heart failure.

Your doctor also will check for swelling in your legs or feet and look for an enlarged thyroid gland or other signs of hyperthyroidism (too much thyroid hormone).

Diagnostic Tests and Procedures

EKG: An EKG is a simple, painless test that records the heart's electrical activity. It's the most useful test for diagnosing AF.

An EKG shows how fast your heart is beating and its rhythm (steady or irregular). It also records the strength and timing of electrical signals as they pass through your heart.

A standard EKG records the heartbeat for only a few seconds. It won't detect AF that doesn't happen during the test. To diagnose paroxysmal AF, your doctor may ask you to wear a portable EKG monitor that can record your heartbeat for longer periods.

Stress test: Some heart problems are easier to diagnose when your heart is working hard and beating fast. During stress testing, you exercise to make your heart work hard and beat fast while heart tests are done. If you can't exercise, you may be given medicine to make your heart work hard and beat fast.

Echocardiography: Echocardiography (echo) uses sound waves to create a moving picture of your heart. The test shows the size and shape of your heart and how well your heart chambers and valves are working.

Echo also can identify areas of poor blood flow to the heart, areas of heart muscle that aren't contracting normally, and previous injury to the heart muscle caused by poor blood flow.

Transesophageal echocardiography: Transesophageal echo, or TEE, uses sound waves to take pictures of your heart through the esophagus. The esophagus is the passage leading from your mouth to your stomach.

Your heart's upper chambers, the atria, are deep in your chest. They often can't be seen very well using transthoracic echo. Your doctor can see the atria much better using TEE.

TEE is used to detect blood clots that may be forming in the atria because of AF.

Chest x-ray: A chest x-ray is a painless test that creates pictures of the structures in your chest, such as your heart and lungs. This test can show fluid buildup in the lungs and signs of other AF complications.

Blood tests: Blood tests check the level of thyroid hormone in your body and the balance of your body's electrolytes. Electrolytes are minerals that help maintain fluid levels and acid-base balance in the body. They're essential for normal health and functioning of your body's cells and organs.

How Is Atrial Fibrillation Treated?

Treatment for atrial fibrillation (AF) depends on how often you have symptoms, how severe they are, and whether you already have heart disease. General treatment options include medicines, medical procedures, and lifestyle changes.

Who Needs Treatment for Atrial Fibrillation?

People who have AF but don't have symptoms or related heart problems may not need treatment. AF may even go back to a normal heart rhythm on its own. (This also can occur in people who have AF with symptoms.)

In some people who have AF for the first time, doctors may choose to use an electrical procedure or medicine to restore a normal heart rhythm.

Repeat episodes of AF tend to cause changes to the heart's electrical system, leading to persistent or permanent AF. Most people who have persistent or permanent AF need treatment to control their heart rate and prevent complications.

Specific Types of Treatment

Blood Clot Prevention

People who have AF are at increased risk for stroke. This is because blood can pool in the heart's upper chambers (the atria), causing a blood clot to form. If the clot breaks off and travels to the brain, it can cause a stroke.

Preventing blood clots from forming is probably the most important part of treating AF. The benefits of this type of treatment have been proven in multiple studies.

Doctors prescribe blood-thinning medicines to prevent blood clots. These medicines include warfarin (Coumadin®), dabigatran, heparin, and aspirin.

People taking blood-thinning medicines need regular blood tests to check how well the medicines are working.

Rate Control

Doctors can prescribe medicines to slow down the rate at which the ventricles are beating. These medicines help bring the heart rate to a normal level.

Rate control is the recommended treatment for most patients who have AF, even though an abnormal heart rhythm continues and the heart doesn't work as well as it should. Most people feel better and can function well if their heart rates are well-controlled.

Medicines used to control the heart rate include beta blockers (for example, metoprolol and atenolol), calcium channel blockers (diltiazem and verapamil), and digitalis (digoxin). Several other medicines also are available.

Rhythm Control

Restoring and maintaining a normal heart rhythm is a treatment approach recommended for people who aren't doing well with rate control treatment. This treatment also may be used for people who have only recently started having AF. The long-term benefits of rhythm control have not been proven conclusively yet.

Doctors use medicines or procedures to control the heart's rhythm. Patients often begin rhythm control treatment in a hospital so that their hearts can be closely watched.

The longer you have AF, the less likely it is that doctors can restore a normal heart rhythm. This is especially true for people who have had AF for six months or more.

Restoring a normal rhythm also becomes less likely if the atria are enlarged or if any underlying heart disease worsens. In these cases, the chance that AF will recur is high, even if you're taking medicine to help convert AF to a normal rhythm.

Medicines: Medicines used to control the heart rhythm include amiodarone, sotalol, flecainide, propafenone, dofetilide, and ibutilide. Sometimes older medicines—such as quinidine, procainamide, and disopyramide—are used.

Your doctor will carefully tailor the dose and type of medicines he or she prescribes to treat your AF. This is because medicines used to treat AF can cause a different kind of arrhythmia.

These medicines also can harm people who have underlying diseases of the heart or other organs. This is especially true for patients who have an unusual heart rhythm problem called Wolff-Parkinson-White syndrome.

Your doctor may start you on a small dose of medicine and then gradually increase the dose until your symptoms are controlled. Medicines used for rhythm control can be given regularly by injection at a doctor's office, clinic, or hospital. Or, you may routinely take pills to try to control AF or prevent repeat episodes.

If your doctor knows how you'll react to a medicine, a specific dose may be prescribed for you to take on an as-needed basis if you have an episode of AF.

Procedures: Doctors use several procedures to restore a normal heart rhythm. For example, they may use electrical cardioversion to treat a fast or irregular heartbeat. For this procedure, low-energy shocks are given to your heart to trigger a normal rhythm. You're temporarily put to sleep before you receive the shocks.

Electrical cardioversion isn't the same as the emergency heart shocking procedure often seen on TV programs. It's planned in advance and done under carefully controlled conditions.

Before doing electrical cardioversion, your doctor may recommend transesophageal echocardiography (TEE). This test can rule out the presence of blood clots in the atria. If clots are present, you may need to take blood-thinning medicines before the procedure. These medicines can help get rid of the clots.

Catheter ablation may be used to restore a normal heart rhythm if medicines or electrical cardioversion don't work. For this procedure, a wire is inserted through a vein in the leg or arm and threaded to the heart.

Radio wave energy is sent through the wire to destroy abnormal tissue that may be disrupting the normal flow of electrical signals. An electrophysiologist usually does this procedure in a hospital. Your doctor may recommend a TEE before catheter ablation to check for blood clots in the atria.

Sometimes doctors use catheter ablation to destroy the atrioventricular (AV) node. The AV node is where the heart's electrical signals pass from the atria to the ventricles (the heart's lower chambers). This procedure requires your doctor to surgically implant a device called a pacemaker, which helps maintain a normal heart rhythm.

Research on the benefits of catheter ablation as a treatment for AF is still ongoing.

Another procedure to restore a normal heart rhythm is called maze surgery. For this procedure, the surgeon makes small cuts or burns in the atria. These cuts or burns prevent the spread of disorganized electrical signals.

This procedure requires open-heart surgery, so it's usually done when a person requires heart surgery for other reasons, such as for heart valve disease (which can increase the risk of AF).

Section 18.2

Atrial Flutter

Atrial flutter (AFL) is a common abnormal heart rhythm, similar to atrial fibrillation (AFib), the most common abnormal heart rhythm. Both conditions are types of supraventricular (above the ventricles) tachycardia (rapid heartbeat). In AFL, the upper chambers (atria) of the heart beat too fast, which results in atrial muscle contractions that are faster than and out of sync with the lower chambers (ventricles).

What Is Atrial Flutter?

The electrical system of the heart is the power source that makes the heart beat. Electrical impulses travel along a pathway in the heart and make the upper and lower chambers of the heart (the atria and the ventricles) work together to pump blood through the heart.

A normal heartbeat begins as a single electrical impulse that comes from the sinoatrial (SA) node, a small bundle of tissue located in the right atrium. The impulse sends out an electrical pulse that causes the atria to contract (squeeze) and move blood into the lower ventricles. The electrical current passes through the atrioventricular (AV) node (the electrical bridge between the upper and lower chambers of the heart), causing the ventricles to squeeze and release in a steady, rhythmic sequence. As the chambers squeeze and release, they draw blood into the heart and push it back out to the rest of the body. This is what causes the pulse we feel on our wrist or neck.

With AFL, the electrical signal travels along a pathway within the right atrium. It moves in an organized circular motion, or "circuit," causing the atria to beat faster than the ventricles of your heart.

AFL is a heart rhythm disorder that is similar to the more common AFib. In AFib, the heart beats fast and in no regular pattern or rhythm. With AFL, the heart beats fast, but in a regular pattern. The fast but regular pattern of AFL is what makes it special. AFL makes a very distinct "sawtooth" pattern on an electrocardiogram (ECG), a test used to diagnose abnormal heart rhythms.

Risk Factors for Atrial Flutter

Some medical conditions increase the risk for developing AFL. These medical conditions include:

- heart failure;
- previous heart attack;
- valve abnormalities or congenital defects;
- high blood pressure;
- recent surgery;
- thyroid dysfunction;
- alcoholism (especially binge drinking);
- chronic lung disease;
- acute (serious) illness;
- diabetes.

Symptoms of Atrial Flutter

The electrical signal that causes AFL circulates in an organized, predictable pattern. This means that people with AFL usually continue to have a steady heartbeat, even though it is faster than normal. It is possible that people with AFL may feel no symptoms at all. Others do experience symptoms, which may include:

- heart palpitations (feeling like your heart is racing, pounding, or fluttering);
- fast, steady pulse;
- shortness of breath;
- trouble with everyday exercises or activities;
- pain, pressure, tightness, or discomfort in your chest;
- dizziness, light-headedness, or fainting.

Complications of Atrial Flutter

AFL itself is not life threatening. If left untreated, the side effects of AFL can be potentially life threatening. AFL makes it harder for the heart to pump blood effectively. With the blood moving more slowly, it is more likely to form clots. If the clot is pumped out of the heart, it could travel to the brain and lead to a stroke or heart attack.

Without treatment, AFL can also cause a fast pulse rate for long periods of time. This means that the ventricles are beating too fast. When the ventricles beat too fast for long periods of time, the heart muscle can become weak. This condition is called cardiomyopathy. This can lead to heart failure and long-term disability.

Without treatment, AFL can also cause another type of arrhythmia called atrial fibrillation. Atrial fibrillation (AFib) is the most common type of abnormal heart rhythm.

Section 18.3

Brugada Syndrome

Excerpted from "Brugada Syndrome,"
Genetics Home Reference, September 9, 2013.

What is Brugada syndrome?

Brugada syndrome is a condition that causes a disruption of the heart's normal rhythm. Specifically, this disorder can lead to uncoordinated electrical activity in the heart's lower chambers (ventricles), an abnormality called ventricular arrhythmia. If untreated, the irregular heartbeats can cause fainting (syncope), seizures, difficulty breathing, or sudden death. These complications typically occur when an affected person is resting or asleep.

Brugada syndrome usually becomes apparent in adulthood, although signs and symptoms, including sudden death, can occur any time from early infancy to old age. The mean age of sudden death is approximately forty years. This condition may explain some cases of sudden infant death syndrome (SIDS), which is a major cause of death in babies younger than one year. It is characterized by sudden and unexplained death, usually during sleep.

Sudden unexplained nocturnal death syndrome (SUNDS) is a condition characterized by unexpected cardiac arrest in young adults, usually at night during sleep. This condition was originally described in Southeast Asian populations, where it is a major cause of death. Researchers have determined that SUNDS and Brugada syndrome are the same disorder.

How common is Brugada syndrome?

The exact prevalence of Brugada syndrome is unknown, although it is estimated to affect five in ten thousand people worldwide. This condition occurs much more frequently in people of Asian ancestry, particularly in Japanese and Southeast Asian populations.

Although Brugada syndrome affects both men and women, the condition appears to be eight to ten times more common in men. Researchers suspect that testosterone, a sex hormone present at much higher levels in men, may be responsible for this difference.

What genes are related to Brugada syndrome?

Mutations in the SCN5A gene cause Brugada syndrome.

Mutations in the SCN5A gene have been identified in fewer than one-third of people with Brugada syndrome. This gene provides instructions for making a sodium channel, which normally transports positively charged sodium atoms (ions) into heart muscle cells. This type of ion channel plays a critical role in maintaining the heart's normal rhythm. Mutations in the SCN5A gene alter the structure or function of the channel, which reduces the flow of sodium ions into cells. A disruption in ion transport alters the way the heart beats, leading to the abnormal heart rhythm characteristic of Brugada syndrome.

In affected people without an identified SCN5A mutation, the cause of Brugada syndrome is often unknown. In some cases, certain drugs may cause a nongenetic (acquired) form of the disorder. Drugs that can induce an altered heart rhythm include medications used to treat some forms of arrhythmia, a condition called angina (which causes chest pain), high blood pressure, depression, and other mental illnesses. Abnormally high blood levels of calcium (hypercalcemia) or potassium (hyperkalemia), as well as unusually low potassium levels (hypokalemia), also have been associated with acquired Brugada syndrome. In addition to causing a nongenetic form of this disorder, these factors may trigger symptoms in people with an underlying SCN5A mutation.

This condition is inherited in an autosomal dominant pattern, which means one copy of the altered gene in each cell is sufficient to cause the disorder. In most cases, an affected person has one parent with the condition. Other cases may result from new mutations in the gene. These cases occur in people with no history of the disorder in their family.

Section 18.4

Heart Block

Heart block is an abnormal heart rhythm where the heart beats too slowly (bradycardia). In this condition, the electrical signals that tell the heart to contract are partially or totally blocked between the upper chambers (atria) and the lower chambers (ventricles). For this reason, it is also called atrioventricular block (AV block).

What Is Heart Block?

A normal heartbeat is initiated by an electrical signal that comes from the heart's natural pacemaker, the sinoatrial (SA) node, located at the top of the right atrium. The electrical signal travels through the atria and reaches the atrioventricular (AV) node. After crossing the AV node, the electrical signal passes through the bundle of His. This bundle then divides into thin, wire-like structures called bundle branches that extend into the right and left ventricles. The electrical signal travels down the bundle branches and eventually reaches the muscle cells of the ventricles, causing them to contract and pump blood to the body. Heart block occurs when this passage of electricity from top to bottom of the heart is delayed or interrupted.

Types of Heart Block

- **First-degree heart block:** The electrical impulses are slowed as they pass through the conduction system, but they all successfully reach the ventricles. First-degree heart block rarely causes symptoms or problems. Well-trained athletes may have first-degree heart block. Medications can also cause this condition. No treatment is generally needed for first-degree heart block.

- **Second-degree heart block (Type I):** The electrical impulses are delayed further and further with each heartbeat until a beat fails to reach to the ventricles entirely. It sometimes causes dizziness and/or other symptoms. People with normal conduction systems may sometimes have type 1 second-degree heart block when they sleep.

- **Second-degree heart block (Type II):** With this condition, some of the electrical impulses are unable to reach the ventricles. This condition is less common than Type I, and is more serious. Usually, your doctor will recommend a pacemaker to treat type II second-degree heart block, as it frequently progresses to third-degree heart block.

- **Third-degree heart block:** With this condition, also called complete heart block, none of the electrical impulses from the atria reach the ventricles. When the ventricles (lower chambers) do not receive electrical impulses from the atria (upper chambers), they may generate some impulses on their own, called junctional or ventricular escape beats. Ventricular escape beats, the heart's naturally occurring backups, are usually very slow. Patients frequently feel poorly in complete heart block, with light-headedness and fatigue.

- **Bundle branch block:** With this condition, the electrical impulses are slowed or blocked as they travel through the specialized conducting tissue in one of the two ventricles.

Symptoms of Heart Block

Some people with heart block will not experience any symptoms. Others will have symptoms that may include the following:

- Fainting (syncope)
- Dizziness or light-headedness
- Chest pain
- Shortness of breath

Risk Factors for Heart Block

Some medical conditions increase the risk for developing heart block. These medical conditions include:

- heart failure;
- prior heart attack;
- heart valve abnormalities;

- heart valve surgery;

- some medications or exposure to toxic substances;

- Lyme disease;

- aging.

Section 18.5

Long QT Syndrome

Excerpted from "Long QT Syndrome," National Heart, Lung, and Blood
Institute, National Institutes of Health, September 21, 2011.

What Is Long QT Syndrome?

Long QT syndrome (LQTS) is a disorder of the heart's electrical
activity. It can cause sudden, uncontrollable, dangerous arrhythmias
in response to exercise or stress. Arrhythmias are problems with the
rate or rhythm of the heartbeat.

People who have LQTS also can have arrhythmias for no known
reason. However, not everyone who has LQTS has dangerous heart
rhythms. When they do occur, though, they can be fatal.

What Does "Long QT" Mean?

The term "long QT" refers to an abnormal pattern seen on an electrocardiogram (EKG). An EKG is a test that detects and records the
heart's electrical activity.

With each heartbeat, an electrical signal spreads from the top of
your heart to the bottom. As it travels, the signal causes the heart to
contract and pump blood. An EKG records electrical signals as they
move through your heart.

Data from the EKG are mapped on a graph so your doctor can
study your heart's electrical activity. Each heartbeat is mapped as five
distinct electrical waves: P, Q, R, S, and T.

The electrical activity that occurs between the Q and T waves is
called the QT interval. This interval shows electrical activity in the
heart's lower chambers, the ventricles.

The timing of the heart's electrical activity is complex, and the body carefully controls it. Normally the QT interval is about a third of each heartbeat cycle. However, in people who have LQTS, the QT interval lasts longer than normal.

A long QT interval can upset the careful timing of the heartbeat and trigger dangerous heart rhythms.

Overview

On the surface of each heart muscle cell are tiny pores called ion channels. Ion channels open and close to let electrically charged sodium, calcium, and potassium atoms (ions) flow into and out of each cell. This generates the heart's electrical activity.

In people who have LQTS, the ion channels may not work well, or there may be too few of them. This may disrupt electrical activity in the heart's ventricles and cause dangerous arrhythmias.

LQTS often is inherited, which means you're born with the condition and have it your whole life. There are seven known types of inherited LQTS. The most common ones are LQTS 1, 2, and 3.

In LQTS 1, emotional stress or exercise (especially swimming) can trigger arrhythmias. In LQTS 2, extreme emotions, such as surprise, can trigger arrhythmias. In LQTS 3, a slow heart rate during sleep can trigger arrhythmias.

You also can acquire LQTS. This means you aren't born with the disorder, but you develop it during your lifetime. Some medicines and conditions can cause acquired LQTS.

Outlook

More than half of the people who have untreated, inherited types of LQTS die within ten years. However, lifestyle changes and medicines can help people who have LQTS prevent complications and live longer.

If you have LQTS, talk with your doctor about which lifestyle changes and treatments are best for you.

What Are the Signs and Symptoms of Long QT Syndrome?

Major Signs and Symptoms

If you have long QT syndrome (LQTS), you can have sudden and dangerous arrhythmias (abnormal heart rhythms). Signs and symptoms of LQTS-related arrhythmias often first occur during childhood and include the following:

- **Unexplained fainting:** This happens because the heart isn't pumping enough blood to the brain. Fainting may occur during physical or emotional stress. Fluttering feelings in the chest may occur before fainting.

- **Unexplained drowning or near drowning:** This may be due to fainting while swimming.

- **Unexplained sudden cardiac arrest (SCA) or death:** SCA is a condition in which the heart suddenly stops beating for no obvious reason. People who have SCA die within minutes unless they receive treatment. In about one out of ten people who have LQTS, SCA or sudden death is the first sign of the disorder.

Other Signs and Symptoms

Often, people who have LQTS 3 develop an abnormal heart rhythm during sleep. This may cause noisy gasping while sleeping.

Silent Long QT Syndrome

Sometimes long QT syndrome doesn't cause any signs or symptoms. This is called silent LQTS. For this reason, doctors often advise family members of people who have LQTS to be tested for the disorder, even if they have no symptoms.

Medical and genetic tests may reveal whether these family members have LQTS and what type of the condition they have.

How Is Long QT Syndrome Diagnosed?

Cardiologists diagnose and treat long QT syndrome (LQTS). Cardiologists are doctors who specialize in diagnosing and treating heart diseases and conditions. To diagnose LQTS, your cardiologist will consider the following things:

- Your electrocardiogram (EKG) results

- Your medical history and the results from a physical exam

- Your genetic test results

How Is Long QT Syndrome Treated?

The goal of treating long QT syndrome (LQTS) is to prevent life-threatening, abnormal heart rhythms and fainting spells.

Treatment isn't a cure for the disorder and may not restore a normal QT interval on an EKG. However, treatment greatly improves the chances of survival.

Specific Types of Treatment

Your doctor will recommend the best treatment for you based on the following things:

- Whether you've had symptoms, such as fainting or sudden cardiac arrest (SCA)

- What type of LQTS you have

- How likely it is that you'll faint or have SCA

- What treatment you feel most comfortable with

People who have LQTS without symptoms may be advised to do the following things:

- Make lifestyle changes that reduce the risk of fainting or SCA. Lifestyle changes may include avoiding certain sports and strenuous exercise, such as swimming, which can cause abnormal heart rhythms.

- Avoid medicines that may trigger abnormal heart rhythms. This may include some medicines used to treat allergies, infections, high blood pressure, high blood cholesterol, depression, and arrhythmias.

- Take medicines such as beta blockers, which reduce the risk of symptoms by slowing the heart rate.

The type of medicine you take will depend on the type of LQTS you have. For example, doctors usually will prescribe sodium channel blocker medicines only for people who have LQTS 3.

If your doctor thinks you're at increased risk for LQTS complications, he or she may suggest more aggressive treatments (in addition to medicines and lifestyle changes). These treatments may include the following:

- A surgically implanted device, such as a pacemaker or implantable cardioverter defibrillator (ICD). These devices help control abnormal heart rhythms.

- Surgery on the nerves that regulate your heartbeat.

People at increased risk are those who have fainted or who have had dangerous heart rhythms from their LQTS.

Section 18.6

Premature Ventricular Contractions

What are premature ventricular contractions?

Premature ventricular contractions (PVCs) are a heart arrhythmia that begins in the heart's lower chambers, or ventricles. PVCs are early extra beats that happen when the ventricles contract too soon. This disrupts the heart's normal rhythm.

What are the signs of premature ventricular contractions?

Many people with PVCs feel no symptoms. Others may notice "missed beats" or a "flopping" in the chest (heart palpitations).

What causes premature ventricular contractions?

Normally, the four chambers of the heart (two atria and two ventricles) beat in a very specific, coordinated manner. This beating is guided by an electrical impulse from the sinoatrial node, the body's natural pacemaker.

An arrhythmia occurs:

- when the sinoatrial node develops an abnormal rate or rhythm;

- when the normal pathway from the sinoatrial node to the heart is interrupted;

- when another part of the heart takes over as pacemaker.

Some people are born with arrhythmias, meaning the condition is congenital. PVCs are often harmless, but they can be a symptom of more serious conditions, such as heart disease or an imbalance in the minerals in your blood and other body fluids (electrolytes).

Other things that may cause PVCs:

- Stress

- Stimulants like caffeine or nicotine

- Excessive smoking and/or alcohol consumption

- Illegal drugs like cocaine

- Some kinds of over-the-counter cough and cold medicines

How does my doctor tell if I have premature ventricular contractions?

Your doctor will want to do a complete physical exam to make sure there are no deeper reasons for your PVCs. He or she may also recommend some of the following tests:

- An electrocardiogram (ECG or EKG) measures the electrical activity of your heart. It helps your doctor see how well your heart beats, and can tell if your heart muscle has been damaged in any way. A technician puts small metal disks—electrodes—on your skin to read the pattern of electrical impulses from your heart. The test only takes a few minutes.

- An echocardiogram uses sound waves to make a picture of your heart. Your doctor sees this image on a television monitor, and can examine how well your heart works. Doctors often use echocardiograms to tell if a person has a heart arrhythmia, or irregular heartbeat. The test takes about forty-five minutes, and is painless.

- In an angiography, the doctor injects dye into the heart arteries and measures the blood flow and blood pressure in the heart chambers. With the patient awake and under pain medicine, the doctor inserts a thin, flexible tube called a catheter into an artery in the leg, and guides it into the heart.

- A Holter monitor provides a nonstop reading of your heart rate and rhythm as you go about your daily activities. You wear the small monitor at all times, and it makes a record of your heart's electrical activity, much like an electrocardiogram. This gives your doctor valuable information about what happens to your heart when you feel an arrhythmia (irregular heartbeat), or chest pain (angina). Holter monitors are most often used for a day or two.

How are premature ventricular contractions treated?

Most people with PVCs only need treatment if symptoms are severe or if the extra beats happen very often. If you have heart disease or a history of ventricular tachycardia, PVCs can cause a more serious arrhythmia.

Lifestyle changes:

- Keep active: talk with your doctor about an ideal exercise program.

- Drink alcohol in moderation, no more than one or two drinks per day.

- If you smoke, try to quit.

- Limit the amount of caffeine you consume, found in drinks such as coffee, tea, and soft drinks.

Medications:

- Beta blockers decrease the heart rate and lower blood pressure by blocking the effects of adrenalin.

- Digitalis medicines control irregular heart rhythms by slowing the signals that start in the sinoatrial node, or natural pacemaker.

Section 18.7

Sick Sinus Syndrome

Sick sinus syndrome (SSS) is a relatively uncommon heart rhythm disorder. SSS is not a specific disease, but rather a group of signs or symptoms that indicate the sinus node, the heart's natural pacemaker, is not functioning properly. A person with SSS may have a heart rhythm that is too slow (bradycardia), too fast (tachycardia), or one that alternates between the fast and slow (bradycardia-tachycardia).

What Is Sick Sinus Syndrome?

The sinus node is a specialized group of cells in the upper chamber of the heart, the atria, that creates electrical signals that regulate the pace and rhythm of the heartbeat. Normally, the sinus node produces a regular, steady pattern of signals. With SSS, the pattern is irregular. Sick sinus syndrome may be due to defects in the heart itself, or it can be related to factors outside the heart.

Symptoms of Sick Sinus Syndrome

Most people with sick sinus syndrome have few or no symptoms. In others, symptoms may come and go. These symptoms can include:

- slower than normal pulse (bradycardia);
- fainting (syncope);
- feeling tired all the time (fatigue);
- weakness;
- shortness of breath (dyspnea);
- chest pain (angina);
- disturbed sleep;
- confusion;
- heart palpitations (feeling like your heart is racing, pounding, or fluttering).

Risk Factors for Sick Sinus Syndrome

While the exact cause of SSS is unknown, some factors, however, often are associated with the condition, such as:

- age;
- previous heart attack (myocardial infarction);
- medications to treat high blood pressure and other heart diseases;
- hyperkalemia (too much potassium in the blood);
- thyroid disease;
- sleep apnea;
- heart surgery.

In rare cases, SSS may be associated with conditions such as:

- diphtheria (an infection that can damage the heart muscle);
- hemochromatosis (excess iron in the blood);

- muscular dystrophy (an inherited condition in which the body's muscles are damaged and weak);

- amyloidosis (a condition in which a protein called amyloid is deposited in tissues or organs).

Section 18.8

Ventricular Fibrillation

Ventricular fibrillation (VF) is a severely abnormal heart rhythm (arrhythmia) that can be life-threatening.

Causes

The heart pumps blood to the lungs, brain, and other organs. Interruption of the heartbeat for only a few seconds can lead to fainting (syncope) or cardiac arrest.

Fibrillation is an uncontrolled twitching or quivering of muscle fibers (fibrils). When it occurs in the lower chambers of the heart, it is called ventricular fibrillation. During ventricular fibrillation, blood is not pumped from the heart. Sudden cardiac death results.

The most common cause of VF is a heart attack. However, VF can occur whenever the heart muscle does not get enough oxygen.

Conditions that can lead to VF include:

- electrocution accidents or injury to the heart;

- heart attack;

- heart disease that is present at birth (congenital);

- heart muscle disease, including cardiomyopathies;

- heart surgery;

- narrowed coronary arteries;

- sudden cardiac death (commotio cordis), typically occurring in athletes after an injury over the surface of the heart.

Most people with VF have no history of heart disease. Yet they often have risk factors for heart disease, such as smoking, high blood pressure, and diabetes.

Symptoms

A person who has a VF episode can suddenly collapse or become unconscious, because the brain and muscles have stopped receiving blood from the heart.

The following symptoms may occur within minutes to one hour before the collapse:

- Chest pain

- Dizziness

- Nausea

- Rapid heartbeat

- Shortness of breath

Exams and Tests

A cardiac monitor will show a very disorganized heart rhythm. Tests will be done to search for the cause of the VF.

Treatment

Ventricular fibrillation is a medical emergency and must be treated immediately to save a person's life.

If a person who is having a VF episode collapses at home or becomes unconscious, call the local emergency number (such as 911):

- While waiting for help, place the person's head and neck in line with the rest of the body to help make breathing easier. Start cardiopulmonary resuscitation (CPR) by doing chest compressions.

- Continue to do this until the person becomes alert or help arrives.

VF is treated by delivering a quick electric shock through the chest using a device called an external defibrillator. The electric shock can immediately restore the heartbeat to a normal rhythm, and should be done as quickly as possible. Many public places now have these machines.

Medicines may be given to control the heartbeat and heart function. An implantable cardioverter defibrillator (ICD) is a device that can be implanted in the chest wall of people who are at risk for this serious rhythm disorder. The ICD can help prevent sudden cardiac death by quickly sending an electrical shock when ventricular fibrillation occurs.

It is a good idea for family members and friends of people who have had VF and heart disease to take a CPR course. CPR courses are available through the American Red Cross, hospitals, or the American Heart Association.

Outlook (Prognosis)

VF will lead to death within a few minutes unless it is treated quickly and effectively. Even then, long-term survival for people who live through a VF attack outside of the hospital is between 2 percent and 25 percent.

People who have survived VF may be in a coma or have long-term damage.

Alternative Names

VF; Fibrillation—ventricular

References

Epstein AE, DiMarco JP, Ellenbogen KA, et al. ACC/AHA/IIRS 2008 Guidelines for Device-Based Therapy of Cardiac Rhythm Abnormalities: A Report of the American College of Cardiology/American Heart Association Task Force on Practice Guidelines (Writing Committee to Revise the ACC/AHA/NASPE 2002 Guideline Update for Implantation of Cardiac Pacemakers and Antiarrhythmia Devices): developed in collaboration with the American Association for Thoracic Surgery and Society of Thoracic Surgeons. *Circulation*. 2008;117:e350–e408.

Myerburg RJ, Castellanos A. Approach to cardiac arrest and life-threatening arrhythmias. In: Goldman L, Schafer AI, eds. *Cecil Medicine. 24th ed.* Philadelphia, Pa: Saunders Elsevier; 2011:chap 63.

Olgin JE, Zipes DP. Specific arrhythmias: diagnosis and treatment. In: Bonow RO, Mann DL, Zipes DP, Libby P, eds. *Braunwald's Heart Disease: A Textbook of Cardiovascular Medicine. 9th ed.* Philadelphia, Pa: Saunders Elsevier; 2011:chap 39.

Stevenson WG. Ventricular arrhythmias. In: Goldman L, Schafer AI, eds. *Cecil Medicine. 24th ed.* Philadelphia, Pa: Saunders Elsevier; 2011:chap 65.

Section 18.9

Ventricular Tachycardia

What is ventricular tachycardia?

Ventricular tachycardia is an arrhythmia. It is a rapid heartbeat that starts in the lower portion of your heart, or ventricles. Because the heart beats too fast to circulate blood properly, a person with this condition can lose consciousness, and possibly die.

What are the signs of ventricular tachycardia?

Patients with ventricular tachycardia may have these symptoms:

- A "flopping" in the chest, or palpitations
- Feeling dizzy or light-headed
- Fainting (syncope), or near-fainting
- Shortness of breath
- Chest pain (angina)
- Loss of consciousness

Symptoms may begin and stop suddenly.

What causes ventricular tachycardia?

Normally, the four chambers of the heart (two atria and two ventricles) beat in a very specific, coordinated manner. This beating is guided by an electrical impulse from the sinoatrial node, the body's natural pacemaker.

Ventricular tachycardia happens when an electrical "short circuit" occurs in ventricular tissue, causing rapid electrical activity and resulting in rapid ventricular contractions.

Some people are born with arrhythmias, meaning the condition is congenital. Other things that can make you more likely to have ventricular tachycardia include:

- coronary heart disease;

- heart attack or heart failure;

- heart valve disease;

- recent heart surgery;

- cardiomyopathy, or a weakening of the heart muscle.

How does my doctor tell if I have ventricular tachycardia?

Your doctor will first listen to your heart with a stethoscope to find an abnormal rhythm. A normal heart beats 60 to 100 times a minute, but a heart with ventricular tachycardia may beat 160 to 240 times a minute. Your doctor also may use some of the following tests:

- An electrocardiogram (ECG or EKG) measures the electrical activity of your heart. It helps your doctor see how well your heart beats, and can tell if your heart muscle has been damaged in any way. A technician puts small metal disks—electrodes—on your skin to read the pattern of electrical impulses from your heart. The test only takes a few minutes.

- A Holter monitor provides a nonstop reading of your heart rate and rhythm as you go about your daily activities. You wear the small monitor at all times, and it makes a record of your heart's electrical activity, much like an electrocardiogram. This gives your doctor valuable information about what happens to your heart when you feel an arrhythmia (irregular heartbeat), or chest pain (angina). Holter monitors are most often used for a day or two.

- A loop recorder is similar to a Holter monitor, in that it provides a reading of your heart rate and rhythm as you go about your daily activities. However, a loop recorder is used for longer periods of time than a Holter monitor. Most record your heart's rate and rhythm only when a button or switch is turned on.

- An electrophysiology study (EPS) shows how your heart reacts to electrical signals. You will be awake, but under a mild sedative, for the procedure. Your doctor first threads a thin, flexible tube—a catheter—from an artery in your leg up into your heart. He or she then uses small electrical impulses to make your heart beat at different speeds. This helps your doctor learn where the arrhythmia starts, and which medicines might help stop your heart's irregular rhythm. You will need to rest in the hospital for a few hours after an electrophysiology study.

How is ventricular tachycardia treated?

Ventricular tachycardia may be an emergency situation and require immediate cardiopulmonary resuscitation (CPR), electrical shock (defibrillation), or anti-arrhythmic medications. Long-term treatment may include:

- Nonsurgical:

  - Radiofrequency ablation uses a thin, flexible tube (catheter) to map the electrical impulses from your heart, and discover which cells are "misfiring." Doctors then use high-frequency radio waves to destroy the pathways causing the arrhythmia. With the patient awake and under local pain medicine, this procedure causes little discomfort.

  - Cryoablation is like radiofrequency ablation, except the surgeon uses a cold probe to destroy the problem cells.

Surgical:

  - Long-term ventricular tachycardias can be treated with an implantable cardioverter defibrillator (ICD). It is placed in the chest and connected with wires to the heart in surgery. The ICD can sense an arrhythmia and give the heart a shock to jolt it back to a regular rhythm.

  - In rare cases, ventricular tachycardia is treated with surgical removal of the abnormal (triggering) heart tissue.

Chapter 19

Heart Valve Disease

Chapter Contents

Section 19.1

Aortic Regurgitation

What Is Aortic Regurgitation?

Aortic regurgitation (AR) is reflux of blood from the aorta (the big vessel carrying blood out of the heart). The problem occurs when some of the blood pumped out falls back into the heart because of an incompetent aortic valve which would normally stop this from happening.

Statistics on Aortic Regurgitation

The disease increases in incidence with increasing age, and the vast majority of people over eighty years of age show evidence of regurgitation on testing with or without symptoms. The disease occurs more commonly in men, but the majority of patients with rheumatic AR are women.

Risk Factors for Aortic Regurgitation

The major predisposing factors are:

1. Rheumatic heart disease, syphilis.

2. Damage to the cusps of the valve secondary to infective endocarditis.

3. Any primary cause of aortic stenosis (progressive narrowing of the aortic valve) can lead to AR when the valve cusps become fixed and cannot close adequately any longer.

Rarer associations include:

*   ankylosing spondylitis;

*   aortic cusp fenestration;

*   Marfan syndrome;

- systemic lupus erythematosus; and
- aortitis.

Progression of Aortic Regurgitation

The regurgitation of blood back into the left ventricle of the heart leads to dilatation of the ventricle. This reflects and attempts to maintain heart output by increasing the volume of blood being pumped out. This dilatation eventually leads to cardiac failure.

Left ventricular dilatation also decreases the amount of blood entering the heart, causing angina, and can also cause atrial fibrillation, infective endocarditis, and mitral regurgitation. However, there are frequently no clinical symptoms until the onset of ventricular failure.

How Is Aortic Regurgitation Diagnosed?

Clinical suspicion should dictate:

- **Electrocardiogram (ECG):** May detect ventricular ischemia. Also associated myocardial infarction and atrial fibrillation.

- **Chest x-ray:** May show calcification of the aortic valve. In late disease, pulmonary edema may be seen.

Prognosis of Aortic Regurgitation

Compensation usually prevents the disease from becoming symptomatic for many years. As many as 85 to 95 percent of patients with mild to moderate regurgitation will live another ten years. However, after the onset of symptoms of heart failure, there is a fairly rapid deterioration within a couple of years.

How Is Aortic Regurgitation Treated?

General

Treatment of underlying causes—such as syphilis and infective endocarditis. Antibiotic prophylaxis against development of infective endocarditis should also be used.

Specific

Surgical replacement of the valve should be undertaken, but timing of the operation is important. Because a significantly enlarged heart will not recover completely, the operation should take place before the development of severe disease. Any heart failure should be treated with drug regimes.

References

1. Schlant RC, Alexander RW, Fuster V (eds). *Hurst's The Heart* (8th edition). New York, NY: McGraw-Hill, 1994.

2. Kumar P, Clark M (eds). *Clinical Medicine* (4th edition). Edinburgh: WB Saunders Company, 1998.

Section 19.2

Mitral Regurgitation

Mitral regurgitation is a disorder in which the heart valve that separates the upper and lower chambers on the left side of the heart does not close properly.

Regurgitation means leaking from a valve that does not close all the way.

Causes

Mitral regurgitation is the most common type of heart valve disorder.

Blood that flows between different chambers of your heart must flow through a valve. The valve between the two chambers on the left side of your heart is called the mitral valve.

When the mitral valve doesn't close all the way, blood flows backward into the upper heart chamber (atrium) from the lower chamber as it contracts. This leads to a decrease in blood flow to the rest of the body. As a result, the heart may try to pump harder. This may lead to congestive heart failure.

Mitral regurgitation may begin suddenly, most often after a heart attack. When the regurgitation does not go away, it becomes long-term (chronic).

Many other diseases or problems can weaken or damage the valve or the heart tissue around the valve and cause mitral regurgitation:

- Coronary heart disease and high blood pressure

- Infection of the heart valves

- Mitral valve prolapse (MVP)

- Rare causes, such as untreated syphilis or Marfan syndrome

- Rheumatic heart disease, a complication of untreated strep throat (which is becoming less common because of effective treatment)

- Swelling of the left lower heart chamber

Risk factors include a personal or family history of any of the disorders mentioned above, and use of fenfluramine or dexfenfluramine (appetite suppressants banned by the U.S. Food and Drug Administration [FDA]) for four or more months.

Symptoms

Symptoms may begin suddenly if:

- a heart attack damages the muscles around the mitral valve;

- the cords that attach the muscle to the valve break;

- an infection of the valve destroys part of the valve.

There are often no symptoms. When symptoms occur, they often develop gradually, and may include:

- cough;

- fatigue, exhaustion, and light-headedness;

- rapid breathing;

- sensation of feeling the heart beat (palpitations) or a rapid heartbeat;

- shortness of breath that increases with activity and when lying down;

- urination, excessive at night.

Exams and Tests

When listening to your heart and lungs, the health care provider may detect:

- a thrill (vibration) over the heart when feeling the chest area;
- an extra heart sound (S4 gallop);
- a distinctive heart murmur;
- crackles in the lungs (if fluid backs up into the lungs).

The physical exam may also reveal ankle swelling, an enlarged liver, bulging neck veins, and other signs of right-sided heart failure.

The following tests may be done to examine the heart valve structure and function:

- Computed tomography (CT) scan of the chest
- Echocardiogram (an ultrasound examination of the heart)
- Magnetic resonance imaging (MRI)

Cardiac catheterization may be done if heart function becomes worse.

Treatment

The choice of treatment depends on the symptoms, and the condition and function of the heart.

Patients with high blood pressure or a weakened heart muscle may be given medications to reduce the strain on the heart and help improve the condition.

The following drugs may be prescribed when mitral regurgitation symptoms get worse:

- Beta blockers or angiotensin-converting enzyme (ACE) inhibitors
- Blood thinners (anticoagulants) to help prevent blood clots in people with atrial fibrillation
- Drugs that help control uneven or abnormal heartbeats
- Water pills (diuretics) to remove excess fluid in the lungs

A low-sodium diet may be helpful. If a person develops symptoms, activity may be restricted.

Once the diagnosis is made, you should make regular visits to your health care provider to follow your symptoms and heart function. Surgical repair or replacement of the valve is recommended if heart function is poor, the heart becomes larger (dilated), and symptoms become more severe.

People with abnormal or damaged heart valves are at risk for an infection called endocarditis. Anything that causes bacteria to get into your bloodstream can lead to this infection. Steps to avoid this problem include:

- Avoid unclean injections.

- Treat strep infections quickly to prevent rheumatic fever.

- Always tell your health care provider and dentist if you have a history of heart valve disease or congenital heart disease before treatment. Guidelines recommend antibiotics for some patients, but only under certain conditions.

Outlook (Prognosis)

The outcome varies. Usually the condition is mild, so no therapy or restriction is needed. Symptoms can usually be controlled with medication.

Possible Complications

Problems that may develop include:

- abnormal heart rhythms, including atrial fibrillation and possibly more serious, or even life-threatening abnormal rhythms;

- clots that may travel to other areas of the body, such as the lungs or brain;

- infection of the heart valve;

- heart failure.

When to Contact a Medical Professional

Call your health care provider if symptoms get worse or do not improve with treatment.

Also call your health care provider if you are being treated for this condition and develop signs of infection, which include:

- chills;
- fever;
- general ill feeling;
- headache;
- muscle aches.

Prevention

Treat strep infections right away to prevent rheumatic fever. Prompt treatment of disorders that can cause mitral regurgitation reduces your risk.

Alternative Names

Mitral valve regurgitation; Mitral valve insufficiency

References

Otto CM, Bonow RO. Valvular heart disease. In: Bonow RO, Mann DL, Zipes DP, Libby P, eds. *Braunwald's Heart Disease: A Textbook of Cardiovascular Medicine. 9th ed.* Philadelphia, Pa: Saunders Elsevier; 2011:chap 66.

Nishimura RA, Carabello BA, Faxon DP, et al. ACC/AHA 2008 Guideline update on valvular heart disease: focused update on infective endocarditis: a report of the American College of Cardiology/American Heart Association Task Force on Practice Guidelines endorsed by the Society of Cardiovascular Anesthesiologists, Society for Cardiovascular Angiography and Interventions, and Society of Thoracic Surgeons. *J Am Coll Cardiol*. 2008;52:676–85.

Section 19.3

Mitral Valve Prolapse

What is mitral valve prolapse?

The mitral valve separates the heart's left upper chamber (atrium) from the left lower chamber (ventricle). The valve opens and shuts to let blood flow from the atrium to the ventricle. The ventricle pumps the blood through the body.

Mitral valve prolapse happens when the valve does not close right, and small amounts of blood flow from the ventricle back into the atrium. This can cause a heart murmur, or a "clicking" sound.

What are the signs of mitral valve prolapse?

In some cases, patients with mitral valve prolapse feel no symptoms. Others may:

- feel their heart beating (palpitations);
- have chest pain;
- have a cough;
- be short of breath after exertion;
- be short of breath after lying flat;
- feel fatigued.

What causes mitral valve prolapse?

Some forms of mitral valve prolapse may be hereditary. It is also happens with certain conditions:

- A hole in the wall that separates the left and right upper heart chambers (atrial septal defect)
- Chest wall deformities and curvature of the spine, especially in women

- Marfan syndrome, a disorder that affects the skeletal system, cardiovascular system, eyes, and skin

- Graves disease, an autoimmune disease that affects the thyroid gland

How does my doctor tell if I have mitral valve prolapse?

With a stethoscope, a doctor may hear a murmur, click, or other unusual sound coming from your heart. Your doctor also may use some of the following tests:

- An echocardiogram uses sound waves to make a picture of your heart. Your doctor sees this image on a television monitor, and can examine how well your heart works. The test takes about forty-five minutes, and is painless.

- A heart catheterization allows a doctor to record information from inside the heart. With the patient awake and under pain medicine, the doctor inserts a thin, flexible tube called a catheter into an artery in the leg, and guides it into the heart. The doctor can then perform many tests, including an angiography, where an injected dye shows the heart and its arteries. A doctor can also use heart catheterization to measure blood pressure and oxygen levels inside the heart, as well as the pumping ability of the heart muscle.

- An electrocardiogram (ECG or EKG) measures the electrical activity of your heart. It helps your doctor see how well your heart beats, and can tell if your heart muscle has been damaged in any way. A technician puts small metal disks—electrodes—on your skin to read the pattern of electrical impulses from your heart. The test only takes a few minutes.

How is mitral valve prolapse treated?

Most patients with mitral valve prolapse do not need treatment and can lead normal lives, as long as they often see a doctor.
Nonsurgical (medication):

- You may need to take antibiotics before dental procedures or general surgery, to prevent the mitral valve from becoming infected.

- Anti-arrhythmic drugs may be used to control irregular heart rhythms, or arrhythmia.

- Vasodilators (drugs that dilate blood vessels) may be used to reduce your heart's workload.

- Diuretics may be used to remove excess fluid in the lungs.

Surgical:

- In a small number of cases, mitral valve prolapse can cause severe leakage of blood through the valve back into the atria. In these situations, surgery to repair or replace the abnormal valve may be necessary.

Chapter 20

Heart Murmurs

What Is a Heart Murmur?

A heart murmur is an extra or unusual sound heard during a heartbeat. Murmurs range from very faint to very loud. Sometimes they sound like a whooshing or swishing noise.

Normal heartbeats make a "lub-DUPP" or "lub-DUB" sound. This is the sound of the heart valves closing as blood moves through the heart. Doctors can hear these sounds and heart murmurs using a stethoscope.

How the Heart Works

The heart is a muscle about the size of your fist. It works like a pump and beats one hundred thousand times a day.

Four valves control the flow of blood from the atria to the ventricles and from the ventricles into the two large arteries connected to the heart.

Valves are like doors that open and close. They open to allow blood to flow through to the next chamber or to one of the arteries. Then they shut to keep blood from flowing backward.

When the heart's valves open and close, they make a "lub-DUB" sound that a doctor can hear using a stethoscope:

Excerpted from "Heart Murmurs," National Heart, Lung, and Blood Institute, National Institutes of Health, September 20, 2012.

- The first sound—the "lub"—is made by the mitral and tricuspid valves closing at the beginning of systole (SIS-toe-lee). Systole is when the ventricles contract, or squeeze, and pump blood out of the heart.

- The second sound—the "DUB"—is made by the aortic and pulmonary valves closing at the beginning of diastole (di-AS-toe-lee). Diastole is when the ventricles relax and fill with blood pumped into them by the atria.

What Causes Heart Murmurs?

Innocent Heart Murmurs

Why some people have innocent heart murmurs and others do not isn't known. Innocent murmurs are simply sounds made by blood flowing through the heart's chambers and valves, or through blood vessels near the heart.

Extra blood flow through the heart also may cause innocent heart murmurs. After childhood, the most common cause of extra blood flow through the heart is pregnancy. This is because during pregnancy, women's bodies make extra blood. Most heart murmurs that occur in pregnant women are innocent.

Abnormal Heart Murmurs

Congenital heart defects or acquired heart valve disease often are the cause of abnormal heart murmurs.

Congenital heart defects: Congenital heart defects are the most common cause of abnormal heart murmurs in children. These defects are problems with the heart's structure that are present at birth. They change the normal flow of blood through the heart.

Congenital heart defects can involve the interior walls of the heart, the valves inside the heart, or the arteries and veins that carry blood to and from the heart. Some babies are born with more than one heart defect.

Heart valve problems, septal defects (also called holes in the heart), and diseases of the heart muscle such as hypertrophic cardiomyopathy are common heart defects that cause abnormal heart murmurs.

Examples of valve problems are narrow valves that limit blood flow or leaky valves that don't close properly. Septal defects are holes in the wall that separates the right and left sides of the heart. This wall is called the septum.

A hole in the septum between the heart's two upper chambers is called an atrial septal defect. A hole in the septum between the heart's two lower chambers is called a ventricular septal defect.

Hypertrophic cardiomyopathy (HCM) occurs if heart muscle cells enlarge and cause the walls of the ventricles (usually the left ventricle) to thicken. The thickening may block blood flow out of the ventricle. If a blockage occurs, the ventricle must work hard to pump blood to the body. HCM also can affect the heart's mitral valve, causing blood to leak backward through the valve.

Acquired heart valve disease: Acquired heart valve disease often is the cause of abnormal heart murmurs in adults. This is heart valve disease that develops as the result of another condition.

Many conditions can cause heart valve disease. Examples include heart conditions and other disorders, age-related changes, rheumatic fever, and infections.

Heart conditions and other disorders. Certain conditions can stretch and distort the heart valves, such as:

- *Damage and scar tissue from a heart attack or injury to the heart.*

- *Advanced high blood pressure and heart failure:* These conditions can enlarge the heart or its main arteries.

- *Age-related changes:* As you get older, calcium deposits or other deposits may form on your heart valves. These deposits stiffen and thicken the valve flaps and limit blood flow. This stiffening and thickening of the valve is called sclerosis.

- *Rheumatic fever:* The bacteria that cause strep throat, scarlet fever, and, in some cases, impetigo also can cause rheumatic fever. This serious illness can develop if you have an untreated or not fully treated streptococcal (strep) infection. Rheumatic fever can damage and scar the heart valves. The symptoms of this heart valve damage often don't occur until many years after recovery from rheumatic fever. Today, most people who have strep infections are treated with antibiotics before rheumatic fever develops. It's very important to take all of the antibiotics your doctor prescribes for strep throat, even if you feel better before the medicine is gone.

- *Infections:* Common germs that enter the bloodstream and get carried to the heart can sometimes infect the inner surface of the heart, including the heart valves. This rare but sometimes life-threatening infection is called infective endocarditis, or IE.

IE is more likely to develop in people who already have abnormal blood flow through a heart valve because of heart valve disease. The abnormal blood flow causes blood clots to form on the surface of the valve. The blood clots make it easier for germs to attach to and infect the valve. IE can worsen existing heart valve disease.

Other Causes

Some heart murmurs occur because of an illness outside of the heart. The heart is normal, but an illness or condition can cause blood flow that's faster than normal. Examples of this type of illness include fever, anemia, and hyperthyroidism.

Anemia is a condition in which the body has a lower than normal number of red blood cells. Hyperthyroidism is a condition in which the body has too much thyroid hormone.

What Are the Signs and Symptoms of a Heart Murmur?

People who have innocent (harmless) heart murmurs don't have any signs or symptoms other than the murmur itself. This is because innocent heart murmurs aren't caused by heart problems.

People who have abnormal heart murmurs may have signs or symptoms of the heart problems causing the murmurs. These signs and symptoms may include the following:

- Poor eating and failure to grow normally (in infants)
- Shortness of breath, which may occur only with physical exertion
- Excessive sweating with minimal or no exertion
- Chest pain
- Dizziness or fainting
- A bluish color on the skin, especially on the fingertips and lips
- Chronic cough
- Swelling or sudden weight gain
- Enlarged liver
- Enlarged neck veins

Signs and symptoms depend on the problem causing the heart murmur and its severity.

How Is a Heart Murmur Diagnosed?

Doctors use a stethoscope to listen to heart sounds and hear heart murmurs. They may detect heart murmurs during routine checkups or while checking for another condition.

If a congenital heart defect causes a murmur, it's often heard at birth or during infancy. Abnormal heart murmurs caused by other heart problems can be heard in patients of any age.

Evaluating Heart Murmurs

When evaluating a heart murmur, your doctor will pay attention to many things, such as the following:

- How faint or loud the sound is. Your doctor will grade the murmur on a scale of 1 to 6 (1 is very faint and 6 is very loud).

- When the sound occurs in the cycle of the heartbeat.

- Where the sound is heard in the chest and whether it also can be heard in the neck or back.

- Whether the sound has a high, medium, or low pitch.

- How long the sound lasts.

- How breathing, physical activity, or a change in body position affects the sound.

Diagnostic Tests and Procedures

If your doctor thinks you or your child has an abnormal heart murmur, he or she may recommend one or more of the following tests:

- Chest x-ray

- Electrocardiogram (EKG)

- Echocardiography

How Is a Heart Murmur Treated?

A heart murmur isn't a disease. It's an extra or unusual sound heard during the heartbeat. Thus, murmurs themselves don't require treatment. However, if an underlying condition is causing a heart murmur, your doctor may recommend treatment for that condition.

Innocent (Harmless) Heart Murmurs

Healthy children who have innocent (harmless) heart murmurs don't need treatment. Their heart murmurs aren't caused by heart problems or other conditions.

Pregnant women who have innocent heart murmurs due to extra blood volume also don't need treatment. Their heart murmurs should go away after pregnancy.

Abnormal Heart Murmurs

If you or your child has an abnormal heart murmur, your doctor will recommend treatment for the disease or condition causing the murmur.

Some medical conditions, such as anemia or hyperthyroidism, can cause heart murmurs that aren't related to heart disease. Treating these conditions should make the heart murmur go away.

If a congenital heart defect is causing a heart murmur, treatment will depend on the type and severity of the defect. Treatment may include medicines or surgery.

If acquired heart valve disease is causing a heart murmur, treatment usually will depend on the type, amount, and severity of the disease.

Currently, no medicines can cure heart valve disease. However, lifestyle changes and medicines can treat symptoms and help delay complications. Eventually, though, you may need surgery to repair or replace a faulty heart valve.

Chapter 21

Infectious Diseases
of the Heart

Chapter Contents

Section 21.1

Endocarditis

Excerpted from "Endocarditis," National Heart, Lung, and
Blood Institute, National Institutes of Health, October 1, 2010.

What Is Endocarditis?

Endocarditis is an infection of the inner lining of the heart chambers
and valves. This lining is called the endocardium. The condition also
is called infective endocarditis (IE).

IE occurs if bacteria, fungi, or other germs invade your bloodstream
and attach to abnormal areas of your heart. The infection can damage
your heart and cause serious and sometimes fatal complications.

What Causes Endocarditis?

A common underlying factor in IE is a structural heart defect, especially faulty heart valves. Usually your immune system will kill germs in
your bloodstream. However, if your heart has a rough lining or abnormal
valves, the invading germs can attach and multiply in the heart.

Other factors also can play a role in causing IE. Common activities,
such as brushing your teeth or having certain dental procedures, can
allow bacteria to enter your bloodstream. This is even more likely to
happen if your teeth and gums are in poor condition.

Having a catheter (tube) or another medical device inserted through
your skin, especially for long periods, also can allow bacteria to enter
your bloodstream. People who use intravenous (IV) drugs also are at
risk for IE because of the germs on needles and syringes.

Bacteria also may spread to the blood and heart from infections in
other parts of the body, such as the gut, skin, or genitals.

Endocarditis Complications

As the bacteria or other germs multiply in your heart, they form
clumps with other cells and matter found in the blood. These clumps
are called vegetations.

As IE worsens, pieces of the vegetations can break off and travel to almost any other organ or tissue in the body. There, the pieces can block blood flow or cause a new infection. As a result, IE can cause a range of complications.

Heart Complications

Heart problems are the most common complication of IE. They occur in one-third to one-half of all people who have the infection. These problems may include a new heart murmur, heart failure, heart valve damage, heart block, or, rarely, a heart attack.

Central Nervous System Complications

These complications occur in as many as 20 to 40 percent of people who have IE. Central nervous system complications most often occur when bits of the vegetation, called emboli, break away and lodge in the brain.

The emboli can cause local infections called brain abscesses. Or, they can cause a more widespread brain infection called meningitis.

Emboli also can cause strokes or seizures. This happens if they block blood vessels or affect the brain's electrical signals. These complications can cause long-term damage to the brain and may even be fatal.

Complications in Other Organs

IE also can affect other organs in the body, such as the lungs, kidneys, and spleen.

Who Is at Risk for Endocarditis?

Infective endocarditis (IE) is an uncommon condition that can affect both children and adults. It's more common in men than women.

IE typically affects people who have abnormal hearts or other conditions that put them at risk for the infection. Sometimes IE does affect people who were healthy before the infection.

Major Risk Factors

The germs that cause IE tend to attach and multiply on damaged, malformed, or artificial (man-made) heart valves and implanted medical devices. Certain conditions put you at higher risk for IE. These include the following:

- Congenital heart defects (defects that are present at birth). Examples include a malformed heart or abnormal heart valves.

- Artificial heart valves, an implanted medical device in the heart (such as a pacemaker wire), or an intravenous (IV) catheter (tube) in a blood vessel for a long time.

- Heart valves damaged by rheumatic fever or calcium deposits that cause age-related valve thickening. Scars in the heart from a previous case of IE also can damage heart valves.

- IV drug use, especially if needles are shared or reused, contaminated substances are injected, or the skin isn't properly cleaned before injection.

What Are the Signs and Symptoms of Endocarditis?

Infective endocarditis (IE) can cause a range of signs and symptoms that can vary from person to person. Signs and symptoms also can vary over time in the same person.

Signs and symptoms differ depending on whether you have an underlying heart problem, the type of germ causing the infection, and whether you have acute or subacute IE.

Signs and symptoms of IE may include the following:

- Flu-like symptoms, such as fever, chills, fatigue (tiredness), aching muscles and joints, night sweats, and headaches.

- Shortness of breath or a cough that won't go away.

- A new heart murmur or a change in an existing heart murmur.

- Skin changes such as the following:
    - Overall paleness.
    - Small, painful, red or purplish bumps under the skin on the fingers or toes.
    - Small, dark, painless flat spots on the palms of the hands or the soles of the feet.
    - Tiny spots under the fingernails, on the whites of the eyes, on the roof of the mouth and inside of the cheeks, or on the chest. These spots are from broken blood vessels.

- Nausea (feeling sick to your stomach), vomiting, a decrease in appetite, a sense of fullness with discomfort on the upper left side of the abdomen, or weight loss with or without a change in appetite.

- Blood in the urine.

- Swelling in the feet, legs, or abdomen.

How Is Endocarditis Diagnosed?

Your doctor will diagnose infective endocarditis (IE) based on your risk factors, your medical history and signs and symptoms, and test results.

Diagnosis of IE often is based on many factors, rather than a single positive test result, sign, or symptom.

Diagnostic tests used include the following:

- Blood tests

- Echocardiogram

- Electrocardiogram (EKG)

How Is Endocarditis Treated?

Infective endocarditis (IE) is treated with antibiotics and sometimes with heart surgery.

Antibiotics

Antibiotics usually are given for two to six weeks through an intravenous (IV) line inserted into a vein. You're often in a hospital for at least the first week or more of treatment. This allows your doctor to make sure the medicine is helping.

Surgery

Sometimes surgery is needed to repair or replace a damaged heart valve or to help clear up IE. For example, IE caused by fungi often requires surgery. This is because this type of IE is harder to treat than IE caused by bacteria.

How Can Endocarditis Be Prevented?

If you're at risk for infective endocarditis (IE), you can take steps to prevent the infection and its complications:

- Be alert to the signs and symptoms of IE. Contact your doctor right away if you have any of these signs or symptoms, especially a persistent fever or unexplained fatigue (tiredness).

- Brush and floss your teeth regularly, and have regular dental checkups. Germs from a gum infection can enter your bloodstream.

- Avoid body piercing, tattoos, and other procedures that may allow germs to enter your bloodstream.

Let your health care providers, including your dentist, know if you're at risk for IE. They can tell you whether you need antibiotics before exams and procedures.

Section 21.2

Myocarditis

Excerpted from "Myocarditis,"
© 2013, A.D.A.M., Inc. Reprinted with permission.

Myocarditis is inflammation of the heart muscle.

Causes

Myocarditis is an uncommon disorder that is usually caused by viral, bacterial, or fungal infections that reach the heart.
Viral infections:

- coxsackie;

- cytomegalovirus;

- hepatitis C;

- herpes;

- human immunodeficiency virus (HIV);

- parvovirus.

Bacterial infections:

- chlamydia;

- mycoplasma;

- streptococcus;

- treponema.

  Fungal infections:

- aspergillus;

- candida;

- coccidioides;

- cryptococcus;

- histoplasma.

When you have an infection, your immune system produces special cells that release chemicals to fight off disease. If the infection affects your heart, the disease-fighting cells enter the heart. However, the chemicals produced by an immune response can damage the heart muscle. As a result, the heart can become thick, swollen, and weak. This leads to symptoms of heart failure.

Other causes of myocarditis may include:

- allergic reactions to certain medications or toxins (alcohol, cocaine, certain chemotherapy drugs, heavy metals, and catecholamines);

- being around certain chemicals;

- certain diseases that cause inflammation throughout the body (rheumatoid arthritis, sarcoidosis).

Symptoms

There may be no symptoms. Symptoms may be similar to the flu. If symptoms occur, they may include:

- abnormal heartbeat;

- chest pain that may resemble a heart attack;

- fatigue;

- fever and other signs of infection including headache, muscle aches, sore throat, diarrhea, or rashes;

- joint pain or swelling;

- leg swelling;

- shortness of breath.

Other symptoms that may occur with this disease:

- fainting, often related to irregular heart rhythms;
- low urine output.

Exams and Tests

A physical examination may show no abnormalities, or may reveal the following:

- abnormal heartbeat or heart sounds (murmurs, extra heart sounds);
- fever;
- fluid in the lungs;
- rapid heartbeat (tachycardia);
- swelling (edema) in the legs.

Tests used to diagnosis myocarditis include:

- blood cultures for infection;
- blood tests for antibodies against the heart muscle and the body itself;
- chest x-ray;
- electrocardiogram (ECG);
- heart muscle biopsy (endomyocardial biopsy);
- red blood cell count;
- ultrasound of the heart (echocardiogram);
- white blood cell count.

Treatment

Treatment is aimed at the cause of the problem, and may involve:

- antibiotics;
- anti-inflammatory medicines to reduce swelling;
- diuretics to remove excess water from the body;

- low-salt diet;
- reduced activity.

If the heart muscle is very weak, your health care provider will prescribe medicines to treat heart failure. Abnormal heart rhythms may require the use of additional medications, a pacemaker, or an implantable cardioverter-defibrillator. If a blood clot is in the heart chamber, you will also receive blood thinning medicine.

Outlook (Prognosis)

How well you do depends on the cause of the problem and your overall health. The outlook varies. Some people may recover completely. Others may have permanent heart failure.

Possible Complications

- Cardiomyopathy
- Heart failure
- Pericarditis

When to Contact a Medical Professional

Call your health care provider if you have symptoms of myocarditis, especially after a recent infection.

Seek immediate medical help if you have severe symptoms or have been diagnosed with myocarditis and have increased:

- chest pain;
- difficulty breathing;
- swelling.

Prevention

Promptly treating conditions that cause myocarditis may reduce the risk.

References

Liu P, Baughman KL. Myocarditis. In: Bonow RO, Mann DL, Zipes DP, Libby P, eds. *Braunwald's Heart Disease: A Textbook of Cardiovascular Medicine. 9th ed.* Philadelphia, Pa: Saunders Elsevier; 2011:chap 70.

McKenna W. Diseases of the myocardium and endocardium. In: Goldman L, Schafer AI, eds. *Cecil Medicine. 24th ed.* Philadelphia, PA: Saunders Elsevier; 2011:chap 60.

Section 21.3

Pericarditis

Excerpted from "Pericarditis," National Heart, Lung, and Blood Institute, National Institutes of Health, September 26, 2012.

What Is Pericarditis?

Pericarditis is a condition in which the membrane, or sac, around your heart is inflamed. This sac is called the pericardium.

The pericardium holds the heart in place and helps it work properly. The sac is made of two thin layers of tissue that enclose your heart. Between the two layers is a small amount of fluid. This fluid keeps the layers from rubbing against each other and causing friction.

In pericarditis, the layers of tissue become inflamed and can rub against the heart. This causes chest pain, a common symptom of pericarditis.

The chest pain from pericarditis may feel like pain from a heart attack. More often, the pain may be sharp and get worse when you inhale, and improve when you are sitting up and leaning forward. If you have chest pain, you should call 9-1-1 right away, as you may be having a heart attack.

What Causes Pericarditis?

In many cases, the cause of pericarditis (both acute and chronic) is unknown.

Viral infections are likely a common cause of pericarditis, although the virus may never be found. Pericarditis often occurs after respiratory infections. Bacterial, fungal, and other infections also can cause pericarditis.

Most cases of chronic, or recurring, pericarditis are thought to be the result of autoimmune disorders. Examples of such disorders include lupus, scleroderma, and rheumatoid arthritis.

With autoimmune disorders, the body's immune system makes antibodies (proteins) that mistakenly attack the body's tissues or cells. Other possible causes of pericarditis include the following:

- Heart attack and heart surgery

- Kidney failure, human immunodeficiency virus (HIV)/acquired immune deficiency syndrome (AIDS), cancer, tuberculosis, and other health problems

- Trauma to the chest or prior radiation therapy to the chest

- Autoimmune diseases, including ulcerative colitis

- Certain medicines, like phenytoin (an antiseizure medicine), warfarin and heparin (blood-thinning medicines), and procainamide (a medicine to treat irregular heartbeats

Who Is at Risk for Pericarditis?

Pericarditis occurs in people of all ages. However, men aged twenty to fifty are more likely to develop it than others.

People who are treated for acute pericarditis may get it again. This may happen in 15 to 30 percent of people who have the condition. A small number of these people go on to develop chronic pericarditis.

What Are the Signs and Symptoms of Pericarditis?

The most common sign of acute pericarditis is sharp, stabbing chest pain. The pain usually comes on quickly. It often is felt in the middle or left side of the chest or over the front of the chest. You also may feel pain in one or both shoulders, the neck, back, and abdomen.

The pain tends to ease when you sit up and lean forward. Lying down and deep breathing worsens it. For some people, the pain feels like a dull ache or pressure in the chest.

The chest pain also may feel like pain from a heart attack. If you have chest pain, you should call 9-1-1 right away, as you may be having a heart attack.

Some people with acute pericarditis develop a fever. Other symptoms are weakness, palpitations, trouble breathing, and coughing. (Palpitations are feelings that your heart is skipping a beat, fluttering, or beating too hard or too fast.)

The most common symptom of chronic pericarditis is chest pain. Chronic pericarditis also often causes tiredness, coughing, and shortness of breath. Severe cases of chronic pericarditis can lead to swelling in the stomach and legs and hypotension (low blood pressure).

Complications of Pericarditis

Two serious complications of pericarditis are cardiac tamponade and chronic constrictive pericarditis.

Cardiac tamponade occurs if too much fluid collects in the pericardium (the sac around the heart). The extra fluid puts pressure on the heart. This prevents the heart from properly filling with blood. As a result, less blood leaves the heart, which causes a sharp drop in blood pressure. If left untreated, cardiac tamponade can be fatal.

Chronic constrictive pericarditis is a rare disease that develops over time. It leads to scar-like tissue forming throughout the pericardium. The sac becomes stiff and can't move properly. In time, the scarred tissue compresses the heart and prevents it from working well.

How Is Pericarditis Diagnosed?

Your doctor will diagnose pericarditis based on your medical history, a physical exam, and test results.

Medical History

Your doctor may ask whether you:

- have had a recent respiratory infection or flu-like illness;
- have had a recent heart attack or injury to your chest;
- have any other medical conditions.

Your doctor also may ask about your symptoms. If you have chest pain, he or she will ask you to describe how it feels, where it's located, and whether it's worse when you lie down, breathe, or cough.

Physical Exam

When the pericardium (the sac around your heart) is inflamed, the amount of fluid between its two layers of tissue increases. As part of the exam, your doctor will look for signs of excess fluid in your chest.

A common sign is the pericardial rub. This is the sound of the pericardium rubbing against the outer layer of your heart. Your doctor will place a stethoscope on your chest to listen for this sound.

Your doctor may hear other chest sounds that are signs of fluid in the pericardium (pericardial effusion) or the lungs (pleural effusion). These are more severe problems related to pericarditis.

Diagnostic Tests

Your doctor may recommend one or more tests to diagnose your condition and show how severe it is. The most common tests are as follows:

- **Electrocardiogram (EKG):** This simple test detects and records your heart's electrical activity. Certain EKG results may suggest pericarditis.

- **Chest x-ray:** A chest x-ray creates pictures of the structures inside your chest, such as your heart, lungs, and blood vessels. The pictures can show whether you have an enlarged heart. This is a sign of excess fluid in your pericardium.

- **Echocardiography:** This painless test uses sound waves to create pictures of your heart. The pictures show the size and shape of your heart and how well your heart is working. This test can show whether fluid has built up in the pericardium.

- **Cardiac computed tomography (CT):** Cardiac CT is a type of x-ray that takes a clear, detailed picture of your heart and pericardium. A cardiac CT helps rule out other causes of chest pain.

- **Cardiac magnetic resonance imaging (MRI):** This test uses powerful magnets and radio waves to create detailed pictures of your organs and tissues. A cardiac MRI can show thickening or other changes in the pericardium.

Your doctor also may recommend blood tests. These tests can help your doctor find out whether you've had a heart attack, the cause of your pericarditis, and how inflamed your pericardium is.

How Is Pericarditis Treated?

Most cases of pericarditis are mild; they clear up on their own or with rest and simple treatment. Other times, more intense treatment is needed to prevent complications. Treatment may include medicines and, less often, procedures or surgery.

Specific Types of Treatment

As a first step in your treatment, your doctor may advise you to rest until you feel better and have no fever. He or she may tell you to take over-the-counter, anti-inflammatory medicines to reduce pain and inflammation. Examples of these medicines include aspirin and ibuprofen.

You may need stronger medicine if your pain is severe. If your pain continues to be severe, your doctor may prescribe a medicine called colchicine and, possibly, prednisone (a steroid medicine).

If an infection is causing your pericarditis, your doctor will prescribe an antibiotic or other medicine to treat the infection.

You may need to stay in the hospital during treatment for pericarditis so your doctor can check you for complications.

The symptoms of acute pericarditis can last from a few days to a few weeks. Chronic pericarditis may last for several months.

Other Types of Treatment

You may need treatment for complications of pericarditis. Two serious complications are cardiac tamponade and chronic constrictive pericarditis.

Cardiac tamponade is treated with a procedure called pericardiocentesis. A needle or tube (called a catheter) is inserted into the chest wall to remove excess fluid in the pericardium. This procedure relieves pressure on the heart.

The only cure for chronic constrictive pericarditis is surgery to remove the pericardium. This is known as a pericardiectomy.

The treatments for these complications require staying in the hospital.

Living with Pericarditis

Many cases of pericarditis are mild and go away on their own. But other cases, if not treated, can lead to chronic pericarditis and serious problems that affect your heart. Some problems can be life threatening.

Sometimes it takes weeks or months to recover from pericarditis. Full recovery is likely with rest and ongoing care.

Chapter 22

Cardiac Tumors

What are cardiac tumors?

Cardiac tumors are abnormal growths in the heart or heart valves. There are many types of cardiac tumors. But, cardiac tumors, in general, are rare. The tumors can be cancerous (malignant) or noncancerous (benign). Tumors that begin growing in the heart and stay there are called primary tumors. Tumors that start in another part of the body and move to the heart (metastasize) are called secondary tumors. Most cardiac tumors are benign. But, even benign tumors can cause problems because of their size and location. Sometimes, small pieces of tumor fall into the bloodstream and are carried to distant blood vessels and get in the way of blood flow to vital organs (embolism).

What causes cardiac tumors?

A small percentage of patients with cardiac tumors have a family history of the condition. Sometimes, the tumors can be part of another health condition, such as NAME syndrome, LAMB syndrome, or Carney syndrome. Most often, the tumor develops without any of those conditions or family history. They are the result of cell overgrowth that either starts in the heart or moves to the heart.

What are the types of cardiac tumors?

Primary tumors: Primary tumors affect only 1 in 1,000 to 100,000 people. The most common type of primary cardiac tumor is myxoma. Most of these are benign. Patients of any age can develop a myxoma. They are more common in women than men. Most times, the tumor grows in the left upper chamber of the heart (left atrium) at the atrial septum, which divides the two upper chambers of the heart. Myxomas can grow in other areas of the heart or in the heart valves, but such growth is rare. About 10 percent of myxomas are hereditary or develop as a result of other diseases (see above).

Other types of benign primary tumors are papillary fibroelastomas, fibromas, rhabdomyomas, hemangiomas, teratomas, lipomas, paragangliomas, and pericardial cysts. Malignant primary tumors include pericardial mesothelioma, primary lymphoma, and sarcoma.

Secondary tumors: Secondary cardiac tumors are much more common than primary tumors. They do not start in the heart. Instead, they move to the heart after developing in another area of the body. Most often, these tumors start in the lungs, breasts, stomach, kidneys, liver, or colon. They can also be tumors related to lymphoma, leukemia, or melanoma.

What are the symptoms of cardiac tumors?

Many times, patients do not know they have a cardiac tumor. They are often found when the patient has an echocardiogram for another reason. If the tumor becomes hardened by calcium deposits (calcified), it may be seen on a chest x-ray. Most primary cardiac tumors are discovered when patients are in their fifties and sixties. However, they can be found in younger patients, too.

Patients with cardiac myxoma in the left atrium may develop symptoms. This is due to blocked blood flow through the mitral valve. The blood flow may be blocked all the time, or just when the patient is in a certain physical position (i.e., lying down). While many patients have no symptoms, if blood flow is blocked and there is increased pressure in the left atrium, it can cause shortness of breath, lightheadedness, or a cough. The inflammation may cause a fever, and the patient may have joint pain or not feel well.

What are the risks of cardiac tumors?

Tumors that block blood flow can cause heart failure, stroke, atrial fibrillation, and blood clots. Another risk is embolism. This means that part of the tumor or a blood clot can travel to other parts of the circulatory system.

How are cardiac tumors diagnosed?

If your doctor thinks you may have a cardiac tumor, the diagnosis can be confirmed using an echocardiogram, computed tomography (CT) scan, magnetic resonance imaging (MRI), or radionuclide imaging.

How are cardiac tumors treated?

Because cardiac tumors can lead to problems with blood flow, surgery to remove the tumor is usually the treatment of choice. But whether surgery is needed depends on the tumor size, whether it causes symptoms, and the patient's overall health.

Removal requires open heart surgery. But in many cases, the surgery can be done robotically or using a minimally invasive technique. During the surgery, the surgeon removes the tumor and the tissue around it to reduce the risk of the tumor returning. Because the surgery is complicated and requires a still heart, a heart-lung machine will be used to take over the work of your heart and lungs during surgery.

Recovery after traditional surgery is usually four to five days in the hospital, and six weeks total recovery time. If the tumor is removed using a robotic or minimally invasive approach, your hospital stay will likely be shorter, and you should make a full recovery in about two to three weeks.

After surgery, you will need to have an echocardiogram every year to make sure that the tumor has not returned and that there are no new growths.

Part Three

Blood Vessel Disorders

Chapter 23

Atherosclerosis

What Is Atherosclerosis?

Atherosclerosis is a disease in which plaque builds up inside your arteries. Arteries are blood vessels that carry oxygen-rich blood to your heart and other parts of your body.

Plaque is made up of fat, cholesterol, calcium, and other substances found in the blood. Over time, plaque hardens and narrows your arteries. This limits the flow of oxygen-rich blood to your organs and other parts of your body.

Atherosclerosis can lead to serious problems, including heart attack, stroke, or even death.

Atherosclerosis-Related Diseases

Atherosclerosis can affect any artery in the body, including arteries in the heart, brain, arms, legs, pelvis, and kidneys. As a result, different diseases may develop based on which arteries are affected.

Coronary heart disease: Coronary heart disease (CHD), also called coronary artery disease, is the number one killer of both men and women in the United States. CHD occurs if plaque builds up in the coronary arteries. These arteries supply oxygen-rich blood to your heart.

Excerpted from "Atherosclerosis," National Heart, Lung, and Blood Institute, National Institutes of Health, July 1, 2011.

Plaque narrows the coronary arteries and reduces blood flow to your heart muscle. Plaque buildup also makes it more likely that blood clots will form in your arteries. Blood clots can partially or completely block blood flow.

If blood flow to your heart muscle is reduced or blocked, you may have angina (chest pain or discomfort) or a heart attack.

Plaque also can form in the heart's smallest arteries. This disease is called coronary microvascular disease (MVD). In coronary MVD, plaque doesn't cause blockages in the arteries as it does in CHD.

Carotid artery disease: Carotid artery disease occurs if plaque builds up in the arteries on each side of your neck (the carotid arteries). These arteries supply oxygen-rich blood to your brain. If blood flow to your brain is reduced or blocked, you may have a stroke.

Peripheral arterial disease: Peripheral arterial disease (PAD) occurs if plaque builds up in the major arteries that supply oxygen-rich blood to your legs, arms, and pelvis.

If blood flow to these parts of your body is reduced or blocked, you may have numbness, pain, and, sometimes, dangerous infections.

Chronic kidney disease: Chronic kidney disease can occur if plaque builds up in the renal arteries. These arteries supply oxygen-rich blood to your kidneys.

Over time, chronic kidney disease causes a slow loss of kidney function. The main function of the kidneys is to remove waste and extra water from the body.

What Causes Atherosclerosis?

The exact cause of atherosclerosis isn't known. However, studies show that atherosclerosis is a slow, complex disease that may start in childhood. It develops faster as you age.

Atherosclerosis may start when certain factors damage the inner layers of the arteries. These factors include the following:

- Smoking

- High amounts of certain fats and cholesterol in the blood

- High blood pressure

- High amounts of sugar in the blood due to insulin resistance or diabetes

Plaque may begin to build up where the arteries are damaged. Over time, plaque hardens and narrows the arteries. Eventually, an area of plaque can rupture (break open).

When this happens, blood cell fragments called platelets stick to the site of the injury. They may clump together to form blood clots. Clots narrow the arteries even more, limiting the flow of oxygen-rich blood to your body.

Depending on which arteries are affected, blood clots can worsen angina (chest pain) or cause a heart attack or stroke.

Who Is at Risk for Atherosclerosis?

Coronary heart disease (atherosclerosis of the coronary arteries) is the number one killer of both men and women in the United States.

The exact cause of atherosclerosis isn't known. However, certain traits, conditions, or habits may raise your risk for the disease. These conditions are known as risk factors. The more risk factors you have, the more likely it is that you'll develop atherosclerosis.

You can control most risk factors and help prevent or delay athero-sclerosis. Other risk factors can't be controlled.

Major Risk Factors

- Unhealthy blood cholesterol levels

- High blood pressure

- Smoking

- Insulin resistance

- Diabetes

- Overweight or obesity

- Lack of physical activity

- Unhealthy diet

- Older age

- Family history of early heart disease

Emerging Risk Factors

Scientists continue to study other possible risk factors for athero-sclerosis.

High levels of a protein called C-reactive protein (CRP) in the blood may raise the risk for atherosclerosis and heart attack. High levels of CRP are a sign of inflammation in the body.

Inflammation is the body's response to injury or infection. Damage to the arteries' inner walls seems to trigger inflammation and help plaque grow.

People who have low CRP levels may develop atherosclerosis at a slower rate than people who have high CRP levels. Research is under way to find out whether reducing inflammation and lowering CRP levels also can reduce the risk for atherosclerosis.

High levels of triglycerides in the blood also may raise the risk for atherosclerosis, especially in women. Triglycerides are a type of fat.

Studies are under way to find out whether genetics may play a role in atherosclerosis risk.

What Are the Signs and Symptoms of Atherosclerosis?

Atherosclerosis usually doesn't cause signs and symptoms until it severely narrows or totally blocks an artery. Many people don't know they have the disease until they have a medical emergency, such as a heart attack or stroke.

Some people may have signs and symptoms of the disease. Signs and symptoms will depend on which arteries are affected.

Coronary Arteries

The coronary arteries supply oxygen-rich blood to your heart. If plaque narrows or blocks these arteries (a disease called coronary heart disease, or CHD), a common symptom is angina. Angina is chest pain or discomfort that occurs when your heart muscle doesn't get enough oxygen-rich blood.

Angina may feel like pressure or squeezing in your chest. You also may feel it in your shoulders, arms, neck, jaw, or back. Angina pain may even feel like indigestion. The pain tends to get worse with activity and go away with rest. Emotional stress also can trigger the pain.

Other symptoms of CHD are shortness of breath and arrhythmias. Arrhythmias are problems with the rate or rhythm of the heartbeat.

Plaque also can form in the heart's smallest arteries. This disease is called coronary microvascular disease (MVD). Symptoms of coronary MVD include angina, shortness of breath, sleep problems, fatigue (tiredness), and lack of energy.

Carotid Arteries

The carotid arteries supply oxygen-rich blood to your brain. If plaque narrows or blocks these arteries (a disease called carotid artery disease), you may have symptoms of a stroke. These symptoms may include the following:

- Sudden weakness
- Paralysis (an inability to move) or numbness of the face, arms, or legs, especially on one side of the body
- Confusion
- Trouble speaking or understanding speech
- Trouble seeing in one or both eyes
- Problems breathing
- Dizziness, trouble walking, loss of balance or coordination, and unexplained falls
- Loss of consciousness
- Sudden and severe headache

Peripheral Arteries

Plaque also can build up in the major arteries that supply oxygen-rich blood to the legs, arms, and pelvis (a disease called peripheral arterial disease).

If these major arteries are narrowed or blocked, you may have numbness, pain, and, sometimes, dangerous infections.

Renal Arteries

The renal arteries supply oxygen-rich blood to your kidneys. If plaque builds up in these arteries, you may develop chronic kidney disease. Over time, chronic kidney disease causes a slow loss of kidney function.

Early kidney disease often has no signs or symptoms. As the disease gets worse it can cause tiredness, changes in how you urinate (more often or less often), loss of appetite, nausea (feeling sick to the stomach), swelling in the hands or feet, itchiness or numbness, and trouble concentrating.

How Is Atherosclerosis Diagnosed?

Your doctor will diagnose atherosclerosis based on your medical and family histories, a physical exam, and test results.

Physical Exam

During the physical exam, your doctor may listen to your arteries for an abnormal whooshing sound called a bruit (broo-E). Your doctor can hear a bruit when placing a stethoscope over an affected artery. A bruit may indicate poor blood flow due to plaque buildup.

Your doctor also may check to see whether any of your pulses (for example, in the leg or foot) are weak or absent. A weak or absent pulse can be a sign of a blocked artery.

Diagnostic Tests

Your doctor may recommend one or more tests to diagnose atherosclerosis. These tests also can help your doctor learn the extent of your disease and plan the best treatment.

Blood tests: Blood tests check the levels of certain fats, cholesterol, sugar, and proteins in your blood. Abnormal levels may be a sign that you're at risk for atherosclerosis.

Electrocardiogram (EKG): An EKG is a simple, painless test that detects and records the heart's electrical activity. The test shows how fast the heart is beating and its rhythm (steady or irregular). An EKG also records the strength and timing of electrical signals as they pass through the heart.

An EKG can show signs of heart damage caused by CHD. The test also can show signs of a previous or current heart attack.

Chest x-ray: A chest x-ray takes pictures of the organs and structures inside your chest, such as your heart, lungs, and blood vessels. A chest x-ray can reveal signs of heart failure.

Ankle/brachial index: This test compares the blood pressure in your ankle with the blood pressure in your arm to see how well your blood is flowing. This test can help diagnose PAD.

Echocardiography: Echocardiography (echo) uses sound waves to create a moving picture of your heart. The test provides information about the size and shape of your heart and how well your heart chambers and valves are working.

Echo also can identify areas of poor blood flow to the heart, areas of heart muscle that aren't contracting normally, and previous injury to the heart muscle caused by poor blood flow.

Computed tomography scan: A computed tomography (CT) scan creates computer-generated pictures of the heart, brain, or other areas of the body. The test can show hardening and narrowing of large arteries.

A cardiac CT scan also can show whether calcium has built up in the walls of the coronary (heart) arteries. This may be an early sign of CHD.

Stress testing: During stress testing, you exercise to make your heart work hard and beat fast while heart tests are done. If you can't exercise, you may be given medicine to make your heart work hard and beat fast.

When your heart is working hard, it needs more blood and oxygen. Plaque-narrowed arteries can't supply enough oxygen-rich blood to meet your heart's needs.

A stress test can show possible signs and symptoms of CHD, such as the following:

- Abnormal changes in your heart rate or blood pressure

- Shortness of breath or chest pain

- Abnormal changes in your heart rhythm or your heart's electrical activity

As part of some stress tests, pictures are taken of your heart while you exercise and while you rest. These imaging stress tests can show how well blood is flowing in various parts of your heart. They also can show how well your heart pumps blood when it beats.

Angiography: Angiography is a test that uses dye and special x-rays to show the inside of your arteries. This test can show whether plaque is blocking your arteries and how severe the blockage is.

A thin, flexible tube called a catheter is put into a blood vessel in your arm, groin (upper thigh), or neck. Dye that can be seen on an x-ray picture is injected through the catheter into the arteries. By looking at the x-ray picture, your doctor can see the flow of blood through your arteries.

How Is Atherosclerosis Treated?

Lifestyle Changes

Making lifestyle changes often can help prevent or treat atherosclerosis. For some people, these changes may be the only treatment needed.

Follow a healthy diet: A healthy diet is an important part of a healthy lifestyle. Following a healthy diet can prevent or reduce high blood pressure and high blood cholesterol and help you maintain a healthy weight.

Be physically active: Regular physical activity can lower many atherosclerosis risk factors, including low-density lipoprotein (LDL, or "bad") cholesterol, high blood pressure, and excess weight.

231

Physical activity also can lower your risk for diabetes and raise your high-density lipoprotein (HDL) cholesterol level. HDL is the "good" cholesterol that helps prevent atherosclerosis.

Maintain a healthy weight: Maintaining a healthy weight can lower your risk for atherosclerosis. A general goal to aim for is a body mass index (BMI) of less than 25.

Quit smoking: If you smoke or use tobacco, quit. Smoking can damage and tighten blood vessels and raise your risk for atherosclerosis. Talk with your doctor about programs and products that can help you quit. Also, try to avoid secondhand smoke.

Manage stress: Research shows that the most commonly reported "trigger" for a heart attack is an emotionally upsetting event—particularly one involving anger. Also, some of the ways people cope with stress—such as drinking, smoking, or overeating—aren't healthy.

Medicines

To slow the progress of plaque buildup, your doctor may prescribe medicines to help lower your cholesterol level or blood pressure. He or she also may prescribe medicines to prevent blood clots from forming.

Medical Procedures and Surgery

If you have severe atherosclerosis, your doctor may recommend a medical procedure or surgery.

Angioplasty is a procedure that's used to open blocked or narrowed coronary (heart) arteries. Angioplasty can improve blood flow to the heart and relieve chest pain. Sometimes a small mesh tube called a stent is placed in the artery to keep it open after the procedure.

Coronary artery bypass grafting (CABG) is a type of surgery. In CABG, arteries or veins from other areas in your body are used to bypass (that is, go around) your narrowed coronary arteries. CABG can improve blood flow to your heart, relieve chest pain, and possibly prevent a heart attack.

Bypass grafting also can be used for leg arteries. For this surgery, a healthy blood vessel is used to bypass a narrowed or blocked artery in one of the legs. The healthy blood vessel redirects blood around the blocked artery, improving blood flow to the leg.

Carotid endarterectomy is surgery to remove plaque buildup from the carotid arteries in the neck. This procedure restores blood flow to the brain, which can help prevent a stroke.

Chapter 24

Carotid Artery Disease

What Is Carotid Artery Disease?

Carotid artery disease is a disease in which a waxy substance called plaque builds up inside the carotid arteries. You have two common carotid arteries, one on each side of your neck. They each divide into internal and external carotid arteries.

The internal carotid arteries supply oxygen-rich blood to your brain. The external carotid arteries supply oxygen-rich blood to your face, scalp, and neck.

Carotid artery disease is serious because it can cause a stroke, also called a "brain attack." A stroke occurs if blood flow to your brain is cut off.

If blood flow is cut off for more than a few minutes, the cells in your brain start to die. This impairs the parts of the body that the brain cells control. A stroke can cause lasting brain damage; long-term disability, such as vision or speech problems or paralysis (an inability to move); or death.

What Causes Carotid Artery Disease?

Carotid artery disease seems to start when damage occurs to the inner layers of the carotid arteries. Major factors that contribute to damage include the following:

Excerpted from "Carotid Artery Disease," National Heart, Lung, and Blood Institute, National Institutes of Health, November 1, 2010.

- Smoking
- High levels of certain fats and cholesterol in the blood
- High blood pressure
- High levels of sugar in the blood due to insulin resistance or diabetes

When damage occurs, your body starts a healing process. The healing may cause plaque to build up where the arteries are damaged.

The plaque in an artery can crack or rupture. If this happens, blood cell fragments called platelets will stick to the site of the injury and may clump together to form blood clots.

The buildup of plaque or blood clots can severely narrow or block the carotid arteries. This limits the flow of oxygen-rich blood to your brain, which can cause a stroke.

Who Is at Risk for Carotid Artery Disease?

The major risk factors for carotid artery disease, listed below, also are the major risk factors for coronary heart disease (also called coronary artery disease) and peripheral arterial disease. They are as follows:

- Unhealthy blood cholesterol levels
- High blood pressure
- Smoking
- Insulin resistance
- Diabetes
- Overweight or obesity
- Metabolic syndrome
- Lack of physical activity
- Unhealthy diet
- Older age
- Family history of atherosclerosis

Having any of these risk factors doesn't guarantee that you'll develop carotid artery disease. However, if you know that you have one or more risk factors, you can take steps to help prevent or delay the disease.

What Are the Signs and Symptoms of Carotid Artery Disease?

Carotid artery disease may not cause signs or symptoms until it severely narrows or blocks a carotid artery. Signs and symptoms may include a bruit, a transient ischemic attack (TIA), or a stroke.

Bruit

During a physical exam, your doctor may listen to your carotid arteries with a stethoscope. He or she may hear a whooshing sound called a bruit. This sound may suggest changed or reduced blood flow due to plaque buildup. To find out more, your doctor may recommend tests.

Not all people who have carotid artery disease have bruits.

Transient Ischemic Attack (Mini-Stroke)

For some people, having a TIA, or "mini-stroke," is the first sign of carotid artery disease. During a mini-stroke, you may have some or all of the symptoms of a stroke. However, the symptoms usually go away on their own within twenty-four hours.

The symptoms may include the following:

- Sudden weakness or numbness in the face or limbs, often on just one side of the body

- The inability to move one or more of your limbs

- Trouble speaking or understanding speech

- Sudden trouble seeing in one or both eyes

- Dizziness or loss of balance

- A sudden, severe headache with no known cause

Even if the symptoms stop quickly, you should see a doctor right away. Call 9-1-1 for help. Do not drive yourself to the hospital. It's important to get checked and to get treatment started as soon as possible.

A mini-stroke is a warning sign that you're at high risk of having a stroke. You shouldn't ignore these symptoms. About one-third of people who have mini-strokes will later have strokes. Getting medical care can help find possible causes of a mini-stroke and help you manage risk factors. These actions might prevent a future stroke.

Stroke

The symptoms of a stroke are the same as those of a mini-stroke, but the results are not. A stroke can cause lasting brain damage; long-term disability, such as vision or speech problems or paralysis (an inability to move); or death. Most people who have strokes have not previously had warning mini-strokes.

Getting treatment for a stroke right away is very important. You have the best chance for full recovery if treatment to open a blocked artery is given within four hours of symptom onset. The sooner treatment occurs, the better your chances of recovery.

Call 9-1-1 for help as soon as symptoms occur. Do not drive yourself to the hospital. It's very important to get checked and to get treatment started as soon as possible.

How Is Carotid Artery Disease Diagnosed?

Your doctor will diagnose carotid artery disease based on your medical history, a physical exam, and test results.

Diagnostic Tests

The following tests are common for diagnosing carotid artery disease. If you have symptoms of a mini-stroke or stroke, your doctor may use other tests as well.

Carotid ultrasound: Carotid ultrasound (also called sonography) is the most common test for diagnosing carotid artery disease. It's a painless, harmless test that uses sound waves to create pictures of the insides of your carotid arteries. This test can show whether plaque has narrowed your carotid arteries and how narrow they are.

A standard carotid ultrasound shows the structure of your carotid arteries. A Doppler carotid ultrasound shows how blood moves through your carotid arteries.

Carotid angiography: Carotid angiography is a special type of x-ray. This test may be used if the ultrasound results are unclear or don't give your doctor enough information.

For this test, your doctor will inject a substance (called contrast dye) into a vein, most often in your leg. The dye travels to your carotid arteries and highlights them on x-ray pictures.

Magnetic resonance angiography: Magnetic resonance angiography (MRA) uses a large magnet and radio waves to take pictures of your carotid arteries. Your doctor can see these pictures on a computer screen.

For this test, your doctor may give you contrast dye to highlight your carotid arteries on the pictures.

Computed tomography angiography: Computed tomography angiography, or CT angiography, takes x-ray pictures of the body from many angles. A computer combines the pictures into two- and three-dimensional images.

For this test, your doctor may give you contrast dye to highlight your carotid arteries on the pictures.

How Is Carotid Artery Disease Treated?

Treatments for carotid artery disease may include lifestyle changes, medicines, and medical procedures. The goals of treatment are to stop the disease from getting worse and to prevent a stroke.

Your treatment will depend on your symptoms, how severe the disease is, and your age and overall health.

Lifestyle Changes

Making lifestyle changes can help prevent carotid artery disease or keep it from getting worse. For some people, these changes may be the only treatment needed:

- Follow a healthy diet to prevent or lower high blood pressure and high blood cholesterol and to maintain a healthy weight.

- Be physically active. Check with your doctor first to find out how much and what kinds of activity are safe for you.

- If you're overweight or obese, lose weight.

- If you smoke, quit. Also, try to avoid secondhand smoke.

Medicines

You may need medicines to treat diseases and conditions that damage the carotid arteries. High blood pressure, high blood cholesterol, and diabetes can worsen carotid artery disease.

Some people can control these risk factors with lifestyle changes. Others also need medicines to achieve and maintain control.

You may need anticlotting medicines to prevent blood clots from forming in your carotid arteries and causing a stroke. Damage and plaque buildup make blood clots more likely.

Aspirin and clopidogrel are two common anticlotting medicines. They stop platelets from clumping together to form clots. These medicines are a mainstay of treatment for people who have known carotid artery disease.

Your health care team will help find a treatment plan that's right for you. Sticking to this plan will help avoid further harm to your carotid arteries.

If you have a stroke due to a blood clot, you may be given a clot-dissolving, or clot-busting, medicine. This type of medicine must be given within four hours of symptom onset.

The sooner treatment occurs, the better your chances of recovery. Thus, it's important to know the signs and symptoms of a stroke and call 9-1-1 right away for emergency care.

Medical Procedures

You may need a medical procedure to treat carotid artery disease. Doctors use one of two methods to open narrowed or blocked carotid arteries: carotid endarterectomy and carotid artery angioplasty and stenting.

Carotid endarterectomy: Carotid endarterectomy is mainly for people whose carotid arteries are blocked 50 percent or more.

For the procedure, a surgeon will make a cut in your neck to reach the narrowed or blocked carotid artery. Next, your surgeon will make a cut in the blocked part of the artery and remove the artery's inner lining.

Finally, your surgeon will close the artery with stitches and stop any bleeding. He or she will then close the cut in your neck.

Carotid artery angioplasty and stenting: Doctors use a procedure called angioplasty to widen the carotid arteries and restore blood flow to the brain.

A thin tube with a deflated balloon on the end is threaded through a blood vessel in your neck to the narrowed or blocked carotid artery. Once in place, the balloon is inflated to push the plaque outward against the wall of the artery.

A stent (a small mesh tube) is then put in the artery to support the inner artery wall. The stent also helps prevent the artery from becoming narrowed or blocked again.

Chapter 25

Stroke

What Is a Stroke?

A stroke occurs if the flow of oxygen-rich blood to a portion of the brain is blocked. Without oxygen, brain cells start to die after a few minutes. Sudden bleeding in the brain also can cause a stroke if it damages brain cells.

If brain cells die or are damaged because of a stroke, symptoms occur in the parts of the body that these brain cells control. Examples of stroke symptoms include sudden weakness; paralysis or numbness of the face, arms, or legs (paralysis is an inability to move); trouble speaking or understanding speech; and trouble seeing.

A stroke is a serious medical condition that requires emergency care. A stroke can cause lasting brain damage, long-term disability, or even death.

If you think you or someone else is having a stroke, call 9-1-1 right away. Do not drive to the hospital or let someone else drive you. Call an ambulance so that medical personnel can begin life-saving treatment on the way to the emergency room. During a stroke, every minute counts.

Types of Stroke

Ischemic stroke: An ischemic stroke occurs if an artery that supplies oxygen-rich blood to the brain becomes blocked. Blood clots often cause the blockages that lead to ischemic strokes.

Excerpted from "Stroke," National Heart, Lung, and Blood Institute, National Institutes of Health, February 1, 2011.

The two types of ischemic stroke are thrombotic and embolic. In a thrombotic stroke, a blood clot (thrombus) forms in an artery that supplies blood to the brain.

In an embolic stroke, a blood clot or other substance (such as plaque, a fatty material) travels through the bloodstream to an artery in the brain. (A blood clot or piece of plaque that travels through the bloodstream is called an embolus.)

With both types of ischemic stroke, the blood clot or plaque blocks the flow of oxygen-rich blood to a portion of the brain.

Hemorrhagic stroke: A hemorrhagic stroke occurs if an artery in the brain leaks blood or ruptures (breaks open). The pressure from the leaked blood damages brain cells.

The two types of hemorrhagic stroke are intracerebral and subarachnoid. In an intracerebral hemorrhage, a blood vessel inside the brain leaks blood or ruptures.

In a subarachnoid hemorrhage, a blood vessel on the surface of the brain leaks blood or ruptures. When this happens, bleeding occurs between the inner and middle layers of the membranes that cover the brain.

In both types of hemorrhagic stroke, the leaked blood causes swelling of the brain and increased pressure in the skull. The swelling and pressure damage cells and tissues in the brain.

What Causes a Stroke?

Ischemic Stroke and Transient Ischemic Attack

An ischemic stroke or transient ischemic attack (TIA) occurs if an artery that supplies oxygen-rich blood to the brain becomes blocked. Many medical conditions can increase the risk of ischemic stroke or TIA.

For example, atherosclerosis is a disease in which a fatty substance called plaque builds up on the inner walls of the arteries. Plaque hardens and narrows the arteries, which limits the flow of blood to tissues and organs (such as the heart and brain).

Plaque in an artery can crack or rupture (break open). Blood platelets, which are disc-shaped cell fragments, stick to the site of the plaque injury and clump together to form blood clots. These clots can partly or fully block an artery.

Plaque can build up in any artery in the body, including arteries in the heart, brain, and neck. The two main arteries on each side of the neck are called the carotid arteries. These arteries supply oxygen-rich blood to the brain, face, scalp, and neck.

When plaque builds up in the carotid arteries, the condition is called carotid artery disease. Carotid artery disease causes many of the ischemic strokes and TIAs that occur in the United States.

An embolic stroke (a type of ischemic stroke) or TIA also can occur if a blood clot or piece of plaque breaks away from the wall of an artery. The clot or plaque can travel through the bloodstream and get stuck in one of the brain's arteries. This stops blood flow through the artery and damages brain cells.

Heart conditions and blood disorders also can cause blood clots that can lead to a stroke or TIA. For example, atrial fibrillation, or AF, is a common cause of embolic stroke.

In AF, the upper chambers of the heart contract in a very fast and irregular way. As a result, some blood pools in the heart. The pooling increases the risk of blood clots forming in the heart chambers.

An ischemic stroke or TIA also can occur because of lesions caused by atherosclerosis. These lesions may form in the small arteries of the brain, and they can block blood flow to the brain.

Hemorrhagic Stroke

Sudden bleeding in the brain can cause a hemorrhagic stroke. The bleeding causes swelling of the brain and increased pressure in the skull. The swelling and pressure damage brain cells and tissues.

Examples of conditions that can cause a hemorrhagic stroke include high blood pressure, aneurysms, and arteriovenous malformations (AVMs).

"Blood pressure" is the force of blood pushing against the walls of the arteries as the heart pumps blood. If blood pressure rises and stays high over time, it can damage the body in many ways.

Aneurysms are balloon-like bulges in an artery that can stretch and burst. AVMs are tangles of faulty arteries and veins that can rupture within the brain. High blood pressure can increase the risk of hemorrhagic stroke in people who have aneurysms or AVMs.

Who Is at Risk for a Stroke?

Certain traits, conditions, and habits can raise your risk of having a stroke or transient ischemic attack (TIA). These traits, conditions, and habits are known as risk factors.

The more risk factors you have, the more likely you are to have a stroke. You can treat or control some risk factors, such as high blood pressure and smoking. Other risk factors, such as age and gender, you can't control.

The major risk factors for stroke include the following:

- High blood pressure
- Smoking
- Diabetes
- Heart diseases
- Brain aneurysms or arteriovenous malformations (AVMs)
- Age and gender
- Race and ethnicity
- Personal or family history of stroke or TIA

Other risk factors for stroke, many of which of you can control, include the following:

- Alcohol and illegal drug use, including cocaine, amphetamines, and other drugs
- Unhealthy cholesterol levels
- Lack of physical activity
- Unhealthy diet
- Obesity
- Stress and depression
- Certain medical conditions, such as sickle cell anemia, vasculitis (inflammation of the blood vessels), and bleeding disorders

Following a healthy lifestyle can lower the risk of stroke. Some people also may need to take medicines to lower their risk.

Sometimes strokes can occur in people who don't have any known risk factors.

What Are the Signs and Symptoms of a Stroke?

The signs and symptoms of a stroke often develop quickly. However, they can develop over hours or even days.

The type of symptoms depends on the type of stroke and the area of the brain that's affected. How long symptoms last and how severe they are vary among different people.

Signs and symptoms of a stroke may include the following:

- Sudden weakness

- Paralysis (an inability to move) or numbness of the face, arms, or legs, especially on one side of the body

- Confusion

- Trouble speaking or understanding speech

- Trouble seeing in one or both eyes

- Problems breathing

- Dizziness, trouble walking, loss of balance or coordination, and unexplained falls

- Loss of consciousness

- Sudden and severe headache

A transient ischemic attack (TIA) has the same signs and symptoms as a stroke. However, TIA symptoms usually last less than one to two hours (although they may last up to twenty-four hours). A TIA may occur only once in a person's lifetime or more often.

At first, it may not be possible to tell whether someone is having a TIA or stroke. All stroke-like symptoms require medical care.

If you think you or someone else is having a TIA or stroke, call 9-1-1 right away. Do not drive to the hospital or let someone else drive you. Call an ambulance so that medical personnel can begin life-saving treatment on the way to the emergency room. During a stroke, every minute counts.

Stroke Complications

After you've had a stroke, you may develop other complications, such as the following:

- **Blood clots and muscle weakness:** Being immobile (unable to move around) for a long time can raise your risk of developing blood clots in the deep veins of the legs. Being immobile also can lead to muscle weakness and decreased muscle flexibility.

- **Problems swallowing and pneumonia:** If a stroke affects the muscles used for swallowing, you may have a hard time eating or drinking. You also may be at risk of inhaling food or drink into your lungs. If this happens, you may develop pneumonia.

- **Loss of bladder control:** Some strokes affect the muscles used to urinate. You may need a urinary catheter (a tube placed into the bladder) until you can urinate on your own. Use of these catheters can lead to urinary tract infections. Loss of bowel control or constipation also may occur after a stroke.

How Is a Stroke Diagnosed?

Your doctor will diagnose a stroke based on your signs and symptoms, your medical history, a physical exam, and test results.

Your doctor will want to find out the type of stroke you've had, its cause, the part of the brain that's affected, and whether you have bleeding in the brain.

If your doctor thinks you've had a transient ischemic attack (TIA), he or she will look for its cause to help prevent a future stroke.

Medical History and Physical Exam

Your doctor will ask you or a family member about your risk factors for stroke. Examples of risk factors include high blood pressure, smoking, heart disease, and a personal or family history of stroke. Your doctor also will ask about your signs and symptoms and when they began.

During the physical exam, your doctor will check your mental alertness and your coordination and balance. He or she will check for numbness or weakness in your face, arms, and legs; confusion; and trouble speaking and seeing clearly.

Your doctor will look for signs of carotid artery disease, a common cause of ischemic stroke. He or she will listen to your carotid arteries with a stethoscope. A whooshing sound called a bruit (broo-E) may suggest changed or reduced blood flow due to plaque buildup in the carotid arteries.

Diagnostic Tests and Procedures

Your doctor may recommend one or more of the following tests to diagnose a stroke or TIA.

Brain computed tomography: A brain computed tomography scan, or brain CT scan, is a painless test that uses x-rays to take clear, detailed pictures of your brain. This test often is done right after a stroke is suspected.

A brain CT scan can show bleeding in the brain or damage to the brain cells from a stroke. The test also can show other brain conditions that may be causing your symptoms.

Magnetic resonance imaging: Magnetic resonance imaging (MRI) uses magnets and radio waves to create pictures of the organs and structures in your body. This test can detect changes in brain tissue and damage to brain cells from a stroke.

An MRI may be used instead of, or in addition to, a CT scan to diagnose a stroke.

Computed tomography arteriogram and magnetic resonance arteriogram: A CT arteriogram (CTA) and magnetic resonance arteriogram (MRA) can show the large blood vessels in the brain. These tests may give your doctor more information about the site of a blood clot and the flow of blood through your brain.

Carotid ultrasound: Carotid ultrasound is a painless and harmless test that uses sound waves to create pictures of the insides of your carotid arteries. These arteries supply oxygen-rich blood to your brain.

Carotid ultrasound shows whether plaque has narrowed or blocked your carotid arteries.

Your carotid ultrasound test may include a Doppler ultrasound. Doppler ultrasound is a special test that shows the speed and direction of blood moving through your blood vessels.

Carotid angiography: Carotid angiography is a test that uses dye and special x-rays to show the insides of your carotid arteries.

For this test, a small tube called a catheter is put into an artery, usually in the groin (upper thigh). The tube is then moved up into one of your carotid arteries.

Your doctor will inject a substance (called contrast dye) into the carotid artery. The dye helps make the artery visible on x-ray pictures.

Heart Tests

Electrocardiogram (EKG): An EKG is a simple, painless test that records the heart's electrical activity. The test shows how fast the heart is beating and its rhythm (steady or irregular). An EKG also records the strength and timing of electrical signals as they pass through each part of the heart.

An EKG can help detect heart problems that may have led to a stroke. For example, the test can help diagnose atrial fibrillation or a previous heart attack.

Echocardiography: Echocardiography, or echo, is a painless test that uses sound waves to create pictures of your heart.

The test gives information about the size and shape of your heart and how well your heart's chambers and valves are working.

Echo can detect possible blood clots inside the heart and problems with the aorta. The aorta is the main artery that carries oxygen-rich blood from your heart to all parts of your body.

Blood tests: Your doctor also may use blood tests to help diagnose a stroke.

A blood glucose test measures the amount of glucose (sugar) in your blood. Low blood glucose levels may cause symptoms similar to those of a stroke.

A platelet count measures the number of platelets in your blood. Blood platelets are cell fragments that help your blood clot. Abnormal platelet levels may be a sign of a bleeding disorder (not enough clotting) or a thrombotic disorder (too much clotting).

Your doctor also may recommend blood tests to measure how long it takes for your blood to clot. Two tests that may be used are called PT and PTT tests. These tests show whether your blood is clotting normally.

How Is a Stroke Treated?

Treatment for a stroke depends on whether it is ischemic or hemorrhagic. Treatment for a transient ischemic attack (TIA) depends on its cause, how much time has passed since symptoms began, and whether you have other medical conditions.

Strokes and TIAs are medical emergencies. If you have stroke symptoms, call 9-1-1 right away. Do not drive to the hospital or let someone else drive you. Call an ambulance so that medical personnel can begin life-saving treatment on the way to the emergency room. During a stroke, every minute counts.

Once you receive initial treatment, your doctor will try to treat your stroke risk factors and prevent complications.

Treating Ischemic Stroke and Transient Ischemic Attack

An ischemic stroke or TIA occurs if an artery that supplies oxygen-rich blood to the brain becomes blocked. Often, blood clots cause the blockages that lead to ischemic strokes and TIAs.

Treatment for an ischemic stroke or TIA may include medicines and medical procedures.

Medicines: A medicine called tissue plasminogen activator (tPA) can break up blood clots in the arteries of the brain. A doctor will inject tPA into a vein in your arm. This medicine must be given within four hours of the start of symptoms to work. Ideally, it should be given as soon as possible.

If, for medical reasons, your doctor can't give you tPA, you may get an antiplatelet medicine. For example, aspirin may be given within forty-eight hours of a stroke. Antiplatelet medicines help stop platelets from clumping together to form blood clots.

Your doctor also may prescribe anticoagulants, or "blood thinners." These medicines can keep blood clots from getting larger and prevent new blood clots from forming.

Medical procedures: If you have carotid artery disease, your doctor may recommend a carotid endarterectomy or carotid artery angioplasty. Both procedures open blocked carotid arteries.

Researchers are testing other treatments for ischemic stroke, such as intra-arterial thrombolysis and mechanical clot (embolus) removal in cerebral ischemia (MERCI).

In intra-arterial thrombolysis, a long, flexible tube called a catheter is put into your groin (upper thigh) and threaded to the tiny arteries of the brain. Your doctor can deliver medicine through this catheter to break up a blood clot in the brain.

MERCI is a device that can remove blood clots from an artery. During the procedure, a catheter is threaded through a carotid artery to the affected artery in the brain. The device is then used to pull the blood clot out through the catheter.

Treating Hemorrhagic Stroke

A hemorrhagic stroke occurs if an artery in the brain leaks blood or ruptures (breaks open). The first steps in treating a hemorrhagic stroke are to find the cause of bleeding in the brain and then control it.

Unlike ischemic strokes, hemorrhagic strokes aren't treated with antiplatelet medicines and blood thinners. This is because these medicines can make bleeding worse.

If you're taking antiplatelet medicines or blood thinners and have a hemorrhagic stroke, you'll be taken off the medicine.

If high blood pressure is the cause of bleeding in the brain, your doctor may prescribe medicines to lower your blood pressure. This can help prevent further bleeding.

Surgery also may be needed to treat a hemorrhagic stroke. The types of surgery used include aneurysm clipping, coil embolization, and arteriovenous malformation (AVM) repair.

Aneurysm clipping and coil embolization: If an aneurysm (a balloon-like bulge in an artery) is the cause of a stroke, your doctor may recommend aneurysm clipping or coil embolization.

Aneurysm clipping is done to block off the aneurysm from the blood vessels in the brain. This surgery helps prevent further leaking of blood from the aneurysm. It also can help prevent the aneurysm from bursting again.

During the procedure, a surgeon will make an incision (cut) in the brain and place a tiny clamp at the base of the aneurysm. You'll be given medicine to make you sleep during the surgery. After the surgery, you'll need to stay in the hospital's intensive care unit for a few days.

Coil embolization is a less complex procedure for treating an aneurysm. The surgeon will insert a tube called a catheter into an artery in the groin. He or she will thread the tube to the site of the aneurysm.

Then, a tiny coil will be pushed through the tube and into the aneurysm. The coil will cause a blood clot to form, which will block blood flow through the aneurysm and prevent it from bursting again.

Coil embolization is done in a hospital. You'll be given medicine to make you sleep during the surgery.

Arteriovenous malformation repair: If an AVM is the cause of a stroke, your doctor may recommend an AVM repair. (An AVM is a tangle of faulty arteries and veins that can rupture within the brain.) AVM repair helps prevent further bleeding in the brain.

Doctors use several methods to repair AVMs. These methods include the following:

• Surgery to remove the AVM

• Injecting a substance into the blood vessels of the AVM to block blood flow

• Using radiation to shrink the blood vessels of the AVM

Treating Stroke Risk Factors

After initial treatment for a stroke or TIA, your doctor will treat your risk factors. He or she may recommend lifestyle changes to help control your risk factors.

Lifestyle changes may include quitting smoking, following a healthy diet, maintaining a healthy weight, and being physically active.

If lifestyle changes aren't enough, you may need medicine to control your risk factors.

Life After a Stroke

The time it takes to recover from a stroke varies—it can take weeks, months, or even years. Some people recover fully, while others have long-term or lifelong disabilities.

Ongoing care, rehabilitation, and emotional support can help you recover and may even help prevent another stroke.

If you've had a stroke, you're at risk of having another one. Know the warning signs of a stroke and transient ischemic attack (TIA) and what to do if they occur. Call 9-1-1 as soon as symptoms start.

Do not drive to the hospital or let someone else drive you. Call an ambulance so that medical personnel can begin life-saving treatment on the way to the emergency room. During a stroke, every minute counts.

Ongoing Care

Lifestyle changes can help you recover from a stroke and may help prevent another one. Examples of these changes include quitting smoking, following a healthy diet, maintaining a healthy weight, and being physically active. Talk with your doctor about the types and amounts of physical activity that are safe for you.

Your doctor also may prescribe medicines to help you recover from a stroke or control your stroke risk factors. Take all of your medicines as your doctor prescribes.

If you had an ischemic stroke, you may need to take anticoagulants, also called blood thinners. These medicines prevent blood clots from getting larger and keep new clots from forming. You'll likely need routine blood tests to check how well these medicines are working.

The most common side effect of blood thinners is bleeding. This happens if the medicine thins your blood too much. This side effect can be life threatening. Bleeding can occur inside your body cavities (internal bleeding) or from the surface of your skin (external bleeding).

Know the warning signs of bleeding so you can get help right away. They include the following:

- Unexplained bruising and/or tiny red or purple dots on the skin

- Unexplained bleeding from the gums and nose

- Increased menstrual flow

- Bright red vomit or vomit that looks like coffee grounds

- Blood in your urine, bright red blood in your stools, or black tarry stools

- Pain in your abdomen or severe pain in your head

A lot of bleeding after a fall or injury or easy bruising or bleeding also may mean that your blood is too thin. Call your doctor right away if you have any of these signs. If you have severe bleeding, call 9-1-1.

Talk with your doctor about how often you should schedule follow-up visits or tests. These visits and tests can help your doctor monitor your stroke risk factors and adjust your treatment as needed.

Rehabilitation

After a stroke, you may need rehabilitation (rehab) to help you recover. Rehab may include working with speech, physical, and occupational therapists.

Language, speech, and memory: You may have trouble communicating after a stroke. You may not be able to find the right words, put complete sentences together, or put words together in a way that makes sense. You also may have problems with your memory and thinking clearly. These problems can be very frustrating.

Speech and language therapists can help you learn ways to communicate again and improve your memory.

Muscle and nerve problems: A stroke may affect only one side of the body or part of one side. It can cause paralysis (an inability to move) or muscle weakness, which can put you at risk for falling.

Physical and occupational therapists can help you strengthen and stretch your muscles. They also can help you relearn how to do daily activities, such as dressing, eating, and bathing.

Bladder and bowel problems: A stroke can affect the muscles and nerves that control the bladder and bowels. You may feel like you have to urinate often, even if your bladder isn't full. You may not be able to get to the bathroom in time. Medicines and a bladder or bowel specialist can help with these problems.

Swallowing and eating problems: You may have trouble swallowing after a stroke. Signs of this problem are coughing or choking during eating or coughing up food after eating.

A speech therapist can help you with these issues. He or she may suggest changes to your diet, such as eating puréed (finely chopped) foods or drinking thick liquids.

Emotional issues and support: After a stroke, you may have changes in your behavior or judgment. For example, your mood may change quickly. Because of these and other changes, you may feel scared, anxious, and depressed. Recovering from a stroke can be slow and frustrating.

Talk about how you feel with your health care team. Talking to a professional counselor also can help. If you're very depressed, your doctor may recommend medicines or other treatments that can improve your quality of life.

Joining a patient support group may help you adjust to life after a stroke. You can see how other people have coped with having strokes. Talk with your doctor about local support groups or check with an area medical center.

Support from family and friends also can help relieve fear and anxiety. Let your loved ones know how you feel and what they can do to help you.

Chapter 26

Aortic Disorders

Chapter Contents

Section 26.1

Aortic Aneurysm

Excerpted from "Aneurysm," National Heart, Lung, and Blood Institute,
National Institutes of Health, April 1, 2011.

What Is an Aneurysm?

An aneurysm is a balloon-like bulge in an artery. Arteries are blood vessels that carry oxygen-rich blood to your body.

Arteries have thick walls to withstand normal blood pressure. However, certain medical problems, genetic conditions, and trauma can damage or injure artery walls. The force of blood pushing against the weakened or injured walls can cause an aneurysm.

An aneurysm can grow large and rupture (burst) or dissect. A rupture causes dangerous bleeding inside the body. A dissection is a split in one or more layers of the artery wall. The split causes bleeding into and along the layers of the artery wall.

Both rupture and dissection often are fatal.

Overview

Most aneurysms occur in the aorta, the main artery that carries oxygen-rich blood from the heart to the body. The aorta goes through the chest and abdomen.

An aneurysm that occurs in the chest portion of the aorta is called a thoracic aortic aneurysm. An aneurysm that occurs in the abdominal portion of the aorta is called an abdominal aortic aneurysm.

Aneurysms also can occur in other arteries, but these types of aneurysm are less common. This section focuses on aortic aneurysms.

About thirteen thousand Americans die each year from aortic aneurysms. Most of the deaths result from rupture or dissection.

Early diagnosis and treatment can help prevent rupture and dissection. However, aneurysms can develop and grow large before causing any symptoms. Thus, people who are at high risk for aneurysms can benefit from early, routine screening.

Types of Aortic Aneurysms

The two types of aortic aneurysm are abdominal aortic aneurysm and thoracic aortic aneurysm. Some people have both types.

Abdominal Aortic Aneurysms

An aneurysm that occurs in the abdominal portion of the aorta is called an abdominal aortic aneurysm (AAA). Most aortic aneurysms are AAAs.

These aneurysms are found more often now than in the past because of computed tomography scans, or CT scans, done for other medical problems.

Small AAAs rarely rupture. However, AAAs can grow very large without causing symptoms. Routine checkups and treatment for an AAA can help prevent growth and rupture.

Thoracic Aortic Aneurysms

An aneurysm that occurs in the chest portion of the aorta (above the diaphragm, a muscle that helps you breathe) is called a thoracic aortic aneurysm (TAA).

TAAs don't always cause symptoms, even when they're large. Only half of all people who have TAAs notice any symptoms. TAAs are found more often now than in the past because of chest CT scans done for other medical problems.

With a common type of TAA, the walls of the aorta weaken and a section close to the heart enlarges. As a result, the valve between the heart and the aorta can't close properly. This allows blood to leak back into the heart.

A less common type of TAA can develop in the upper back, away from the heart. A TAA in this location may result from an injury to the chest, such as from a car crash.

What Causes an Aneurysm?

The force of blood pushing against the walls of an artery combined with damage or injury to the artery's walls can cause an aneurysm.

Many conditions and factors can damage and weaken the walls of the aorta and cause aortic aneurysms. Examples include aging, smoking, high blood pressure, and atherosclerosis. Atherosclerosis is the hardening and narrowing of the arteries due to the buildup of a waxy substance called plaque.

Rarely, infections—such as untreated syphilis (a sexually transmitted infection)—can cause aortic aneurysms. Aortic aneurysms also can occur as a result of diseases that inflame the blood vessels, such as vasculitis.

A family history of aneurysms also may play a role in causing aortic aneurysms.

In addition to the factors above, certain genetic conditions may cause thoracic aortic aneurysms (TAAs). Examples of these conditions include Marfan syndrome, Loeys-Dietz syndrome, Ehlers-Danlos syndrome (the vascular type), and Turner syndrome.

These genetic conditions can weaken the body's connective tissues and damage the aorta. People who have these conditions tend to develop aneurysms at a younger age than other people. They're also at higher risk for rupture and dissection.

Trauma, such as a car accident, also can damage the walls of the aorta and lead to TAAs.

Who Is at Risk for an Aneurysm?

Certain factors put you at higher risk for an aortic aneurysm. These factors include the following:

- **Male gender:** Men are more likely than women to have aortic aneurysms.

- **Age:** The risk for abdominal aortic aneurysms increases as you get older. These aneurysms are more likely to occur in people who are aged sixty-five or older.

- **Smoking:** Smoking can damage and weaken the walls of the aorta.

- **A family history of aortic aneurysms:** People who have family histories of aortic aneurysms are at higher risk for the condition, and they may have aneurysms before the age of sixty-five.

- **A history of aneurysms in the arteries of the legs.**

- **Certain diseases and conditions that weaken the walls of the aorta:** Examples include high blood pressure and atherosclerosis.

Having a bicuspid aortic valve can raise the risk of having a thoracic aortic aneurysm. A bicuspid aortic valve has two leaflets instead of the typical three.

Car accidents or trauma also can injure the arteries and increase the risk for aneurysms.

If you have any of these risk factors, talk with your doctor about whether you need screening for aneurysms.

What Are the Signs and Symptoms of an Aneurysm?

The signs and symptoms of an aortic aneurysm depend on the type and location of the aneurysm. Signs and symptoms also depend on whether the aneurysm has ruptured (burst) or is affecting other parts of the body.

Aneurysms can develop and grow for years without causing any signs or symptoms. They often don't cause signs or symptoms until they rupture, grow large enough to press on nearby body parts, or block blood flow.

Abdominal Aortic Aneurysms

Most abdominal aortic aneurysms (AAAs) develop slowly over years. They often don't cause signs or symptoms unless they rupture. If you have an AAA, your doctor may feel a throbbing mass while checking your abdomen.

When symptoms are present, they can include the following:

- A throbbing feeling in the abdomen

- Deep pain in your back or the side of your abdomen

- Steady, gnawing pain in your abdomen that lasts for hours or days

If an AAA ruptures, symptoms may include sudden, severe pain in your lower abdomen and back; nausea (feeling sick to your stomach) and vomiting; constipation and problems with urination; clammy, sweaty skin; light-headedness; and a rapid heart rate when standing up.

Internal bleeding from a ruptured AAA can send you into shock. Shock is a life-threatening condition in which blood pressure drops so low that the brain, kidneys, and other vital organs can't get enough blood to work well. Shock can be fatal if it's not treated right away.

Thoracic Aortic Aneurysms

A thoracic aortic aneurysm (TAA) may not cause symptoms until it dissects or grows large. If you have symptoms, they may include the following:

- Pain in your jaw, neck, back, or chest
- Coughing and/or hoarseness
- Shortness of breath and/or trouble breathing or swallowing

A dissection is a split in one or more layers of the artery wall. The split causes bleeding into and along the layers of the artery wall.

If a TAA ruptures or dissects, you may feel sudden, severe, sharp or stabbing pain starting in your upper back and moving down into your abdomen. You may have pain in your chest and arms and you can quickly go into shock.

If you have any symptoms of TAA or aortic dissection, call 9-1-1. If left untreated, these conditions may lead to organ damage or death.

How Is an Aneurysm Diagnosed?

If you have an aortic aneurysm but no symptoms, your doctor may find it by chance during a routine physical exam. More often, doctors find aneurysms during tests done for other reasons, such as chest or abdominal pain.

If you have an abdominal aortic aneurysm (AAA), your doctor may feel a throbbing mass in your abdomen. A rapidly growing aneurysm about to rupture (burst) can be tender and very painful when pressed. If you're overweight or obese, it may be hard for your doctor to feel even a large AAA.

If you have an AAA, your doctor may hear rushing blood flow instead of the normal whooshing sound when listening to your abdomen with a stethoscope.

Diagnostic Tests and Procedures

To diagnose and study an aneurysm, your doctor may recommend one or more of the following tests:

• Ultrasound and echocardiography

• Computed tomography scan

• Magnetic resonance imaging

• Angiography

How Is an Aneurysm Treated?

Aortic aneurysms are treated with medicines and surgery. Small aneurysms that are found early and aren't causing symptoms may not need treatment. Other aneurysms need to be treated.

Treatment for an aortic aneurysm is based on its size. Your doctor may recommend routine testing to make sure an aneurysm isn't getting bigger. This method usually is used for aneurysms that are smaller than five centimeters (about two inches) across.

How often you need testing (for example, every few months or every year) is based on the size of the aneurysm and how fast it's growing. The larger it is and the faster it's growing, the more often you may need to be checked.

Medicines

If you have an aortic aneurysm, your doctor may prescribe medicines before surgery or instead of surgery. Medicines are used to lower blood pressure, relax blood vessels, and lower the risk that the aneurysm will rupture (burst). Beta blockers and calcium channel blockers are the medicines most commonly used.

Surgery

Your doctor may recommend surgery if your aneurysm is growing quickly or is at risk of rupture or dissection.

The two main types of surgery to repair aortic aneurysms are open abdominal or open chest repair and endovascular repair.

Open abdominal or open chest repair: The standard and most common type of surgery for aortic aneurysms is open abdominal or open chest repair. This surgery involves a major incision (cut) in the abdomen or chest.

During the surgery, the aneurysm is removed. Then, the section of aorta is replaced with a graft made of material such as Dacron® or Teflon.® The surgery takes three to six hours; you'll remain in the hospital for five to eight days.

If needed, repair of the aortic heart valve also may be done during open abdominal or open chest surgery.

It often takes a month to recover from open abdominal or open chest surgery and return to full activity. Most patients make a full recovery.

Endovascular repair: In endovascular repair, the aneurysm isn't removed. Instead, a graft is inserted into the aorta to strengthen it. Surgeons do this type of surgery using catheters (tubes) inserted into the arteries; it doesn't require surgically opening the chest or abdomen.

The surgeon first inserts a catheter into an artery in the groin (upper thigh) and threads it to the aneurysm. Then, using an x-ray to see the artery, the surgeon threads the graft (also called a stent graft) into the aorta to the aneurysm.

The graft is then expanded inside the aorta and fastened in place to form a stable channel for blood flow. The graft reinforces the weakened section of the aorta. This helps prevent the aneurysm from rupturing.

The recovery time for endovascular repair is less than the recovery time for open abdominal or open chest repair. However, doctors can't repair all aortic aneurysms with endovascular repair. The location or size of an aneurysm may prevent the use of a stent graft.

How Can an Aneurysm Be Prevented?

The best way to prevent an aortic aneurysm is to avoid the factors that put you at higher risk for one. You can't control all aortic aneurysm risk factors, but lifestyle changes can help you lower some risks. If you smoke, try to quit; follow a healthy diet; be as physically active as you can; and work with your doctor to control medical conditions such as high blood pressure and high blood cholesterol.

Screening for Aneurysms

Although you may not be able to prevent an aneurysm, early diagnosis and treatment can help prevent rupture and dissection.

Aneurysms can develop and grow large before causing any signs or symptoms. Thus, people who are at high risk for aneurysms may benefit from early, routine screening.

Section 26.2

Aortic Dissection

Excerpted from "Aortic Dissection," © 2013 A.D.A.M., Inc.
Reprinted with permission.

Aortic dissection is a serious condition in which there is a separation of the aorta walls. The small tear can become larger. It can lead to bleeding into and along the wall of the aorta, the major artery carrying blood out of the heart.

Causes

When it leaves the heart, the aorta first moves up through the chest toward the head (the ascending aorta). It then bends or arches, and finally moves down through the chest and abdomen (the descending aorta).

Aortic dissection most often happens because of a tear or damage to the inner wall of the aorta. This usually occurs in the chest (thoracic) part of the artery, but it may also occur in the abdominal part.

When a tear occurs, it creates two channels:

- One in which blood continues to travel
- Another where blood stays still

If the channel with nontraveling blood gets bigger, it can push on other branches of the aorta. This can narrow the other branches and reduce blood flow through them.

An aortic dissection may also cause abnormal widening or ballooning of the aorta (aneurysm).

The exact cause is unknown, but more common risks include:

- aging;
- atherosclerosis;
- blunt trauma to the chest, such as hitting the steering wheel of a car during an accident;
- high blood pressure.

Other risk factors and conditions associated with the development of aortic dissection include:

- bicuspid aortic valve;
- coarctation (narrowing) of the aorta;
- connective tissue disorders;
- heart surgery or procedures;
- Marfan syndrome and rare genetic disorders;
- pregnancy;
- swelling of the blood vessels due to conditions such as arteritis and syphilis.

Aortic dissection occurs in about two out of every ten thousand people. It can affect anyone, but is most often seen in men ages forty to seventy.

Symptoms

The symptoms usually begin suddenly, and include severe chest pain. The pain may feel like a heart attack, and can:

- be described as sharp, stabbing, tearing, or ripping;

- be felt below the chest bone, then move under the shoulder blades or to the back;
- move to the shoulder, neck, arm, jaw, abdomen, or hips;
- change position—pain typically moves to the arms and legs as the aortic dissection gets worse.

Symptoms are caused by a decrease of blood flowing to the rest of the body, and can include:

- anxiety and a feeling of doom;
- fainting or dizziness;
- heavy sweating (clammy skin);
- nausea and vomiting;
- pale skin (pallor);
- rapid, weak pulse;
- shortness of breath—trouble breathing when lying flat (orthopnea).

Other symptoms may include:

- pain in the abdomen;
- stroke symptoms;
- swallowing difficulties from pressure on the esophagus.

Exams and Tests

The health care provider will take your family history and listen to your heart, lungs, and abdomen with a stethoscope. The examination may find:

- a "blowing" murmur over the aorta, heart murmur, or other abnormal sound;
- a difference in blood pressure between the right and left arms, or between the arms and legs;
- low blood pressure;
- signs resembling a heart attack;
- signs of shock, but with normal blood pressure.

Aortic dissection or aortic aneurysm may be seen on:

- aortic angiography;
- chest x-ray;
- chest magnetic resonance imaging (MRI);
- computed tomography (CT) scan of chest with dye;
- Doppler ultrasonography (occasionally performed);
- echocardiogram;
- transesophageal echocardiogram (TEE).

Blood work to rule out a heart attack is needed.

Treatment

Aortic dissection is a life-threatening condition and needs to be treated right away:

- Dissections that occur in the part of the aorta that is leaving the heart (ascending) are treated with surgery.
- Dissections that occur in other parts of the aorta (descending) may be managed with surgery or medications.

Two different techniques may be used for surgery:

- **Standard, open surgery:** A surgical cut is made in the chest or abdomen.
- **Endovascular aortic repair:** Surgery is done without any major surgical cut.

Drugs that lower blood pressure may be prescribed. These drugs may be given through a vein (intravenously). Beta blockers are the first drugs of choice. Strong pain relievers are usually needed.

If the aortic valve is damaged, valve replacement is needed. If the heart arteries are involved, a coronary bypass is also performed.

Outlook (Prognosis)

Aortic dissection is life threatening. The condition can be managed with surgery if it is done before the aorta ruptures. Less than half of patients with a ruptured aorta survive.

Those who survive will need lifelong, aggressive treatment of high blood pressure. They will need to be followed up with CT scans every few months to monitor the aorta.

Possible Complications

Aortic dissection may decrease or stop the blood flow to many different parts of the body. This may result in short-term or long-term problems, or damage to the:

- brain;
- heart;
- intestines or bowels;
- kidneys;
- legs.

When to Contact a Medical Professional

If you have symptoms of aortic dissection or severe chest pain, call 911 or your local emergency number, or go to the emergency room as quickly as possible.

Prevention

Proper treatment and control of hardening of the arteries (atherosclerosis) and high blood pressure may reduce your risk of aortic dissection. It is very important for patients at risk for dissection to tightly control their blood pressure.

Take safety precautions to prevent injuries, which can cause dissections.

Many cases of aortic dissection cannot be prevented.

If you have been diagnosed with Marfan or Ehlers-Danlos syndrome, make sure you regularly follow-up with your doctor.

Chapter 27

Disorders of the Peripheral Arteries

Chapter Contents

Section 27.1

Fibromuscular Dysplasia

What is fibromuscular dysplasia?

Fibromuscular dysplasia (FMD) is the abnormal development or growth of cells in the walls of the body's arteries. As a result of this growth, areas of the arteries can thicken, narrow, and even enlarge, making it difficult for blood to flow through them.

FMD most often affects the renal arteries, which supply the kidneys with blood. It also occurs in the carotid arteries, which bring blood to the brain. Less commonly, FMD develops in the arteries of the abdomen (mesenteric arteries) or the arteries of the arms and legs. In nearly one-third of people with FMD, more than one artery is affected.

Depending on which arteries are affected, FMD can increase the risk of high blood pressure, impaired kidney function, aneurysm, stroke, and other complications. FMD affects between 1 and 5 percent of Americans, typically women under age fifty.

What causes fibromuscular dysplasia?

The cause of FMD is still unknown. However, several factors may play a role in its development. A combination of these factors is likely responsible:

- **Genetics:** Research suggests that about 10 percent of cases appear in families. People who have a family member with FMD may develop the condition in different arteries than their relative, experience a more or less severe version of the disease, or may not develop FMD at all.

- **Hormones:** FMD is three to four times more common in premenopausal women than in men, suggesting that sex hormones may be involved in its development.

- **Abnormal arteries:** A lack of oxygen to the artery walls may cause them to form abnormally. Arteries may also be located abnormally within the body, predisposing them to FMD.

What conditions are associated with fibromuscular dysplasia?

FMD can increase risk of several conditions, including:

- **High blood pressure:** When the arteries become narrowed, blood pressure can increase. High blood pressure (hypertension) is the most common complication of FMD.

- **Kidney dysfunction or failure:** Reduced blood flow to the kidneys can impair kidney function and, in rare cases, lead to kidney failure.

- **Pain or cramping in lower legs (intermittent claudication):** FMD that affects the arteries in the legs can cause discomfort or pain when walking and exercising.

- **A tear in the artery (dissection):** The lining of the artery wall may tear, causing blood to leak into the wall.

- **Aneurysm:** The pressure of blood flow through a narrowed artery can create a weakened area or bulge in the artery wall called an aneurysm. An aneurysm may rupture, resulting in a life-threatening situation.

- **Stroke:** A stroke may occur if an aneurysm in one of the carotid arteries ruptures or if one of the carotid arteries dissects, disrupting the flow of blood to the brain.

What are the risk factors for fibromuscular dysplasia?

Risk factors for FMD include:

- **Gender:** FMD affects more women than men.

- **Age:** FMD is most common in premenopausal women younger than age fifty.

- **Family history:** FMD appears to have a genetic basis. About 10 percent of people with FMD have a relative with the condition.

What are the symptoms of fibromuscular dysplasia?

Many people with FMD do not develop symptoms. When symptoms do occur, they depend on the location of the affected arteries. In the renal arteries, FMD can cause:

- high blood pressure;
- shrinkage (atrophy) of the kidney, which is often painless;
- impaired kidney function.

In the carotid arteries, FMD can cause:

- dizziness;
- ringing in the ears;
- headache;
- blurred vision or temporary loss of vision;
- neck pain.

In the mesenteric arteries, FMD can cause:

- abdominal pain after eating;
- unintended weight loss.

In the arteries of the arms and legs, FMD can cause:

- numbness;
- weakness;
- discomfort when moving the limb.

How is fibromuscular dysplasia diagnosed?

In addition to a complete medical history and physical examination, physicians may use one or more the following tests to diagnose FMD:

- **Computed tomography angiography (CTA):** This test uses a combination of x-rays, contrast dye, and computer technology to produce cross-sectional images (often called slices) of the body.

- **Duplex ultrasonography:** This technique uses high-frequency sound waves and a computer to create images of blood vessels, tissues, and organs. Duplex ultrasonography is used to measure and assess the flow of blood.

- **Magnetic resonance angiography (MRA):** This noninvasive procedure uses a combination of a large magnet, radiofrequencies, and a computer to produce detailed images of organs and structures within the body.

What is the treatment for fibromuscular dysplasia?

Even though there is no cure for FMD, it can be controlled. A multidisciplinary team of physicians will determine the best treatment based on the patient's individual case. Treatment for FMD includes:

- **Medical therapy:** The physician may prescribe medications to help control high blood pressure, including angiotensin-converting enzyme (ACE) inhibitors, beta blockers, and calcium channel blockers. People with FMD may also need to take antiplatelet drugs, such as aspirin, to prevent blood clots.

- **Interventional therapy:** Physicians may use percutaneous transluminal angioplasty (PTA) to open narrowed sections of arteries. In this technique, a balloon-tipped catheter (thin, flexible tube) is threaded through the affected artery to expand it. A stent, which is a tiny metal-mesh tube, rarely needs to be inserted to keep the artery open in patients with FMD. PTA is less invasive than open surgery and results in faster recovery times.

- **Surgery:** This intervention reroutes blood flow around the diseased artery and may be used in severe cases or when PTA is not an option.

- **Genetic counseling:** Because FMD appears to run in families, women of childbearing age may receive counseling for the genetic basis of the condition. There is not yet a genetic test for FMD.

- **Psychosocial treatment:** FMD often affects young, otherwise healthy women, and coping with it can be difficult. Psychologists or other mental health professionals can offer counseling to help patients deal with the stress and anxiety that may accompany having FMD.

- **Obstetrics/gynecological care:** Specialists in obstetrics and gynecology can advise patients with FMD about the use of oral contraceptives, estrogen therapy, and other hormone-based medications, which can affect blood flow in the arteries.

How long will treatment for FMD continue?

Although FMD can be managed successfully, it can recur in some patients. For this reason, people with FMD should continue to be monitored by their physicians even after interventional or surgical treatments are completed. Patients may be seen for follow-up visits every few months or once or twice a year, depending on their individual case. Physicians will monitor patients' medications and assess signs of possible recurrence.

Section 27.2

Peripheral Aneurysm

A peripheral aneurysm is an aneurysm that occurs in an artery other than the aortic artery. An aneurysm is a weakened area of an artery wall that bulges or expands.

What Is Peripheral Aneurysm?

Peripheral aneurysms develop in arteries other than the aorta (largest artery in your body). Peripheral aneurysms most commonly develop in the popliteal artery, which runs down the lower part of your thigh and knee. Though not as common, peripheral aneurysms can also develop in the:

- femoral artery (located in the groin);
- carotid artery (located in the neck);
- arteries in the arms;
- arteries supplying blood to the kidneys or bowel (a visceral aneurysm).

Peripheral aneurysms are not as likely to rupture as aortic aneurysms. More often, blood clots develop that may block blood flow to your arms, legs, or brain. If it is large enough, a peripheral aneurysm can press on a nerve or vein, causing pain, swelling, or numbness.

What Causes Peripheral Aneurysm?

The specific cause of a peripheral aneurysm is not clear; injury, infection, and aging can be factors. Researchers believe that atherosclerosis (hardening of the arteries) plays an important role. Atherosclerosis occurs when plaque builds up on the artery walls, narrowing them and slowing blood flow. Risk factors that contribute to atherosclerosis include:

- family history of heart or vascular disease;
- high blood pressure;
- high cholesterol;
- obesity;
- smoking.

If a peripheral aneurysm is found in one leg, you are at greater risk of having one in the other leg. Peripheral aneurysm also increases your risk of aortic aneurysm.

Diagnosis of Peripheral Aneurysm

Most people do not feel any symptoms with a peripheral aneurysm, especially if it is small. The warning signs that you may have an aneurysm depend on where it is and its size. Symptoms may include:

- a throbbing lump you can feel in your neck, leg, arm, or groin;
- claudication (cramping in the legs with exercise);
- leg or arm pain even at rest;
- sores on your fingers or toes that will not heal;
- numbness or pain that radiates in your leg or arm;
- gangrene (tissue death).

Tests your physician can use to confirm whether you have an aneurysm include:

- **CT scan (computed tomography scan, also called CAT scan):** An imaging procedure that uses x-rays and computer technology to produce cross-sectional, detailed images of the body, including bones, muscles, fat, and organs.

- **MRI (magnetic resonance imaging):** A noninvasive, sophisticated imaging procedure that uses large magnets and a computer to produce detailed images of organs and structures inside the body.

- **Ultrasound:** A test that uses high-frequency sound waves to evaluate blood flow in a vessel.

Treatment of Peripheral Aneurysm

Surgery

A peripheral aneurysm requires surgical repair because of the risk of a sudden blockage or a dislodged clot obstructing blood flow. If the aneurysm is small and you have no symptoms, your physician will monitor its size to determine when surgery is needed.

There are generally two types of aneurysm repair surgeries:

- Endovascular repair makes use of a catheter that guides a stent graft through small incisions in the groin. The graft is inserted into the aneurysm and seals the aneurysm from within.

- Open surgical repair of a peripheral aneurysm may be recommended if the aneurysm anatomy does not allow for endovascular repair. In this procedure, the damaged area is removed and replaced with a graft (tube).

Medications

If a blood clot is blocking the aneurysm, thrombolytic therapy (the use of drugs to dissolve or break up blood clots) may be used before surgery.

Section 27.3

Peripheral Arterial Disease

Excerpted from "Peripheral Arterial Disease," National Heart, Lung, and
Blood Institute, National Institutes of Health, April 1, 2011.

What Is Peripheral Arterial Disease?

Peripheral arterial disease (P.A.D.) is a disease in which plaque builds up in the arteries that carry blood to your head, organs, and limbs. Plaque is made up of fat, cholesterol, calcium, fibrous tissue, and other substances in the blood.

When plaque builds up in the body's arteries, the condition is called atherosclerosis. Over time, plaque can harden and narrow the arteries. This limits the flow of oxygen-rich blood to your organs and other parts of your body.

P.A.D. usually affects the arteries in the legs, but it also can affect the arteries that carry blood from your heart to your head, arms, kidneys, and stomach. This section focuses on P.A.D. that affects blood flow to the legs.

Other Names for Peripheral Arterial Disease

- Atherosclerotic peripheral arterial disease
- Claudication
- Hardening of the arteries
- Leg cramps from poor circulation
- Peripheral vascular disease
- Poor circulation
- Vascular disease

What Causes Peripheral Arterial Disease?

The most common cause of peripheral arterial disease (P.A.D.) is atherosclerosis. Atherosclerosis is a disease in which plaque builds up in your arteries. The exact cause of atherosclerosis isn't known.

The disease may start if certain factors damage the inner layers of the arteries. These factors include the following:

- Smoking

- High amounts of certain fats and cholesterol in the blood

- High blood pressure

- High amounts of sugar in the blood due to insulin resistance or diabetes

When damage occurs, your body starts a healing process. The healing may cause plaque to build up where the arteries are damaged.

Eventually, a section of plaque can rupture (break open), causing a blood clot to form at the site. The buildup of plaque or blood clots can severely narrow or block the arteries and limit the flow of oxygen-rich blood to your body.

Who Is at Risk for Peripheral Arterial Disease?

Peripheral arterial disease (P.A.D.) affects millions of people in the United States. The disease is more common in African Americans than any other racial or ethnic group.

The major risk factors for P.A.D. are smoking, older age, and having certain diseases or conditions.

Smoking

Smoking is the main risk factor for P.A.D. Your risk of P.A.D. increases four times if you smoke or have a history of smoking.

On average, people who smoke and develop P.A.D. have symptoms ten years earlier than people who don't smoke and develop P.A.D.

Quitting smoking slows the progress of P.A.D. Smoking even one or two cigarettes a day can interfere with P.A.D. treatments. People who smoke and people who have diabetes are at highest risk for P.A.D. complications, such as gangrene (tissue death) in the leg from decreased blood flow.

Older Age

Older age also is a risk factor for P.A.D. Plaque builds up in your arteries as you age. About one in every twenty Americans over the age of fifty has P.A.D. The risk continues to rise as you get older.

Older age combined with other risk factors, such as smoking or diabetes, also puts you at higher risk for P.A.D.

Diseases and Conditions

Many diseases and conditions can raise your risk of P.A.D., including the following:

- Diabetes. About one in three people older than fifty who has diabetes also has P.A.D.

- High blood pressure or a family history of it.

- High blood cholesterol or a family history of it.

- Coronary heart disease (CHD) or a family history of it.

- Stroke or a family history of it.

- Metabolic syndrome (a group of risk factors that raise your risk of CHD and other health problems, such as P.A.D., stroke, and diabetes).

What Are the Signs and Symptoms of Peripheral Arterial Disease?

Many people who have peripheral arterial disease (P.A.D.) don't have any signs or symptoms. Others may have many signs and symptoms.

Even if you don't have signs or symptoms, ask your doctor whether you should get checked for P.A.D. if you're:

- aged seventy or older;

- aged fifty or older and have a history of smoking or diabetes;

- younger than fifty and have diabetes and one or more risk factors for atherosclerosis.

Intermittent Claudication

People who have P.A.D. may have symptoms when walking or climbing stairs. These symptoms may include pain, numbness, aching, or heaviness in the leg muscles.

Symptoms also may include cramping in the affected leg(s) and in the buttocks, thighs, calves, and feet. Symptoms may ease after resting.

These symptoms are called intermittent claudication. During physical activity, your muscles need increased blood flow. If your blood vessels are narrowed or blocked, your muscles won't get enough blood, which will lead to symptoms. When resting, the muscles need less blood flow, so the symptoms will go away.

About 10 percent of people who have P.A.D. have claudication. This symptom is more likely in people who also have atherosclerosis in other arteries.

Other Signs and Symptoms

Other signs and symptoms of P.A.D. include the following:

- Weak or absent pulses in the legs or feet

- Sores or wounds on the toes, feet, or legs that heal slowly, poorly, or not at all

- A pale or bluish color to the skin

- A lower temperature in one leg compared to the other leg

- Poor nail growth on the toes and decreased hair growth on the legs

- Erectile dysfunction, especially among men who have diabetes

How Is Peripheral Arterial Disease Diagnosed?

Peripheral arterial disease (P.A.D.) is diagnosed based on your medical and family histories, a physical exam, and test results.

P.A.D. often is diagnosed after symptoms are reported. A correct diagnosis is important because people who have P.A.D. are at higher risk for coronary heart disease (CHD), heart attack, stroke, and transient ischemic attack ("mini-stroke"). If you have P.A.D., your doctor also may want to check for signs of these diseases and conditions.

Physical Exam

During the physical exam, your doctor will look for signs of P.A.D. He or she may check the blood flow in your legs or feet to see whether you have weak or absent pulses.

Your doctor also may check the pulses in your leg arteries for an abnormal whooshing sound called a bruit. He or she can hear this sound with a stethoscope. A bruit may be a warning sign of a narrowed or blocked artery.

Your doctor may compare blood pressure between your limbs to see whether the pressure is lower in the affected limb. He or she also may check for poor wound healing or any changes in your hair, skin, or nails that may be signs of P.A.D.

Diagnostic Tests

Ankle-brachial index: A simple test called an ankle-brachial index (ABI) often is used to diagnose P.A.D. The ABI compares blood pressure in your ankle to blood pressure in your arm. This test shows how well blood is flowing in your limbs.

ABI can show whether P.A.D. is affecting your limbs, but it won't show which blood vessels are narrowed or blocked.

A normal ABI result is 1.0 or greater (with a range of 0.90 to 1.30). The test takes about ten to fifteen minutes to measure both arms and both ankles. This test may be done yearly to see whether P.A.D. is getting worse.

Doppler ultrasound: A Doppler ultrasound looks at blood flow in the major arteries and veins in the limbs. During this test, a handheld device is placed on your body and passed back and forth over the affected area. A computer converts sound waves into a picture of blood flow in the arteries and veins.

The results of this test can show whether a blood vessel is blocked. The results also can help show the severity of P.A.D.

Treadmill test: A treadmill test can show the severity of symptoms and the level of exercise that brings them on. You'll walk on a treadmill for this test. This shows whether you have any problems during normal walking.

You may have an ABI test before and after the treadmill test. This will help compare blood flow in your arms and legs before and after exercise.

Magnetic resonance angiogram: A magnetic resonance angiogram (MRA) uses magnetic and radio wave energy to take pictures of your blood vessels. This test is a type of magnetic resonance imaging (MRI).

An MRA can show the location and severity of a blocked blood vessel. If you have a pacemaker, man-made joint, stent, surgical clips, mechanical heart valve, or other metallic devices in your body, you might not be able to have an MRA. Ask your doctor whether an MRA is an option for you.

Arteriogram: An arteriogram provides a "road map" of the arteries. Doctors use this test to find the exact location of a blocked artery.

For this test, dye is injected through a needle or catheter (tube) into one of your arteries. This may make you feel mildly flushed. After the dye is injected, an x-ray is taken. The x-ray can show the location, type, and extent of the blockage in the artery.

Some doctors use a newer method of arteriogram that uses tiny ultrasound cameras. These cameras take pictures of the insides of the blood vessels. This method is called intravascular ultrasound.

Blood tests: Your doctor may recommend blood tests to check for P.A.D. risk factors. For example, blood tests can help diagnose conditions such as diabetes and high blood cholesterol.

How Is Peripheral Arterial Disease Treated?

Treatments for peripheral arterial disease (P.A.D.) include lifestyle changes, medicines, and surgery or procedures.

Lifestyle Changes

Treatment often includes making long-lasting lifestyle changes, such as the following:

- **Quitting smoking:** Your risk of P.A.D. increases four times if you smoke. Smoking also raises your risk for other diseases, such as coronary heart disease (CHD). Talk with your doctor about programs and products that can help you quit smoking. Also, try to avoid secondhand smoke.

- **Lowering blood pressure:** This lifestyle change can help you avoid the risk of stroke, heart attack, heart failure, and kidney disease.

- **Lowering high blood cholesterol:** Lowering cholesterol can delay or even reverse the buildup of plaque in your arteries.

- **Lowering blood glucose (sugar) levels if you have diabetes:** A hemoglobin A1C test can show how well you have controlled your blood sugar level over the past three months.

- **Being physically active:** Talk with your doctor about taking part in a supervised exercise program. This type of program has been shown to reduce P.A.D. symptoms.

Follow a healthy eating plan that's low in total fat, saturated fat, trans fat, cholesterol, and sodium (salt). Include fruits, vegetables, and low-fat dairy products in your diet. If you're overweight or obese, work with your doctor to create a reasonable weight-loss plan.

Two examples of healthy eating plans are Therapeutic Lifestyle Changes (TLC) and Dietary Approaches to Stop Hypertension (DASH).

Medicines

Your doctor may prescribe medicines to do the following things:

- Treat unhealthy cholesterol levels and high blood pressure
- Prevent blood clots from forming due to low blood flow
- Help ease leg pain that occurs when you walk or climb stairs

Surgery or Procedures

Bypass grafting: Your doctor may recommend bypass grafting surgery if blood flow in your limb is blocked or nearly blocked. For this surgery, your doctor uses a blood vessel from another part of your body or a man-made tube to make a graft.

This graft bypasses (that is, goes around) the blocked part of the artery. The bypass allows blood to flow around the blockage.

This surgery doesn't cure P.A.D., but it may increase blood flow to the affected limb.

Angioplasty and stenting: Your doctor may recommend angioplasty to restore blood flow through a narrowed or blocked artery.

During this procedure, a catheter (thin tube) with a balloon at the tip is inserted into a blocked artery. The balloon is then inflated, which pushes plaque outward against the artery wall. This widens the artery and restores blood flow.

A stent (a small mesh tube) may be placed in the artery during angioplasty. A stent helps keep the artery open after angioplasty is done. Some stents are coated with medicine to help prevent blockages in the artery.

Atherectomy: Atherectomy is a procedure that removes plaque buildup from an artery. During the procedure, a catheter is used to insert a small cutting device into the blocked artery. The device is used to shave or cut off plaque.

The bits of plaque are removed from the body through the catheter or washed away in the bloodstream (if they're small enough).

Doctors also can do atherectomy using a special laser that dissolves the blockage.

Other Types of Treatment

Researchers are studying cell and gene therapies to treat P.A.D. However, these treatments aren't yet available outside of clinical trials.

Section 27.4

Raynaud Phenomenon

Reprinted from "What Is Raynaud's Phenomenon?" National Institute of
Arthritis and Musculoskeletal and Skin Diseases, National Institutes of
Health, April 2009. Reviewed by David A. Cooke, M.D., FACP, October 2013.

Raynaud phenomenon is a disorder that affects blood vessels, mostly in
the fingers and toes. It causes the blood vessels to narrow when you are:

- cold;

- feeling stress.

Primary Raynaud phenomenon happens on its own. Secondary
Raynaud phenomenon happens along with some other health problem.

Who Gets Raynaud Phenomenon?

People of all ages can have Raynaud phenomenon. Raynaud phenomenon may run in families, but more research is needed.

The primary form is the most common. It most often starts between age fifteen and twenty-five. It is most common in the following
populations:

- Women

- People living in cold places

The secondary form tends to start after age thirty-five to forty.
It is most common in people with connective tissue diseases, such
as scleroderma, Sjögren syndrome, and lupus. Other possible causes
include the following:

- Carpal tunnel syndrome, which affects nerves in the wrists

- Blood vessel disease

- Some medicines used to treat high blood pressure, migraines, or
  cancer

- Some over-the-counter cold medicines

- Some narcotics

People with certain jobs may be more likely to get the secondary form:

- Workers who are around certain chemicals
- People who use tools that vibrate, such as a jackhammer

What Are the Symptoms of Raynaud Phenomenon?

The body saves heat when it is cold by slowing the supply of blood to the skin. It does this by making blood vessels narrower.

With Raynaud phenomenon, the body's reaction to cold or stress is stronger than normal. It makes blood vessels narrow faster and tighter than normal. When this happens, it is called an "attack."

During an attack, the fingers and toes can change colors. They may go from white to blue to red. They may also feel cold and numb from lack of blood flow. As the attack ends and blood flow returns, fingers or toes can throb and tingle. After the cold parts of the body warm up, normal blood flow returns in about fifteen minutes.

What Is the Difference between Primary and Secondary Raynaud Phenomenon?

Primary Raynaud phenomenon is often so mild a person never seeks treatment.

Secondary Raynaud phenomenon is more serious and complex. It is caused when diseases reduce blood flow to fingers and toes.

How Does a Doctor Diagnose Raynaud Phenomenon?

It is fairly easy to diagnose Raynaud phenomenon. But it is harder to find out whether a person has the primary or the secondary form of the disorder.

Doctors will diagnose which form it is using a complete history, an exam, and tests. Tests may include the following:

- Blood tests
- Looking at fingernail tissue with a microscope

What Is the Treatment for Raynaud Phenomenon?

Treatment aims to do the following things:

- Reduce how many attacks you have
- Make attacks less severe
- Prevent tissue damage
- Prevent loss of finger and toe tissue

Primary Raynaud phenomenon does not lead to tissue damage, so nondrug treatment is used first. Treatment with medicine is more common with secondary Raynaud.

Severe cases of Raynaud can lead to sores or gangrene (tissue death) in the fingers and toes. These cases can be painful and hard to treat. In severe cases that cause skin ulcers and serious tissue damage, surgery may be used.

Nondrug Treatments and Self-Help Measures

To reduce how long and severe attacks are, do the following things:

- Keep your hands and feet warm and dry.
- Warm your hands and feet with warm water.
- Avoid air conditioning.
- Wear gloves to touch frozen or cold foods.
- Wear many layers of loose clothing and a hat when it's cold.
- Use chemical warmers, such as small heating pouches that can be placed in pockets, mittens, boots, or shoes.
- Talk to your doctor before exercising outside in cold weather.
- Don't smoke.
- Avoid medicines that make symptoms worse.
- Control stress.
- Exercise regularly.

See a doctor if any of the following are true:

- You worry about attacks.
- You have questions about self-care.
- Attacks happen on just one side of your body.
- You have sores or ulcers on your fingers or toes.

Treatment with Medications

People with secondary Raynaud phenomenon are often treated with the following types of medication:

- Blood pressure medicines.

- Medicines that relax blood vessels. One kind can be put on the fingers to heal ulcers.

If blood flow doesn't return and finger loss is a risk, you will need other medicines.

Pregnant woman should not take these medicines. Sometimes Raynaud phenomenon gets better or goes away when a woman is pregnant.

What Research Is Being Conducted to Help People Who Have Raynaud Phenomenon?

Current research is being done on:

- New ways to find and treat the problem

- New medicines to improve blood flow

- Supplements and herbal treatments, but these have been found ineffective in most studies

- Causes

Section 27.5

Thromboangiitis Obliterans

What is thromboangiitis obliterans?

Thromboangiitis obliterans is also known as Buerger disease. It is a smoking-related condition that results in blood clot formation (thrombosis) in small- and medium-sized arteries, and less commonly veins. The affected areas are most commonly the hands and feet.

Who gets it?

Thromboangiitis obliterans occurs almost exclusively in smokers. It is most common in Eastern Europe, the Middle East, and Asia. Most patients are between twenty and forty-five years old consuming homemade cigarettes. The incidence appears to have decreased over recent years as smoking has decreased. American statistics estimate approximately ten to twenty cases per one hundred thousand.

Thromboangiitis obliterans has also been reported to affect long-term cannabis smokers.

What are the symptoms?

The most common presentation of thromboangiitis obliterans is of painful purple/blue areas on the fingers or toes. It is often one-sided and may involve isolated fingers or toes. Often the pain is worse at night, with exercise, and in cool weather. With time, the areas may ulcerate or become black secondary to death of the involved skin (gangrene). The disease progresses in patients who continue to smoke and may lead to complete loss of digits or limbs. On examination, the hand and foot pulses are often lost at an early stage. Other associated problems may include recurrent venous thrombosis (superficial or deep veins), erythema nodosum, and rarely involvement of the blood supply to internal organs such as the kidneys, heart, and brain.

What causes it?

The cause of the disease is not fully understood but it is probable that the smoking triggers thrombosis in the blood vessels, leading to a lack of oxygen and nutrients to the affected tissue. Research has demonstrated the presence of immunoglobulins and endothelial cell antibodies suggesting an immunological mechanism. The blood level of these antibodies can be used as a marker of disease activity. Response to acetylcholine (a chemical which leads to relaxation of blood vessels) has also been shown to be decreased in Buerger patients compared to normal subjects.

In some cases, thromboangiitis obliterans has been associated with chronic arsenic poisoning.

What tests are necessary?

A skin biopsy can be helpful although the features are not specific for thromboangiitis obliterans. The histology usually shows intraluminal thrombosis (blood clot within the vessel) with associated micro-abscess formation. A mixed infiltrate of white bloods cells and giant cells may be seen in all layers of the vessel wall, although the internal elastic lamina is classically spared and helps distinguish thromboangiitis obliterans from other types of vasculitis.

Tests to rule out the presence of other diseases such as diabetes, clotting disorders, connective tissue disease, atherosclerosis, and embolism are usually performed.

A scan of the limb arteries (arteriogram) may be performed and is likely to show normal proximal vessels (these are the ones closest to the body) but multiple narrowings and occlusions distally (closest to the hands and feet). Many new bypass-vessels (corkscrew collaterals) often develop in an attempt to maintain blood supply.

How is thromboangiitis obliterans treated?

- It is essential to stop smoking.

- Keep the hands and feet warm and protected from trauma and infection.

Although no single treatment is considered definitive, consideration of an intravenous infusion of iloprost (a medication that helps relax blood vessel walls and reduce clotting), sympathectomy (ablation of the nerves causing blood vessel constriction), and removal of gangrenous tissue may be necessary.

There is little evidence that systemic steroids or anticoagulants are helpful.

Chapter 28

Peripheral Venous Disorders

Chapter Contents

Section 28.1

Chronic Venous Insufficiency

Venous insufficiency is a condition in which the veins have problems sending blood from the legs back to the heart.

Causes

Normally, valves in your deeper leg veins keep your blood flowing back toward the heart so it does not collect in one place. But the valves in varicose veins are either damaged or missing. This causes the veins to stay filled with blood, especially when you are standing.

Chronic venous insufficiency is a long-term condition. It occurs because a vein is partly blocked, or blood is leaking around the valves of the veins.

Risk factors for venous insufficiency include:

- age;
- being female (related to levels of the hormone progesterone);
- being tall;
- genetic factors;
- history of deep vein thrombosis in the legs;
- obesity;
- pregnancy;
- sitting or standing for a long time.

Symptoms

- Dull aching, heaviness, or cramping in legs
- Itching and tingling
- Pain that gets worse when standing

- Pain that gets better when legs are raised
- Swelling of the legs

  People with chronic venous insufficiency may also have:
- redness of the legs and ankles;
- skin color changes around the ankles;
- varicose veins on the surface (superficial);
- thickening and hardening of the skin on the legs and ankles (lipodermatosclerosis);
- ulcers on the legs and ankles.

Treatment

Take the following steps to help manage venous insufficiency:

- Use compression stockings to decrease swelling.
- Avoid long periods of sitting or standing. Even moving your legs slightly will help the blood in your veins return to your heart.
- Care for wounds if you have any open sores or infections.

Surgery (varicose vein stripping) or other treatments for varicose veins may be recommended if you have:

- leg pain, which may make your legs feel heavy or tired;
- skin sores caused by poor blood flow in the veins;
- thickening and hardening of the skin on the legs and ankles (lipodermatosclerosis).

Alternative Names

Chronic venous insufficiency

References

Bergan JJ, Schmid-Schonbein GW, Smith PD, et al. Chronic venous disease. *N Engl J Med.* 2006;355(5):488–98.

Freischlag JA, Heller JA. Venous disease. In: Townsend CM, Beauchamp RD, Evers BM, Mattox KL, eds. *Sabiston Textbook of Surgery. 19th ed.* Philadelphia, Pa: Saunders Elsevier; 2012: chap 65.

Section 28.2

Deep Vein Thrombosis

Excerpted from "Deep Vein Thrombosis," National Heart, Lung, and
Blood Institute, National Institutes of Health, October 28, 2011.

Deep vein thrombosis, or DVT, is a blood clot that forms in a vein deep
in the body. Blood clots occur when blood thickens and clumps together.

Most deep vein blood clots occur in the lower leg or thigh. They also
can occur in other parts of the body.

A blood clot in a deep vein can break off and travel through the
bloodstream. The loose clot is called an embolus. It can travel to an
artery in the lungs and block blood flow. This condition is called pulmonary embolism, or PE.

PE is a very serious condition. It can damage the lungs and other
organs in the body and cause death.

Blood clots in the thighs are more likely to break off and cause PE
than blood clots in the lower legs or other parts of the body. Blood clots
also can form in veins closer to the skin's surface. However, these clots
won't break off and cause PE.

What Causes Deep Vein Thrombosis?

Blood clots can form in your body's deep veins if any of the following is true:

- **A vein's inner lining is damaged:** Injuries caused by physical,
  chemical, or biological factors can damage the veins. Such factors
  include surgery, serious injuries, inflammation, and immune re-
  sponses.

- **Blood flow is sluggish or slow:** Lack of motion can cause sluggish or slow blood flow. This may occur after surgery, if you're ill
  and in bed for a long time, or if you're traveling for a long time.

- **Your blood is thicker or more likely to clot than normal:**
  Some inherited conditions (such as factor V Leiden) increase the
  risk of blood clotting. Hormone therapy or birth control pills also
  can increase the risk of clotting.

Who Is at Risk for Deep Vein Thrombosis?

The risk factors for deep vein thrombosis (DVT) include the following:

- A history of DVT.

- Conditions or factors that make your blood thicker or more likely to clot than normal. Some inherited blood disorders (such as factor V Leiden) will do this. Hormone therapy or birth control pills also increase the risk of clotting.

- Injury to a deep vein from surgery, a broken bone, or other trauma.

- Slow blood flow in a deep vein due to lack of movement. This may occur after surgery, if you're ill and in bed for a long time, or if you're traveling for a long time.

- Pregnancy and the first six weeks after giving birth.

- Recent or ongoing treatment for cancer.

- A central venous catheter. This is a tube placed in a vein to allow easy access to the bloodstream for medical treatment.

- Older age. Being older than sixty is a risk factor for DVT, although DVT can occur at any age.

- Overweight or obesity.

- Smoking.

Your risk for DVT increases if you have more than one of the risk factors listed above.

What Are the Signs and Symptoms of Deep Vein Thrombosis?

The signs and symptoms of deep vein thrombosis (DVT) might be related to DVT itself or pulmonary embolism (PE). See your doctor right away if you have signs or symptoms of either condition. Both DVT and PE can cause serious, possibly life-threatening problems if not treated.

Deep Vein Thrombosis

Only about half of the people who have DVT have signs and symptoms. These signs and symptoms occur in the leg affected by the deep vein clot. They include the following:

- Swelling of the leg or along a vein in the leg
- Pain or tenderness in the leg, which you may feel only when standing or walking
- Increased warmth in the area of the leg that's swollen or painful
- Red or discolored skin on the leg

Pulmonary Embolism

Some people aren't aware of a deep vein clot until they have signs and symptoms of PE. Signs and symptoms of PE include the following:

- Unexplained shortness of breath
- Pain with deep breathing
- Coughing up blood

Rapid breathing and a fast heart rate also may be signs of PE.

How Is Deep Vein Thrombosis Diagnosed?

Your doctor will diagnose deep vein thrombosis (DVT) based on your medical history, a physical exam, and test results. He or she will identify your risk factors and rule out other causes of your symptoms.

For some people, DVT might not be diagnosed until after they receive emergency treatment for pulmonary embolism (PE).

Medical History

To learn about your medical history, your doctor may ask about the following things:

- Your overall health
- Any prescription medicines you're taking
- Any recent surgeries or injuries you've had
- Whether you've been treated for cancer

Physical Exam

Your doctor will check your legs for signs of DVT, such as swelling or redness. He or she also will check your blood pressure and your heart and lungs.

Diagnostic Tests

Your doctor may recommend tests to find out whether you have DVT.

Common tests: The most common test for diagnosing deep vein blood clots is ultrasound. This test uses sound waves to create pictures of blood flowing through the arteries and veins in the affected leg.

Your doctor also may recommend a D-dimer test or venography.

A D-dimer test measures a substance in the blood that's released when a blood clot dissolves. If the test shows high levels of the substance, you may have a deep vein blood clot. If your test results are normal and you have few risk factors, DVT isn't likely.

Your doctor may suggest venography if an ultrasound doesn't provide a clear diagnosis. For venography, dye is injected into a vein in the affected leg. The dye makes the vein visible on an x-ray image. The x-ray will show whether blood flow is slow in the vein, which may suggest a blood clot.

Other tests: Other tests used to diagnose DVT include magnetic resonance imaging (MRI) and computed tomography, or CT, scanning. These tests create pictures of your organs and tissues.

You may need blood tests to check whether you have an inherited blood clotting disorder that can cause DVT. This may be the case if you have repeated blood clots that are not related to another cause. Blood clots in an unusual location (such as the liver, kidney, or brain) also may suggest an inherited clotting disorder.

If your doctor thinks that you have PE, he or she may recommend more tests, such as a lung ventilation perfusion scan (VQ scan). A lung VQ scan shows how well oxygen and blood are flowing to all areas of the lungs.

How Is Deep Vein Thrombosis Treated?

Doctors treat deep vein thrombosis (DVT) with medicines and other devices and therapies. The main goals of treating DVT are to do the following things:

- Stop the blood clot from getting bigger

- Prevent the blood clot from breaking off and moving to your lungs

- Reduce your chance of having another blood clot

Medicines

Your doctor may prescribe medicines to prevent or treat DVT.

Anticoagulants: Anticoagulants are the most common medicines for treating DVT. They're also known as blood thinners.

These medicines decrease your blood's ability to clot. They also stop existing blood clots from getting bigger. However, blood thinners can't break up blood clots that have already formed. (The body dissolves most blood clots with time.)

Blood thinners can be taken as a pill, an injection under the skin, or through a needle or tube inserted into a vein (called intravenous, or IV, injection).

Warfarin and heparin are two blood thinners used to treat DVT. Warfarin is given in pill form. (Coumadin® is a common brand name for warfarin.) Heparin is given as an injection or through an IV tube. There are different types of heparin. Your doctor will discuss the options with you.

Your doctor may treat you with both heparin and warfarin at the same time. Heparin acts quickly. Warfarin takes two to three days before it starts to work. Once the warfarin starts to work, the heparin is stopped.

Thrombin inhibitors: These medicines interfere with the blood clotting process. They're used to treat blood clots in patients who can't take heparin.

Thrombolytics: Doctors prescribe these medicines to quickly dissolve large blood clots that cause severe symptoms. Because thrombolytics can cause sudden bleeding, they're used only in life-threatening situations.

Other Types of Treatment

Vena cava filter: If you can't take blood thinners or they're not working well, your doctor may recommend a vena cava filter.

The filter is inserted inside a large vein called the vena cava. The filter catches blood clots before they travel to the lungs, which prevents pulmonary embolism. However, the filter doesn't stop new blood clots from forming.

Graduated compression stockings: Graduated compression stockings can reduce leg swelling caused by a blood clot. These stockings are worn on the legs from the arch of the foot to just above or below the knee.

Compression stockings are tight at the ankle and become looser as they go up the leg. This creates gentle pressure up the leg. The pressure keeps blood from pooling and clotting.

There are three types of compression stockings. One type is support pantyhose, which offer the least amount of pressure.

The second type is over-the-counter compression hose. These stockings give a little more pressure than support pantyhose. Over-the-counter compression hose are sold in medical supply stores and pharmacies.

Prescription-strength compression hose offer the greatest amount of pressure. They also are sold in medical supply stores and pharmacies. However, a specially trained person needs to fit you for these stockings.

Talk with your doctor about how long you should wear compression stockings.

Section 28.3

Varicose Veins and Spider Veins

"Varicose Veins and Spider Veins Fact Sheet," U.S. Department of Health and Human Services, Office on Women's Health, June 2, 2010.

What are varicose veins and spider veins?

Varicose veins are enlarged veins that can be blue, red, or flesh-colored. They often look like cords and appear twisted and bulging. They can be swollen and raised above the surface of the skin. Varicose veins are often found on the thighs, backs of the calves, or the inside of the leg. During pregnancy, varicose veins can form around the vagina and buttocks.

Spider veins are like varicose veins but smaller. They also are closer to the surface of the skin than varicose veins. Often, they are red or blue. They can look like tree branches or spider webs with their short, jagged lines. They can be found on the legs and face and can cover either a very small or very large area of skin.

What causes varicose veins and spider veins?

Varicose veins can be caused by weak or damaged valves in the veins. The heart pumps blood filled with oxygen and nutrients to the whole body through the arteries. Veins then carry the blood from the body back to the heart. As your leg muscles squeeze, they push blood back to the heart from your lower body against the flow of gravity. Veins have valves that act as one-way flaps to prevent blood from flowing backwards as it moves up your legs. If the valves become weak, blood can leak back into the veins and collect there. (This problem is called venous insufficiency.) When backed-up blood makes the veins bigger, they can become varicose.

Spider veins can be caused by the backup of blood. They can also be caused by hormone changes, exposure to the sun, and injuries.

How common are abnormal leg veins?

About 50 to 55 percent of women and 40 to 45 percent of men in the United States suffer from some type of vein problem. Varicose veins affect half of people fifty years old and older.

What factors increase my risk of varicose veins and spider veins?

Many factors increase a person's chances of developing varicose or spider veins. These include the following:

- **Increasing age:** As you get older, the valves in your veins may weaken and not work as well.

- **Medical history:** Being born with weak vein valves increases your risk. Having family members with vein problems also increases your risk. About half of all people who have varicose veins have a family member who has them too.

- **Hormonal changes:** These occur during puberty, pregnancy, and menopause. Taking birth control pills and other medicines containing estrogen and progesterone also may contribute to the forming of varicose or spider veins.

- **Pregnancy:** During pregnancy, there is a huge increase in the amount of blood in the body. This can cause veins to enlarge. The growing uterus also puts pressure on the veins. Varicose veins usually improve within three months after delivery. More varicose veins and spider veins usually appear with each additional pregnancy.

- **Obesity:** Being overweight or obese can put extra pressure on your veins. This can lead to varicose veins.

- **Lack of movement:** Sitting or standing for a long time may force your veins to work harder to pump blood to your heart. This may be a bigger problem if you sit with your legs bent or crossed.

- **Sun exposure:** This can cause spider veins on the cheeks or nose of a fair-skinned person.

Why do varicose veins and spider veins usually appear in the legs?

Most varicose and spider veins appear in the legs due to the pressure of body weight, force of gravity, and task of carrying blood from the bottom of the body up to the heart.

Compared with other veins in the body, leg veins have the toughest job of carrying blood back to the heart. They endure the most pressure. This pressure can be stronger than the one-way valves in the veins.

What are the signs of varicose veins?

Varicose veins can often be seen on the skin. Some other common symptoms of varicose veins in the legs include the following:

- Aching pain that may get worse after sitting or standing for a long time
- Throbbing or cramping
- Heaviness
- Swelling
- Rash that's itchy or irritated
- Darkening of the skin (in severe cases)
- Restless legs

Are varicose veins and spider veins dangerous?

Spider veins rarely are a serious health problem, but they can cause uncomfortable feelings in the legs. If there are symptoms from spider veins, most often they will be itching or burning. Less often, spider veins can be a sign of blood backup deeper inside that you can't see on the skin. If so, you could have the same symptoms you would have with varicose veins.

Varicose veins may not cause any problems, or they may cause aching pain, throbbing, and discomfort. In some cases, varicose veins can lead to more serious health problems. These include the following:

- Sores or skin ulcers due to chronic (long-term) backing up of blood. These sores or ulcers are painful and hard to heal.

Sometimes they cannot heal until the backward blood flow in the vein is repaired.

- Bleeding. The skin over the veins becomes thin and easily injured. When an injury occurs, there can be significant blood loss.

- Superficial thrombophlebitis, which is a blood clot that forms in a vein just below the skin. Symptoms include skin redness; a firm, tender, warm vein; and sometimes pain and swelling.

- Deep vein thrombosis, which is a blood clot in a deeper vein. It can cause a "pulling" feeling in the calf, pain, warmth, redness, and swelling. However, sometimes it causes no significant symptoms. If the blood clot travels to the lungs, it can be fatal.

Should I see a doctor about varicose veins?

You should see a doctor about varicose veins if any of the following are true:

- The vein has become swollen, red, or very tender or warm to the touch

- There are sores or a rash on the leg or near the ankle

- The skin on the ankle and calf becomes thick and changes color

- One of the varicose veins begins to bleed

- Your leg symptoms are interfering with daily activities

- The appearance of the veins is causing you distress

If you're having pain, even if it's just a dull ache, don't hesitate to get help. Also, even if you don't need to see a doctor about your varicose veins, you should take steps to keep them from getting worse.

How are varicose veins diagnosed?

Your doctor may diagnose your varicose veins based on a physical exam. Your doctor will look at your legs while you're standing or sitting with your legs dangling. He or she may ask you about your symptoms, including any pain you're having. Sometimes, you may have other tests to find out the extent of the problem and to rule out other disorders.

You might have an ultrasound, which is used to see the veins' structure, check the blood flow in your veins, and look for blood clots. This test uses sound waves to create pictures of structures in your body.

Although less likely, you might have a venogram. This test can be used to get a more detailed look at blood flow through your veins.

If you seek help for your varicose veins, there are several types of doctors you can see, including the following:

- A phlebologist, which is a vein specialist

- A vascular medicine doctor, who focuses on the blood system

- A vascular surgeon, who can perform surgery and do other procedures

- An interventional radiologist, who specializes in using imaging tools to see inside the body and do treatments with little or no cutting

- A dermatologist, who specializes in skin conditions

Each of these specialists do some or all of the procedures for treating varicose veins. You might start out by asking your regular doctor which specialist he or she recommends. You also might check with your insurance plan to see if it would pay for a particular provider or procedure.

How are varicose and spider veins treated?

Varicose veins are treated with lifestyle changes and medical treatments. These can do the following things:

- Relieve symptoms

- Prevent complications

- Improve appearance

Your doctor may recommend lifestyle changes if your varicose veins don't cause many symptoms. If symptoms are more severe, your doctor may recommend medical treatments. Some treatment options are listed here.

Compression stockings: Compression stockings put helpful pressure on your veins.

There are 3 kinds of compression stockings:

- Support pantyhose, which offer the least amount of pressure. These also often are not "gradient" or "graduated." That means they provide pressure all over instead of where it is needed most.

- Over-the-counter gradient compression hose, which give a little more pressure. They are sold in medical supply and drugstores.

- Prescription-strength gradient compression hose, which offer the greatest amount of pressure. They are sold in medical supply and drugstores. You need to be fitted for them by someone who has been trained to do this.

Sclerotherapy: Sclerotherapy is the most common treatment for both spider veins and varicose veins. The doctor uses a needle to inject a liquid chemical into the vein. The chemical causes the vein walls to swell, stick together, and seal shut. This stops the flow of blood, and the vein turns into scar tissue. In a few weeks, the vein should fade. This treatment does not require anesthesia and can be done in your doctor's office. You can return to normal activity right after treatment.

The same vein may need to be treated more than once. Treatments are usually done every four to six weeks. You may be asked to wear gradient compression stockings after sclerotherapy to help with healing and decrease swelling. This treatment is very effective when done correctly.

Possible side effects include the following:

- Stinging, red and raised patches of skin, or bruises where the injection was made. These usually go away shortly after treatment.

- Spots, brown lines, or groups of fine red blood vessels around the treated vein. These also usually go away shortly after treatment.

- Lumps of blood that get trapped in veins and cause inflammation. This is not dangerous. You can relieve swelling by applying heat and taking aspirin. Your doctor can drain the trapped blood with a small pinprick at a follow-up visit.

There is a type of sclerotherapy called ultrasound-guided sclerotherapy (or echo-sclerotherapy). This type of sclerotherapy uses ultrasound imaging to guide the needle. It can be useful in treating veins that cannot be seen on the skin's surface. It may be used after surgery or endovenous techniques if the varicose veins return. This procedure can be done in a doctor's office. Possible side effects include skin sores, swelling, injection into an artery by mistake, or deep vein thrombosis (a potentially dangerous blood clot).

Surface laser treatments: In some cases, laser treatments can effectively treat spider veins and smaller varicose veins. This technique sends very strong bursts of light through the skin onto the vein. This makes the vein slowly fade and disappear. Not all skin types and colors can be safely treated with lasers.

No needles or incisions are used, but the heat from the laser can be quite painful. Cooling helps reduce the pain. Laser treatments last for fifteen to twenty minutes. Generally, two to five treatments are needed to remove spider veins in the legs. Laser therapy usually isn't effective for varicose veins larger than three millimeters (about a tenth of an inch). You can return to normal activity right after treatment.

Possible side effects of lasers include the following:

- Redness or swelling of the skin right after the treatment that disappears within a few days

- Discolored skin that will disappear within one to two months

- Burns and scars from poorly performed laser surgery, though this is rare

Endovenous techniques (radiofrequency and laser): These methods for treating the deeper veins of the legs, called the saphenous veins, have replaced surgery for most patients with severe varicose veins. These techniques can be done in a doctor's office.

The doctor puts a very small tube, called a catheter, into the vein. A small probe is placed through the tube. A device at the tip of the probe heats up the inside of the vein and closes it off. The device can use radiofrequency or laser energy to seal the vein. The procedure can be done using just local anesthesia. You might have slight bruising after treatment.

Healthy veins around the closed vein take over the normal flow of blood. The symptoms from the varicose vein improve. Usually, veins on the surface of the skin that are connected to the treated varicose vein will also shrink after treatment. If they don't, these connected veins can be treated with sclerotherapy or other techniques.

Surgery: Surgery is used mostly to treat very large varicose veins. Types of surgery for varicose veins include the following:

- *Surgical ligation and stripping:* With this treatment, problem veins are tied shut and completely removed from the leg through small cuts in the skin. Removing the veins does not affect the circulation of blood in the leg. Veins deeper in the leg take care of the larger volumes of blood. This surgery requires general anesthesia and must be done in an operating room. It takes between one and four weeks to recover from the surgery. This surgery is generally safe. Pain in the leg is the most common side effect. Other possible problems include the following:

- A risk of heart and breathing problems from anesthesia.

- Bleeding and congestion of blood. However, the collected blood usually settles on its own and does not require any further treatment.

- Wound infection, inflammation, swelling, and redness.

- Permanent scars.

- Damage of nerve tissue around the treated vein. It's hard to avoid harming small nerve branches when veins are removed. This damage can cause numbness, burning, or a change in feeling around the scar.

- A deep vein blood clot. These clots can travel to the lungs and heart. The medicine heparin may be used to reduce the chance of these dangerous blood clots. But, heparin also can increase the normal amount of bleeding and bruising after surgery.

- *PIN stripping:* In this treatment, an instrument called a PIN stripper is inserted into a vein. The tip of the PIN stripper is sewn to the end of the vein, and when it is removed, the vein is pulled out. This procedure can be done in an operating room or an outpatient center. General or local anesthesia can be used.

- *Ambulatory phlebectomy:* With ambulatory phlebectomy, tiny cuts are made in the skin, and hooks are used to pull the vein out of the leg. Only the parts of your leg that are being pricked will be numbed with anesthesia. The vein is usually removed in one treatment. Very large varicose veins can be removed with this treatment while leaving only very small scars. Patients can return to normal activity the day after treatment. Possible side effects of the treatment include slight bruising and temporary numbness.

How can I prevent varicose veins and spider veins?

Not all varicose and spider veins can be prevented. But there are some steps you can take to reduce your chances of getting new varicose and spider veins. These same things can help ease discomfort from the ones you already have:

- Wear sunscreen to protect your skin from the sun and to limit spider veins on the face.

- Exercise regularly to improve your leg strength, circulation, and vein strength. Focus on exercises that work your legs, such as walking or running.

- Control your weight to avoid placing too much pressure on your legs.

- Don't cross your legs for long times when sitting. It's possible to injure your legs that way, and even a minor injury can increase the risk of varicose veins.

- Elevate your legs when resting as much as possible.

- Don't stand or sit for long periods of time. If you must stand for a long time, shift your weight from one leg to the other every few minutes. If you must sit for long periods of time, stand up and move around or take a short walk every thirty minutes.

- Wear elastic support stockings and avoid tight clothing that constricts your waist, groin, or legs.

- Avoid wearing high heels for long periods of time. Lower-heeled shoes can help tone your calf muscles to help blood move through your veins.

- Eat a low-salt diet rich in high-fiber foods. Eating fiber reduces the chances of constipation, which can contribute to varicose veins. High-fiber foods include fresh fruits and vegetables and whole grains, like bran. Eating less salt can help with the swelling that comes with varicose veins.

Can varicose and spider veins return even after treatment?

Current treatments for varicose veins and spider veins have very high success rates compared to traditional surgical treatments. Over a period of years, however, more abnormal veins can develop because there is no cure for weak vein valves. Ultrasound can be used to keep track of how badly the valves are leaking (venous insufficiency). Ongoing treatment can help keep this problem under control.

The single most important thing you can do to slow down the development of new varicose veins is to wear gradient compression support stockings as much as possible during the day.

Chapter 29

Vasculitis

Vasculitis refers to inflammation of the blood vessels. There are many types of vasculitis. Most types of vasculitis are rare, and the causes are generally not known. Vasculitis can affect persons of both sexes and a broad range of ages.

Fast Facts

- Vasculitis is a term for a group of rare diseases that have in common inflammation of blood vessels.

- There are many types of vasculitis, and they may vary greatly in symptoms, severity, and duration.

- Vasculitis can range from mild to life threatening.

- Early detection and treatment of severe vasculitis can prevent permanent damage.

- Glucocorticoids (prednisone and others) are the main treatment.

- Patients also may be prescribed other medicines that suppress the immune system. These can help severe disease or let patients take lower doses of glucocorticoids.

What Is Vasculitis?

Vasculitis refers to inflammation of the blood vessels. These vessels include arteries and veins.

Vasculitis can result in poor blood flow to tissues throughout the body, such as the lungs, nerves, and skin. Thus, vasculitis has a wide range of signs and symptoms (what you see and feel), such as:

- shortness of breath and cough;

- numbness or weakness in a hand or foot;

- red spots on the skin ("purpura"), lumps ("nodules"), or sores ("ulcers").

On the other hand, vasculitis of the kidneys may produce no symptoms at first but is still a serious problem.

Vasculitis can be mild or disabling, or even lead to death. Patients can have one episode of vasculitis or have repeated episodes over several years. Most types of vasculitis are rare.

What Causes Vasculitis?

We do not know what causes most types of vasculitis. Genetic factors (different genes) appear be somewhat important in the disease. Vasculitis is thought to be an autoimmune disease, which means the body comes under attack by its own immune system. In vasculitis, the immune system attacks blood vessels.

Some cases of vasculitis are caused by reactions to medicines. Also, some chronic (long-term) infections, including with hepatitis C or hepatitis B virus, can cause vasculitis.

Vasculitis can be a part of other rheumatic diseases, mainly including systemic lupus erythematosus, rheumatoid arthritis, and Sjögren syndrome. Most patients with vasculitis have none of these diseases.

Who Gets Vasculitis?

Vasculitis affects persons of both sexes and all ages. A few forms of vasculitis affect certain groups of people. For instance, Kawasaki disease occurs only in children. IgA vasculitis (Henoch-Schönlein) is much more common in children than adults. On the other hand, giant cell arteritis occurs only in adults over fifty years old.

How Is Vasculitis Diagnosed?

Physicians suspect vasculitis when a patient has symptoms and abnormal results of the physical exam, lab tests, or both, and there is no other clear cause.

The most common tests are:

- **Biopsy:** Surgical removal of a small piece of tissue for inspection under a microscope.

- **Angiography:** A type of x-ray to look for abnormalities of blood vessels.

- **Blood tests.**

For most patients, doctors can detect the type of vasculitis based on the size of the affected blood vessels (see Table 29.1) and the organs involved. To find small-vessel vasculitis, doctors most often do a biopsy, such as of the skin or a kidney. Detection of medium-vessel vasculitis happens by either biopsy (for instance, of skin, nerve, or brain) or angiography. Angiography also is the test that often finds large-vessel vasculitis. Detecting giant cell arteritis often involves a biopsy of an artery in the scalp.

A few forms of vasculitis, such as Behçet disease and Kawasaki disease, are usually detected on the basis of a collection of clinical findings rather than biopsy or angiography.

Some blood tests are so suggestive of a certain type of vasculitis that a positive (abnormal) test can be enough evidence to help doctors make the diagnosis. The most useful of these tests is for "antineutrophil cytoplasmic antibodies"—often referred to as ANCA. A positive ANCA test can help detect these types of vasculitis: granulomatosis with polyangiitis (Wegener), microscopic polyangiitis or eosinophilic granulomatosis with polyangiitis (Churg-Strauss). Other lab tests can show damage to organs, but the tests are not enough to prove vasculitis.

How Is Vasculitis Treated?

Glucocorticoids: Glucocorticoids (prednisone, prednisolone, or others), often referred to as "steroids," are an important part of treating most forms of vasculitis. The dose and length of treatment depend on how bad the disease is and how long the patient has had it. These drugs help reduce inflammation but can have long-term side effects.

Other drugs: Doctors sometimes prescribe immune-suppressing drugs because their side effects may be less serious than those of glucocorticoids. This is called "steroid-sparing" treatment. Cyclophosphamide is the strongest of these drugs, and doctors may prescribe it when severe disease endangers vital organs.

For less serious vasculitis, patients may receive methotrexate, azathioprine, or other immune-suppressing drugs. Doctors often prescribe these drugs to treat other rheumatic diseases, but they are useful for vasculitis, too.

Table 29.1. Types of Vasculitis

Largest arteries: aorta and major branches	Giant cell arteritis
	Takayasu arteritis
	Aortitis in Cogan syndrome
	Aortitis in spondyloarthropathies
	Isolated aortitis
Medium-sized arteries	Kawasaki disease
	Polyarteritis nodosa
Small and medium-sized arteries	ANCA-associated vasculitis
	Granulomatosis with polyangiitis (former name: Wegener granulomatosis)
	Microscopic polyangiitis
	Eosinophilic granulomatosis with polyangiitis (Churg-Strauss)
	Primary angiitis of the central nervous system
Small arteries	IgA Vasculitis (Henoch-Schönlein)
	Vasculitis related to rheumatoid arthritis, systemic lupus erythematosus and Sjögren syndrome
	Cryoglobulinemic vasculitis
	Anti-GBM disease (Goodpasture)
	Drug-induced vasculitis
Arteries and veins of various sizes	Behçet disease
	Relapsing polychondritis

Notes: Abbreviations: ANCA, antineutrophil cytoplasmic antibodies; GBM, glomerular basement membrane.

This list is not complete. It does not include some forms of vasculitis related to infection or diseases such as cancer.

Newer drugs designed to treat other autoimmune and inflammatory diseases may also help vasculitis. Researchers found that one of these drugs, rituximab, effectively treats severe cases of certain forms of vasculitis. These include granulomatosis with polyangiitis, microscopic polyangiitis, and cryoglobulinemic vasculitis. Some patients with the most severe cases of these diseases may receive plasma exchange ("plasmapheresis") or intravenous immunoglobulin (often called "IVIg").

Surgery. Damage from severe vasculitis sometimes requires surgery. This may involve vascular bypass grafting (a surgery to redirect blood flow around a blockage in a blood vessel). Depending on where the damage is, other possible operations are sinus surgery or a kidney transplant.

Living with Vasculitis

Vasculitis can be short term or lifelong. Doctors often focus, with good reason, on preventing permanent damage to vital organs (such as the lungs, kidneys, and brain) and the nerves. It is crucial, of course, to prevent death and long-term disability from vasculitis. Yet, other issues often trouble patients. These include fatigue (feeling very tired), pain, arthritis, nose and sinus problems, and many other problems.

Side effects from medications, especially glucocorticoids, also can be troubling. Patients taking immunosuppressants are at risk of infections. Follow your doctor's advice on how to reduce your infection risk.

Fortunately, with current treatments, the outcome for patients with vasculitis is often good.

Points to Remember

- Vasculitic diseases are inflammatory health problems that often need treatment with immunosuppressive drugs. The most common medication used is glucocorticoids.

- Though there are many types of vasculitis, most are rare.

- Detection of vasculitis most often requires biopsy of affected tissue or angiography.

Part Four

Cardiovascular Disorders in Specific Populations

Chapter 30

Cardiovascular Disease in Children

Chapter Contents

Section 30.1

Youth and Cardiovascular Disease: Some Statistics

Excerpted from "Youth and Cardiovascular Diseases," reprinted with permission from www.heart.org. © 2013 American Heart Association, Inc. All rights reserved.

Out-of-Hospital Cardiac Arrest

- Survival to hospital discharge among children with emergency medical service (EMS)–treated, nontraumatic cardiac arrest is 7.8 percent and of bystander-witnessed ventricular fibrillation is 57.1 percent.

- Most sudden deaths in athletes were attributable to cardiovascular disease, or CVD (56 percent). Of the cardiovascular deaths that occurred, 29 percent occurred in blacks, 54 percent in high school students, and 82 percent with physical exertion during competition/training, and only 11 percent occurred in females, although this proportion has increased over time.

- A longitudinal study of students seventeen to twenty-four years of age participating in National Collegiate Athletic Association sports showed that the incidence of nontraumatic out-of-hospital cardiac arrest was one per 22,903 athlete participant years. The incidence of cardiac arrest tended to be higher among blacks than whites and among men than women.

Stroke in Children

- The incidence of stroke in children has been stable over the past ten years.

- The prevalence of perinatal strokes is 29 per 100,000 live births, or 1 per 3,500 live births.

- Boys have a 1.28-fold higher risk of stroke and a higher case-fatality rate for ischemic stroke than girls.

- Compared with the stroke risk of white children, black children have a two-fold higher risk, Hispanics have a lower relative risk of 0.76, and Asians have a similar risk.

- From 1979 to 1998 in the United States, childhood mortality resulting from stroke declined by 58 percent overall, with reductions in all major subtypes.

- Although children with sickle cell disease and congenital heart defects are at high risk for ischemic stroke, the most common cause in a previously healthy child is a cerebral arteriopathy, or disease of arteries in the brain, found in more than half of all cases.

High Blood Pressure (HBP)

- Blood pressure (BP), pre–high blood pressure (pre-HBP) and HBP trends in children and adolescents ages eight to seventeen, were downward from 1963 to 1988 and upward thereafter.

- Pre-HBP and HBP increased 2.3 percent and 1 percent, respectively, between 1988 and 1999.

- Blood pressure and HBP reversed their downward trends ten years after the increase in the prevalence of obesity.

- An ethnic and gender gap appeared in 1988 for pre-HBP and 1999 for HBP; non-Hispanic blacks and Mexican-Americans had a greater prevalence of HBP and pre-HBP than non-Hispanic whites, and males greater than females.

Congenital Cardiovascular Defects

- An estimated minimum of thirty-two thousand infants are expected to be affected each year in the United States. Of these, an approximate 25 percent, or 2.4 per 1,000 live births, require invasive treatment in the first year of life.

- The most commonly reported incidence of congenital heart defects in the United States is between 4 and 10 per 1,000, clustering around 8 per 1,000 live births.

- Congenital cardiovascular defects are the most common cause of infant death resulting from birth defects; 27 percent of infants who die of a birth defect have a heart defect.

- The 2009 death rate attributable to congenital cardiovascular defects was 1.0. Death rates were 1.1 for white males, 1.4 for black males, 0.9 for white females, and 1.2 for black females. Infant mortality rates (less than one year of age) were 31.4 for white infants and 42.2 for black infants.

- Between 1997 and 2004, hospitalization rates increased by 28.5 percent for cardiac and circulatory congenital anomalies.

- In 2009, fifty-two thousand U.S. adults and children (twenty-five thousand males; twenty-seven thousand females) diagnosed with congenital heart defects were discharged from short-stay hospitals.

Cardiomyopathy

- Since 1996, the National Heart, Lung, and Blood Institute (NHLBI)–sponsored Pediatric Cardiomyopathy Registry has collected data on all children with newly diagnosed cardiomyopathy in New England and the Central Southwest (Texas, Oklahoma, and Arkansas):

  - The overall incidence of cardiomyopathy is 1.13 cases per 100,000 in children less than eighteen years of age.

  - In children less than one year of age, the incidence is 8.34, and in children one to eighteen years of age, it is 0.70 per 100,000.

  - The annual incidence is lower in white than in black children, higher in boys than in girls, and higher in New England (1.44 per 100,000) than in the Central Southwest (0.98 per 100,000).

- Hypertrophic cardiomyopathy (HCM) is the most common inherited heart defect, occurring in 1 of 500 individuals. In the United States, about 500,000 people have HCM, yet most are unaware of it.

Section 30.2

Signs and Symptoms of Heart Defects in Children

Parents should be alert to the following symptoms in infancy:

- Tires easily during feeding (i.e., falls asleep before feeding finishes)
- Sweating around the head, especially during feeding
- Fast breathing when at rest or sleeping
- Pale or bluish skin color
- Poor weight gain
- Sleeps a lot—not playful or curious for any length of time
- Puffy face, hands, and/or feet
- Often irritable, difficult to console

Some children with congenital heart defects (CHDs) may not have any symptoms until later in childhood. Things to look for include:

- gets out of breath during play;
- difficulty "keeping up" with playmates;
- tires easily/sleeps a lot;
- change in color during active play or sports (looks pale or has a bluish tint around mouth and nose);
- frequent colds and respiratory illnesses;
- slow growth and weight gain/poor appetite;
- complains of chest pain and/or heart pounding.

If your child has two or more of these symptoms, talk to your pediatrician about a referral to a pediatric cardiologist.

Section 30.3

Basic Facts about Congenital Heart Defects

About 35,000 infants (1 out of every 125) are born with heart defects each year in the United States.[1] The defect may be so slight that the baby appears healthy for many years after birth, or so severe that his life is in immediate danger.

Heart defects are among the most common birth defects and are the leading cause of birth defect-related deaths.[2] However, advances in diagnosis and surgical treatment have led to dramatic increases in survival for children with serious heart defects. In the United States, about 1.4 million children and adults live with congenital heart defects today.[3] Almost all are able to lead active, productive lives.[1]

What is a congenital heart defect?

A congenital heart defect is an abnormality in any part of the heart that is present at birth. Heart defects originate in the early weeks of pregnancy when the heart is forming.

How does the heart work?

The heart is a muscle that pumps blood to the body. It is divided into four hollow parts called chambers. Two chambers are located on the right side of the heart, and two are on the left. Within the heart are four valves (one-way openings) that let the blood go forward and keep it from going back. Blood goes from the heart to the lungs where it picks up oxygen. From the lungs, the blood carrying oxygen, which appears bright red, goes back to the heart. The heart then pumps the oxygen-rich blood through the body by way of arteries. As the oxygen is used up by the body's tissues and organs, the blood becomes dark and returns by way of veins to the heart, where the process starts over again.

How do heart defects affect a child?

Some babies and children with heart defects experience no symptoms. The heart defect may be diagnosed if the health care provider hears an abnormal sound, called a murmur. Children with normal hearts also can have heart murmurs, called innocent or functional murmurs. A provider may suggest tests to rule out a heart defect.

Certain heart defects can cause congestive heart failure. In this condition, the heart can't pump adequate blood to the lungs or other parts of the body. It can lead to fluid buildup in the heart, lungs, and other parts of the body. An affected child may experience a rapid heartbeat and breathing difficulties, especially during exercise. Infants may experience these difficulties during feeding, sometimes resulting in poor weight gain. Affected infants and children also may have swelling of the legs or abdomen or around the eyes.

Some heart defects result in a pale grayish or bluish coloring of the skin called cyanosis. This usually appears soon after birth or during infancy and should be evaluated immediately by a health care provider. On occasion, cyanosis may be delayed until later in childhood. Cyanosis is a sign of defects that prevent the blood from getting enough oxygen. Children with cyanosis may tire easily. Symptoms, such as shortness of breath and fainting, often worsen when the child exerts himself. Some youngsters may squat frequently to ease their shortness of breath.

What tests are used to diagnose heart defects?

Babies and children who are suspected of having a heart defect are usually referred to a pediatric cardiologist (children's heart disease specialist). This doctor can do a physical examination and often recommends one or more of the following tests:

- Chest x-ray

- Electrocardiogram, a test that records heart rate patterns

- Echocardiogram, a special form of ultrasound that uses sound waves to take pictures of the heart

All of these tests are painless and noninvasive (nothing enters the child's body). Some children with heart disease also may need to undergo a procedure called cardiac catheterization. In this procedure, a thin, flexible tube is inserted into the heart after the child is given medications to make him sleepy. This test provides detailed information about the heart and how it is working.

What causes congenital heart defects?

In most cases, scientists do not know what makes a baby's heart develop abnormally. Genetic and environmental factors appear to play roles.

Scientists are making progress in understanding the genetics of heart defects. Since the 1990s, they have identified about ten gene mutations (changes) that can cause isolated (not accompanied by other birth defects) heart defects.[3] For example, a March of Dimes grantee identified a gene that can cause a heart defect called an atrial septal defect (a hole between the upper chambers of the heart), and one that may contribute to hypoplastic left heart syndrome (underdevelopment of the heart's main pumping chamber).[4, 5]

Environmental factors can contribute to congenital heart defects. Women who contract rubella (German measles) during the first three months of pregnancy have a high risk of having a baby with a heart defect. Other viral infections, such as the flu, also may contribute, as may exposure to certain industrial chemicals (solvents).[2] Some studies suggest that drinking alcohol or using cocaine in pregnancy may increase the risk of heart defects.[2]

Certain medications increase the risk. These include:[2]

- the acne medication isotretinoin (Accutane and other brand names);

- thalidomide (approved only for a rare, severe skin disorder, but sometimes used for other conditions);

- certain anti-seizure medications.

Some studies suggest that first-trimester use of trimethoprim-sulfonamide (a combination of antibiotics sometimes used to treat urinary tract infections) may increase the risk of heart defects.[2]

Certain chronic illnesses in the mother, such as diabetes, may contribute to heart defects.[2] However, women with diabetes can reduce their risk by making sure their blood sugar levels are well controlled before becoming pregnant.

Heart defects can be part of a wider pattern of birth defects. For example, at least 30 percent of children with chromosomal abnormalities, such as Down syndrome (intellectual disabilities and physical birth defects) and Turner syndrome (short stature and lack of sexual development), have heart defects.[3] Children with Down syndrome, Turner syndrome, and certain other chromosomal abnormalities should be routinely evaluated for heart defects.

Heart defects also are common in children with a variety of inherited disorders, including Noonan syndrome (short stature, learning disabilities), velocardiofacial syndrome (craniofacial defects and immune deficiencies), Holt-Oram syndrome (limb defects), and Alagille syndrome (liver, skeletal, and eye defects).[3]

What are some of the most common heart defects, and how are they treated?

Patent ductus arteriosus (PDA): Before birth, a large artery (ductus arteriosus) lets the blood bypass the lungs because the fetus gets its oxygen through the placenta. The ductus normally closes soon after birth so that blood can travel to the lungs and pick up oxygen. If it doesn't close, the baby may develop heart failure. This problem occurs most frequently in premature babies. Treatment with medicine during the early days of life often can close the ductus. If that doesn't work, surgery is needed.

Septal defect: This is a hole in the wall (septum) that divides the right and left sides of the heart. A hole in the wall between the heart's two upper chambers is called an atrial septal defect, while a hole between the lower chambers is called a ventricular septal defect. These defects can cause the blood to circulate improperly, so the heart has to work harder. Some atrial septal defects can be repaired without surgery by inserting a thin, flexible tube into the heart and then releasing a device that plugs the hole. A surgeon also can close an atrial or ventricular septal defect by sewing or patching the hole. Small holes may heal by themselves or not need repair at all.

Coarctation of the aorta: Part of the aorta, the large artery that sends blood from the heart to the rest of the body, may be too narrow for the blood to flow evenly. A surgeon can cut away the narrow part and sew the open ends together, replace the constricted section with man-made material, or patch it with part of a blood vessel taken from elsewhere in the body. Sometimes, this narrowed area can be widened by inflating a balloon on the tip of a catheter (tube) inserted through an artery.

Heart valve abnormalities: Some babies are born with heart valves that do not close normally or are narrowed or blocked, so blood can't flow smoothly. Surgeons usually can repair the valves or replace them with man-made ones. Balloons on catheters also are frequently used to fix faulty valves.

Tetralogy of Fallot: This combination of four heart defects keeps some blood from getting to the lungs. As a result, the blood that is pumped to the body may not have enough oxygen. Affected babies

319

have episodes of cyanosis and may grow poorly. This defect is usually surgically repaired in the early months of life.

Transposition of the great arteries: Transposition occurs when the positions of the two major arteries leaving the heart are reversed, so that each arises from the wrong pumping chamber. Affected newborns suffer from severe cyanosis due to a lack of oxygen in the blood. Recent surgical advances make it possible to correct this serious defect in the newborn period.

Hypoplastic left heart syndrome: This combination of defects results in a left ventricle (the heart's main pumping chamber) that is too small to support life. Without treatment, this defect is usually fatal in the first few weeks of life. However, over the last twenty-five years, survival rates have dramatically improved with new surgical procedures and, less frequently, heart transplants.[6]

At what age do children have surgery to repair heart defects?

Many children who require surgical repair of heart defects now undergo surgery in the first months of life. Until recently, it was often necessary to make temporary repairs and postpone corrective surgery until later in childhood. Now, early corrective surgery often prevents development of additional complications and allows the child to live a normal life.

Following surgery, children should have periodic heart checkups with a cardiologist. Children and adults with certain heart defects, even after surgical repair, remain at increased risk of infection involving the heart and its valves. Parents of children with heart defects and adults with repaired heart defects should discuss with their provider whether they need to take antibiotics before dental visits and other procedures to prevent these infections. Antibiotic treatment is recommended only for those considered at highest risk for infection, including those with man-made heart valves.[7]

Is there a prenatal test for congenital heart defects?

Echocardiography can be used before birth to accurately identify many heart defects. If this test shows that a fetus's heart is beating too fast or too slowly (called an arrhythmia), the mother can be treated with medications that may restore a normal heart rhythm in the fetus. This treatment often prevents fetal heart failure. In other cases, where the heart defect can't be treated before birth, parents and providers can plan the delivery so that the baby can receive necessary evaluation and treatment soon after birth.

Can congenital heart defects be prevented?

Most congenital heart defects cannot be prevented. However, there are some steps a woman can take before and during pregnancy that may help reduce the risk of having a baby with a heart defect:

- Take a multivitamin containing 400 micrograms of folic acid daily, starting before pregnancy. This helps to prevent serious birth defects of the brain and spinal cord and may also help prevent heart defects.

- Go for a preconception visit with her health care provider. At this visit, a woman should be tested for immunity to rubella and be vaccinated if she is not immune. Women with chronic health conditions, such as diabetes and phenylketonuria (PKU), should discuss adjusting their medications and/or eating habits to keep these conditions under control before and during pregnancy.

- Discuss all medications with their provider, even over-the-counter or herbal medicines.

- Avoid people who have the flu or other illnesses with fever.

- Avoid exposure to organic solvents, used in products such as paints, varnishes, and degreasing/cleaning agents.

Are heart defects likely to recur in another pregnancy?

Parents who have already had a child with a heart defect do have an increased risk of having other affected children, often with the same heart defect. In many cases, the risk is low. Some heart defects have about a 2 to 3 percent chance of happening again.[8] However, the risk may differ, depending on the specific heart defect. If a child's heart defect is part of a syndrome of other birth defects, the recurrence risk in another pregnancy may be much higher.

Parents who have had a child with a heart defect should consult their pediatric cardiologist and can consult a genetic counselor to find out the risks to any future children. Parents who themselves have a heart defect also are at increased risk of having an affected child and should consider consulting a genetic counselor.

Is pregnancy safe for women with heart defects?

Many women with congenital heart defects can safely become pregnant and have healthy babies. However, women with congenital heart defects always should check with their cardiologist before they become pregnant. Pregnancy can be risky for women with certain types of heart disease (including those with poorly functioning ventricles or high blood pressure in the lungs).[9]

In some cases, the mother's heart disease or the medications she takes to treat it can affect the fetus, causing poor growth, premature delivery, or other problems.[9] Some women with heart disease may need careful monitoring by a high-risk obstetrician, as well as their cardiologist, throughout pregnancy.

References

1. National Heart, Lung and Blood Institute. Congenital Heart Defects. December 2007.

2. Congenital Cardiovascular Defects: Current Knowledge: A Scientific Statement From the American Heart Association Council on Cardiovascular Disease in the Young. *Circulation*, volume 115, June 12, 2007, pages 2995–3014.

3. Pierpont, M.E., et al. Genetic Basis for Congenital Heart Defects: Current Knowledge: A Scientific Statement From the American Heart Association Congenital Cardiac Defects Committee, Council on Cardiovascular Disease in the Young. *Circulation*, volume 115, June 12, 2007, pages 3015–38.

4. Garg, V., et al. GATA4 Mutations Cause Human Congenital Heart Defects and Reveal an Interaction with TBX5. *Nature*, volume 424, July 24, 2003, pages 443–47.

5. Garg, V., et al. Mutations in NOTCH1 Cause Aortic Valve Disease. *Nature*, volume 437, September 8, 2005, pages 270–74.

6. Johnston, M.V. Congenital Heart Disease and Brain Injury. *New England Journal of Medicine*, volume 357, number 19, November 2, 2007, pages 1971–73.

7. American Heart Association. Congenital Heart Defects. Accessed 3/24/08.

8. Gill, H.K., et al. Patterns of Recurrence of Congenital Heart Disease. *Journal of the American College of Cardiology*, volume 42, number 5, September 3, 2003, pages 923–29.

9. Uebing, A., et al. Pregnancy and Congenital Heart Disease. *British Medical Journal*, volume 332, February 18, 2006, pages 401–6.

Section 30.4

Kawasaki Disease: A Disorder with Cardiovascular Implications

Kawasaki disease is an illness that involves the skin, mouth, and lymph nodes, and most often affects kids under age five. The cause is unknown, but if the symptoms are recognized early, kids with Kawasaki disease can fully recover within a few days. Untreated, it can lead to serious complications that can affect the heart.

Kawasaki disease occurs in nineteen out of every one hundred thousand kids in the United States. It is most common among children of Japanese and Korean descent, but can affect all ethnic groups.

Signs and Symptoms

Kawasaki disease can't be prevented, but usually has telltale symptoms and signs that appear in phases.

The first phase, which can last for up to two weeks, usually involves a persistent fever higher than 104°F (39°C) and lasts for at least five days.

Other symptoms that typically develop include:

- severe redness in the eyes;

- a rash on the stomach, chest, and genitals;

- red, dry, cracked lips;

- swollen tongue with a white coating and big red bumps;

- sore, irritated throat;

- swollen palms of the hands and soles of the feet with a purple-red color;

- swollen lymph nodes.

323

During the second phase, which usually begins within two weeks of when the fever started, the skin on the hands and feet may begin to peel in large pieces. The child also may experience joint pain, diarrhea, vomiting, or abdominal pain. If your child shows any of these symptoms, call your doctor.

Complications

Doctors can manage the symptoms of Kawasaki disease if they catch it early. Symptoms often disappear within just two days of the start of treatment. If Kawasaki disease is treated within ten days of the onset of symptoms, heart problems usually do not develop.

Cases that go untreated can lead to more serious complications, such as vasculitis, an inflammation of the blood vessels. This can be particularly dangerous because it can affect the coronary arteries, which supply blood to the heart.

In addition to the coronary arteries, the heart muscle, lining, valves, and the outer membrane that surrounds the heart can become inflamed. Arrhythmias (changes in the normal pattern of the heartbeat) or abnormal functioning of some heart valves also can occur.

Diagnosis

No single test can detect Kawasaki disease, so doctors usually diagnose it by evaluating the symptoms and ruling out other conditions.

Most kids diagnosed with Kawasaki disease will have a fever lasting five or more days and at least four of these symptoms:

- redness in both eyes;
- changes around the lips, tongue, or mouth;
- changes in the fingers and toes, such as swelling, discoloration, or peeling;
- a rash in the trunk or genital area;
- a large swollen lymph node in the neck;
- red, swollen palms of hands and soles of feet.

If Kawasaki disease is suspected, the doctor may order tests to monitor heart function (such as an echocardiogram) and might take blood and urine samples to rule out other conditions, such as scarlet fever, measles, Rocky Mountain spotted fever, juvenile rheumatoid arthritis, or an allergic drug reaction.

Treatment

Treatment should begin as soon as possible, ideally within ten days of when the fever begins. Usually, a child is treated with intravenous doses of gamma globulin (purified antibodies), an ingredient of blood that helps the body fight infection. The child also might be given a high dose of aspirin to reduce the risk of heart problems.

Section 30.5

Rheumatic Heart Disease Is More Common in Children Than in Adults

Excerpted from "What About My Child and Rheumatic Fever?" reprinted with permission from www.heart.org. © 2013 American Heart Association, Inc. All rights reserved.

Rheumatic fever is an inflammatory reaction that can occur after a streptococcal infection of the throat ("strep throat"). Most strep throat infections don't lead to rheumatic fever. When they do, the time between the strep throat and rheumatic fever is about two to four weeks. Rheumatic fever is not contagious; however, the strep infection that comes before it is. If a strep throat infection is treated, rheumatic fever can almost always be prevented. Anyone can get rheumatic fever, but those who do are often five to fifteen years old.

What are the common symptoms of rheumatic fever?

- Sudden onset of a sore throat, especially with painful swallowing
- Fever
- Tender, swollen glands under the jaw angle

The symptoms may be mild in some children. If your child has a sore throat, you can't know for sure if it's strep throat unless you take him or her to a doctor.

How does rheumatic fever affect the body?

It may affect many parts of the body. It can affect the heart and produce inflamed or scarred heart valves. It can also cause painful, swollen joints; skin rash, especially on the chest or abdomen; abnormal movements; or bumps under the skin.

Does rheumatic fever always affect the heart?

No. When it does, the damage may either disappear or remain. When rheumatic fever causes permanent heart damage, it's called rheumatic heart disease.

Is there a cure for rheumatic fever?

There's no "miracle drug" to cure it. An attack of rheumatic fever usually subsides within a few weeks to a few months, but heart damage may last for life. That's why prevention is so important.

If my child has had rheumatic fever, must I restrict his or her activities?

Most children don't need to have their activities restricted after the acute stage of this illness. But talk to your doctor because the answer varies from child to child.

Can you get rheumatic fever more than once?

Yes. Your child is much more likely than others to have another "attack." Taking an antibiotic (usually penicillin) regularly for many years can prevent most recurrences. The antibiotic prevents strep throat and protects the patient from getting rheumatic fever again.

If my child has rheumatic heart disease, how can I protect him or her from more problems?

People with rheumatic heart disease are at risk of developing an infection on their damaged heart valves. This infection is called "bacterial endocarditis" or "infective endocarditis." You can help reduce the risk for this problem by keeping teeth clean and cavities filled. In the past, the American Heart Association recommended that people with rheumatic heart disease take a dose of antibiotics before certain dental or surgical procedures. However, our association does not suggest this type of preventive treatment any longer for people with rheumatic heart disease unless they have a history of endocarditis, an artificial heart valve, certain congenital heart defects, or have had a heart transplant and have heart valve problems.

Chapter 31

Cardiovascular Disease in Men

Chapter Contents

327

Section 31.1

Men and Cardiovascular Disease: A Statistical Overview

Cardiovascular Disease

- More than one in three adult men has some form of CVD.

- In 2009, CVD caused the deaths of 386,436 males. Males represent 49.0 percent of deaths from CVD.

- The 2009 overall death rate from CVD was 236.1. Death rates were 281.4 for white males, 387.0 for black males.

- In 2010, CVD was the first listed diagnosis of 3,021,000 males discharged from short-stay hospitals.

- In 2010, 74.9 percent of bypass and 67.1 percent of PCI patients were male. 68.7 percent of heart transplant patients in 2011 were male.

Coronary Heart Disease (CHD)

- About 8.8 million men alive today have CHD. Of these, 5.0 million have a history of myocardial infarction (MI, or heart attack).

- Among men age twenty and older, 8.2 percent of non-Hispanic whites, 6.8 percent of non-Hispanic blacks, and 6.7 percent of Mexican Americans have CHD.

- Each year new and recurrent MI and fatal CHD will impact an estimated 535,000 men.

- CHD killed 210,069 males in 2009. 68,814 died from MI.

- The 2009 overall CHD death rate was 116.1. Death rates were 155.9 for white males and 181.1 for black males.

- 828,000 males diagnosed with CHD were discharged from short-stay hospitals in 2010.

Angina Pectoris

- Among men age twenty and older, 3.3 percent of non-Hispanic whites, 2.4 percent of non-Hispanic blacks, and 3.4 percent of Mexican Americans have angina.

- Each year about 320,000 men over age forty-five are diagnosed with stable angina.

Congenital Cardiovascular Defects

- The 2009 overall death rate for congenital cardiovascular defects was 1.0. Death rates were 1.1 for white males and 1.4 for black males.

- Twenty-five thousand males were discharged from short-stay hospitals in 2009 with a diagnosis of congenital cardiovascular defects.

Stroke

- An estimated 3.0 million male stroke survivors are alive today.

- Among men age twenty and older, the following have had a stroke: 2.4 percent of non-Hispanic whites, 4.3 percent of non-Hispanic blacks, and 2.3 percent of Mexican Americans.

- In 2009, stroke caused the death of 52,073 males (40.4 percent of total stroke deaths).

- The 2009 overall death rate for stroke was 38.9. Death rates were 37.8 for white males, 60.1 for black males, 30.9 for Hispanic males, 34.1 for Asian/Pacific Islander males, and 29.2 for American Indian/Alaska Native males.

- In 2010, 485,000 males were discharged from short-stay hospitals after having a stroke.

High Blood Pressure (HBP)

- One in three U.S. adults has HBP.

- A higher percentage of men than women have hypertension until age forty-five. From forty-five to fifty-four years of age and fifty-five to sixty-four years of age, the percentages of men and women with hypertension are similar. After that, a much higher percentage of women have hypertension than men.

- Among men age twenty and older, 33.4 percent of non-Hispanic whites, 42.6 percent of non-Hispanic blacks, and 30.1 percent of Mexican Americans have HBP.

- In 2009, 27,668 males died from HBP. They represented 44.8 percent of deaths from HBP.

- The 2009 overall death rate from HBP was 18.5. Death rates were 17.0 for white males and 51.6 for black males.

- 216,000 males diagnosed with HBP were discharged from short-stay hospitals in 2010.

Heart Failure (HF)

- About 2.7 million males alive today have HF. Each year, about 350,000 new cases are diagnosed in males.

- In 2010, the overall prevalence for people age twenty and older is 2.1 percent. Among men, the following have HF: 2.2 percent of non-Hispanic whites, 4.1 percent of non-Hispanic blacks, and 1.9 percent of Mexican Americans.

- In 2009, there were 23,563 male deaths from HF (41.8 percent of HF deaths).

- The 2009 overall any-mention death rate from HF was 82.3. Death rates were 98.3 for white males and 104.5 for black males.

- 501,000 males diagnosed with HF were discharged from short-stay hospitals in 2010.

Smoking

- In 2011:
  - Male students (grades nine to twelve) were more likely than female students to smoke cigarettes (19.9 percent vs.16.1 percent), smoke cigars (17.8 percent vs. 8.0 percent), or use smokeless tobacco (12.8 percent vs. 2.2 percent).

  - Among adults, 21.3 percent of men and 16.7 percent of women smoke cigarettes.

High Blood Cholesterol and Other Lipids

- Among children four to eleven years of age, the mean total blood cholesterol level is 161.9 mg/dL. For boys, it is 162.3 mg/ dL; for girls, it is 161.5 mg/dL.

- Among adolescents twelve to nineteen years of age, the mean total blood cholesterol level is 158.2 mg/dL. For boys, it is 156.1 mg/dL; for girls, it is 160.3 mg/dL.

- Among adults age twenty and older:
  - 41.3 percent of men and 44.9 percent of women have total cholesterol levels of 200 mg/dL or higher.
  - 12.7 percent of men and 14.7 percent of women have levels of 240 mg/dL or higher.
  - 31.9 percent of men and 30.0 percent of women have an low-density lipoprotein (LDL) cholesterol level of 130 mg/dL or higher.
  - 31.8 percent of men and 12.3 percent of women have high-density lipoprotein (HDL) cholesterol level less than 40 mg/dL.

Physical Inactivity

- Boys are less likely than girls to report inactivity (10.0 percent vs. 17.7 percent).

- In a study of 12,812 youth nine to eighteen years of age, the physical activity level in boys and girls declined starting at the age of thirteen, with a significantly greater decline in activity among girls.

- Only 24.9 percent of adult men met the 2008 Federal Physical Activity Guidelines in 2011.

Overweight and Obesity

- An estimated 33.0 percent of boys age two to nineteen are over-weight or obese; 30.1 percent non-Hispanic whites, 36.9 percent non-Hispanic blacks, and 40.5 percent Mexican Americans.

- Of these boys, 18.6 percent are obese; 16.1 percent non-Hispanic whites, 24.3 percent non-Hispanic blacks, and 24.0 percent Mexican Americans.

- An estimated 72.9 percent of men age twenty and older are over-weight or obese; 73.1 percent non-Hispanic whites, 68.7 percent non-Hispanic blacks, and 81.3 percent Mexican Americans.

- Of these men, 33.6 percent are obese; 33.8 percent non-Hispanic whites, 37.9 percent non-Hispanic blacks, and 36.0 percent Mexican Americans.

Diabetes Mellitus (DM)

- Of the estimated 19.7 million American adults with physician-diagnosed diabetes, about 9.6 million are men; 7.7 percent of non-Hispanic whites, 13.5 percent of non-Hispanic blacks, and 11.4 percent of Mexican Americans.

- Of the estimated 8.2 million Americans with undiagnosed diabetes, about 5.3 million are men; 4.5 percent of non-Hispanic whites, 4.8 percent of non-Hispanic blacks, and 6.6 percent of Mexican Americans.

- Of the estimated 87.3 million Americans with pre-diabetes, about 50.7 million are men; 47.7 percent of non-Hispanic whites, 35.7 percent of non-Hispanic blacks, and 47.0 percent of Mexican Americans.

- In 2009, diabetes killed 35,054 males. The overall death rate from diabetes was 20.9. Death rates were 23.3 for white males and 44.2 for black males.

- 311,000 males diagnosed with diabetes were discharged from short-stay hospitals in 2010.

Section 31.2

Cardiovascular Implications of Erectile Dysfunction

"Erectile Dysfunction May Signal Hidden Heart Disease,"
by Randy Dotinga, January 29, 2013. Copyright © 2013 HealthDay
(www.healthday.com). All rights reserved. Reprinted with permission.

Doctors should look more closely at the overall health of impotent men, a large new study suggests.

Men with even mild erectile dysfunction—but no known heart problems—face a major extra risk of developing cardiovascular conditions in the future. And as erectile dysfunction becomes more pronounced, signs of hidden heart disease and earlier death risk grow.

Not surprisingly, men already known to have a heart condition along with severe erectile dysfunction fare worst of all, the Australian researchers found.

Among men aged forty-five and up without diagnosed heart disease, those with moderate or severe erectile dysfunction were up to 50 percent more likely to be hospitalized for heart problems, according to an adjusted analysis. Erectile dysfunction boosted the risk for hospitalization even more when men had a history of cardiovascular disease.

Erectile problems, which become more likely as men grow older, aren't a guarantee of heart problems. Still, men with erectile dysfunction should "take action by seeing a health professional and asking for a heart check," said study lead author Dr. Emily Banks. "Men with erectile dysfunction need to be assessed for their future risk of cardiovascular disease, and any identified risk must be managed appropriately."

Banks is a professor of epidemiology at the Australian National University's National Center for Epidemiology and Population Health.

Banks said an estimated 60 percent of men aged seventy and up suffer from moderate to severe erectile dysfunction. The condition can place major limits on sexual activity and require the use of drugs like Viagra that can come with side effects and awkward challenges when it comes to the timing of doses.

A variety of causes can contribute to impotence, but "it is widely acknowledged that erectile dysfunction is predominantly the result of underlying cardiovascular disease," Banks said.

Doctors already believe that erectile dysfunction is an early warning sign of heart problems, but it's not clear why. It's possible, Banks said, that the arteries of the penis are smaller than those of other parts of the body and may be more likely to reveal problems when their lining deteriorates.

The new study aims to gain more insight into how the severity of erectile dysfunction translates into a higher risk of cardiovascular disease. The researchers tracked more than ninety-five thousand men aged forty-five and up, and compared data collected between 2006 and 2009 to data collected in 2010.

The researchers adjusted their statistics so they wouldn't be thrown off by factors like high or low numbers of men who smoked or drank alcohol, or were wealthy or poor. They found that the men with severe erectile dysfunction, compared to those with no problem, were eight times more likely to have heart failure, 60 percent more likely to have heart disease and almost twice as likely to die of any cause.

What does this mean in the big picture?

"Heart problems are very common, so even a relatively moderate increase in risk translates into quite a number of affected individuals," Banks said. "Among men with no past history of cardiovascular disease, an estimated six per one thousand men per year who did not have erectile dysfunction went on to be admitted to the hospital for coronary heart disease. This compares with eight per one thousand men per year with moderate erectile dysfunction and nine per one thousand men per year among those with severe erectile dysfunction."

Also, she said, "among men with a past history of cardiovascular disease, an estimated twenty per one thousand men per year of those without erectile dysfunction went on to be admitted to the hospital for coronary artery disease. This compares with twenty-eight per one thousand men per year with moderate erectile dysfunction and thirty-four per one thousand men per year with severe erectile dysfunction."

Could drugs for erectile dysfunction, such as Viagra, actually help men with undiagnosed heart problems? Maybe.

"Medications to treat erectile dysfunction have proven benefits in treating [lung] hypertension and are being evaluated as a treatment for heart failure," said Dr. Gregg Fonarow, a professor of cardiology at the University of California, Los Angeles. "However, there are no proven benefits for reducing the risk of heart attack or stroke."

Fonarow agreed with the study's conclusion that men with erectile dysfunction should get their hearts checked, especially since cardio-vascular disease can have no symptoms.

The study authors said, however, that more research is needed before the presence of erectile dysfunction can be considered a clinical predictor of heart disease risk.

The study appears in the January 2013 issue of the journal *PLoS Medicine*.

Section 31.3

Sleep Apnea Tied to Increased Risk of Stroke in Men

"Sleep Apnea Tied to Increased Risk of Stroke,"
National Institutes of Health, April 8, 2010.

Obstructive sleep apnea is associated with an increased risk of stroke in middle-aged and older adults, especially men, according to new results from a landmark study supported by the National Heart, Lung, and Blood Institute (NHLBI) of the National Institutes of Health. Overall, sleep apnea more than doubles the risk of stroke in men. Obstructive sleep apnea is a common disorder in which the upper airway is intermittently narrowed or blocked, disrupting sleep and breathing during sleep.

Researchers from the Sleep Heart Health Study (SHHS) report that the risk of stroke appears in men with mild sleep apnea and rises with the severity of sleep apnea. Men with moderate to severe sleep apnea were nearly three times more likely to have a stroke than men without sleep apnea or with mild sleep apnea. The risk from sleep apnea is independent of other risk factors such as weight, high blood pressure, race, smoking, and diabetes.

They also report for the first time a link between sleep apnea and increased risk of stroke in women. Obstructive Sleep Apnea Hypopnea

335

and Incident Stroke: The Sleep Heart Health Study, was published online March 25, 2010, ahead of print in the *American Journal of Respiratory and Critical Care Medicine.*

Stroke is the second leading cause of death worldwide. "Although scientists have uncovered several risk factors for stroke—such as age, high blood pressure and atrial fibrillation, and diabetes—there are still many cases in which the cause or contributing factors are unknown," noted NHLBI Acting Director Susan B. Shurin, M.D. "This is the largest study to date to link sleep apnea with an increased risk of stroke. The time is right for researchers to study whether treating sleep apnea could prevent or delay stroke in some individuals."

Conducted in nine medical centers across the United States, the SHHS is the largest and most comprehensive prospective, multicenter study on the risk of cardiovascular disease and other conditions related to sleep apnea. In the latest report, researchers studied stroke risk in 5,422 participants aged forty years and older without a history of stroke. At the start of the study, participants performed a standard at-home sleep test, which determined whether they had sleep apnea and, if so, the severity of the sleep apnea.

Researchers followed the participants for an average of about nine years. They report that during the study, 193 participants had a stroke—85 men (of 2,462 men enrolled) and 108 women (out of 2,960 enrolled).

After adjusting for several cardiovascular risk factors, the researchers found that the effect of sleep apnea on stroke risk was stronger in men than in women. In men, a progressive increase in stroke risk was observed as sleep apnea severity increased from mild levels to moderate to severe levels. In women, however, the increased risk of stroke was significant only with severe levels of sleep apnea.

The researchers suggest that the differences between men and women might be because men are more likely to develop sleep apnea at younger ages. Therefore, they tend to have untreated sleep apnea for longer periods of time than women. "It's possible that the stroke risk is related to cumulative effects of sleep apnea adversely influencing health over many years," said Susan Redline, M.D., MPH, professor of medicine, pediatrics, and epidemiology and biostatistics at Case Western Reserve University in Cleveland and lead author of the paper.

"Our findings provide compelling evidence that obstructive sleep apnea is a risk factor for stroke, especially in men," noted Redline. "Overall, the increased risk of stroke in men with sleep apnea is comparable to adding ten years to a man's age. Importantly, we found that increased stroke risk in men occurs even with relatively mild levels of sleep apnea."

"Research on the effects of sleep apnea not only increases our understanding of how lapses of breathing during sleep affects our health and well being, but it can also provide important insight into how cardiovascular problems such as stroke and high blood pressure develop," noted Michael J. Twery, Ph.D., director of the NIH National Center on Sleep Disorders Research, an office administered by the NHLBI.

The new results support earlier findings that have linked sleep apnea to stroke risk. SHHS researchers have also reported that untreated sleep apnea is associated with an increased risk of high blood pressure, heart attack, irregular heartbeats, heart failure, and death from any cause. Other studies have also linked untreated sleep apnea with overweight and obesity and diabetes. It is also linked to excessive daytime sleepiness, which lowers performance in the workplace and at school and increases the risk of injuries and death from drowsy driving and other accidents.

More than twelve million American adults are believed to have sleep apnea, and most are not diagnosed or treated. Treatments to restore regular breathing during sleep include mouthpieces, surgery, and breathing devices, such as continuous positive airway pressure, or CPAP. In people who are overweight or obese, weight loss can also help.

These treatments can help improve breathing and reduce the severity of symptoms such as loud snoring and excessive daytime sleepiness, thereby improving sleep-related quality of life and performance at work or in school. Randomized clinical trials to test whether treating sleep apnea lowers the risk of stroke, other cardiovascular diseases, or death are needed.

"We now have abundant evidence that sleep apnea is associated with cardiovascular risk factors and diseases. The next logical step is to determine if treating sleep apnea can lower a person's risk of these leading killers," said Redline. "With stimulus funds, our research group is now developing the additional research and resources to begin answering this important question."

Chapter 32

Cardiovascular Disease in Women

Chapter Contents

Section 32.1

Women and Heart Disease: Some Gender Differences

Cardiovascular disease—disease of the heart and blood vessels—is by far the top cause of death among American women. According to the American Heart Association, one in 2.5 women will die of heart disease or stroke, compared with one in 30 from breast cancer.

People once thought that cardiovascular disease only affected men. We now know that cardiovascular disease is more common in women than men, partially because women live longer. The risk of getting cardiovascular disease goes up as you age.

What Doctors Know about Women and Cardiovascular Disease

At one time, cardiovascular disease was only studied in men. Doctors are still learning how heart problems affect women:

- During a heart attack, a woman may feel a burning in her stomach, lightheadedness, and sweating instead of the intense chest pain common in a man. A woman sometimes ignores these lesser-known symptoms of a heart attack.

- Heart attacks are generally more severe in women. A woman is 50 percent more likely to die in the first year after a heart attack than a man. And in the first six years after a heart attack, a woman is almost twice as likely as a man to have another heart attack.

- Women often have heart attacks later in life than men. This explains why women are more likely to die after a heart attack. Also, age-related diseases such as arthritis and osteoporosis can hide heart attack symptoms in women.

- Some tests for finding cardiovascular disease, such as a treadmill stress test, may be less accurate in women than in men.

- After menopause, a woman's chances of getting heart disease rise. Some think this is because a woman's estrogen levels decrease during menopause. Estrogen is associated with higher levels of "good cholesterol," which can help ward off a heart attack.

- People with diabetes are more likely to get cardiovascular disease. Diabetes is more common in women. It also cancels the protective effects of estrogen.

- Oral contraceptives (birth control pills) may increase a woman's chances of getting cardiovascular disease, especially if the woman smokes. Birth control pills may raise blood pressure and blood sugar levels in some women, and increase the risk of blood clots, which can cause a heart attack or stroke.

Section 32.2

Basic Facts about Heart Disease in Women

"Heart Disease in Women," U.S. Food and Drug Administration, June 13, 2012.

A lot of people think that women do not get heart disease. More women die from heart disease than from anything else. Any woman can get heart disease.

When you think about heart disease, you probably think about chest pain. Women might not have chest pain. If they do, they might call it an achy, tight, or "heavy" feeling instead of pain. The pain might even be in the back between the shoulder blades, instead of the chest.

Women might think these signs are no big deal because they don't "sound" like a heart attack. Don't ignore these signs. Go to your doctor or clinic right away.

What Are the Signs of Heart Disease in Women?

The most important sign is feeling really tired—even if after enough sleep. Other signs of heart disease in women are as follows:

- Trouble breathing

- Trouble sleeping

- Feeling sick to the stomach

- Feeling scared or nervous

- New or worse headaches

- An ache in the chest

- Feeling "heavy" or "tight" in the chest

- A burning feeling in the chest

- Pain in the back, between the shoulders

- Pain or tightness in the chest that spreads to the jaw, neck, shoulders, ear, or the inside of the arms

- Pain in the belly, above the belly button

There is good news: You can take steps to keep your heart healthy.

Don't wait to get help! Go to your doctor or clinic if you have any warning signs.

Lower Your Risk of Heart Disease

- Find out if heart disease runs in your family.

- Visit your doctor or clinic often. Find out if you are at risk.

- Don't smoke. Stay away from other people who are smoking.

- Get your blood pressure checked often. You might need medicine to keep it at the right level.

- Control your diabetes.

- Get your cholesterol checked often.

- Stay active. Walking every day can lower your chances of a heart attack.

- Eat right and keep a healthy weight.

- Eat less salt.

- If you take birth control pills, don't smoke.

- Hormones for menopause should not be used to prevent heart attacks.

- Being stressed, angry, or sad a lot may add to your risk of heart attack.

- If you've had a heart attack, talk to your doctor about medicine. Some medicines can help cut down the risk of having another heart attack.

High Blood Pressure

- High blood pressure adds to the chance of having heart disease.

- High blood pressure is called the "silent killer." Most people who have it do not feel sick and don't know that they have it.

- Have your blood pressure checked each time you go to the doctor or clinic.

Section 32.3

Birth Control Pills and Cardiovascular Disease Risk

Excerpted from "Your Guide to a Healthy Heart," National Heart, Lung, and Blood Institute, National Institutes of Health, December 2005. Reviewed by David A. Cooke, M.D., FACP, October 2013.

Studies show that women who use high-dose birth control pills (oral contraceptives) are more likely to have a heart attack or stroke because blood clots are more likely to form in the blood vessels. These risks are lessened once the birth control pill is stopped. Using the pill also may worsen the effects of other risk factors, such as smoking, high blood pressure, diabetes, high blood cholesterol, and overweight.

Much of this information comes from studies of birth control pills containing higher doses of hormones than those commonly used today. Still, the risks of using low-dose pills are not fully known. Therefore, if you are now taking any kind of birth control pill or are considering using one, keep these guidelines in mind:

Don't mix smoking and the "pill": If you smoke cigarettes, stop smoking or choose a different form of birth control. Cigarette smoking raises the risk of serious health problems from birth control pill use, especially the risk of blood clots. For women over thirty-five, the risk is particularly high. Women who use birth control pills should not smoke.

Pay attention to diabetes: Levels of glucose, or blood sugar, sometimes change dramatically in women who take birth control pills. If you are diabetic or have a close relative who is, be sure to have regular blood sugar tests if you take birth control pills.

Watch your blood pressure: After starting to take birth control pills, your blood pressure may go up. If your blood pressure increases to 140/90 mmHg or higher, ask your doctor about changing pills or switching to another form of birth control. Be sure to get your blood pressure checked at least once a year.

Talk with your doctor: If you have heart disease or another heart problem, or if you have suffered a stroke, birth control pills may not be a safe choice. Be sure your doctor knows about these and any other serious health conditions before prescribing birth control pills for you.

Section 32.4

Heart Disease and Pregnancy

Women with a heart condition may need to take special precautions before and during pregnancy. Some heart conditions may increase a woman's risk for complications during pregnancy. In addition, some women may have heart or blood vessel conditions that are not identified until pregnancy.

If You Have a Heart Condition, What Should You Do Before Planning a Pregnancy?

If you have a heart condition, such as those listed below, you should be evaluated by a cardiologist (a heart specialist) before you start planning a pregnancy:

- Hypertension (high blood pressure) or high cholesterol.

- Prior diagnosis of any type of heart or blood vessel disease, including aorta disease, arrhythmia, heart murmur, cardiomyopathy, heart failure, Marfan syndrome, or rheumatic fever.

- Prior cardiac event (transient ischemic attack or stroke).

- Poor functional status, defined as NYHA class III or IV. The New York Heart Association (NYHA) functional status is a set of clinical classifications that rank patients as class I-II-III-IV according to the degree of symptomatic or functional limits or cyanosis (a blue tint to the skin, indicates the body is not receiving enough oxygen-rich blood).

- Severe narrowing of the mitral or aortic valve or aortic outflow tract, as determined by echocardiography.

- Ejection fraction of less than 40 percent. Ejection fraction is the amount of blood pumped out of the left ventricle during each heartbeat. The ejection fraction evaluates how well the heart is pumping. A normal ejection fraction ranges from 50 to 70 percent.

The cardiologist can review your health history and perform a physical exam and order diagnostic tests, as needed, to evaluate your heart function and the severity and extent of your condition. After reviewing the test results, the cardiologist can talk to you about the safety of pregnancy, based on your health condition. The cardiologist will discuss your potential risk of complications during pregnancy, including potential fetal risks and possible long-term health risks to you and your baby. The cardiologist can discuss whether medications or other treatments may be needed before pregnancy.

Be sure to discuss all of your medications (including heart medications and any over-the-counter medications you take routinely) with your doctor so your medication dosages can be changed, if necessary, or different medications can be prescribed that may be safer to take during pregnancy.

By preparing for pregnancy and following up regularly with your cardiologist during pregnancy, most women with a heart condition can safely become pregnant and have a healthy baby.

Preexisting Cardiovascular Conditions and Pregnancy

Congenital Heart Conditions and Pregnancy

Atrial (ASD) and ventricular septal defects (VSD), and patent ductus arteriosus (PDA) are the most common congenital heart defects. With these heart defects, there is an opening in the septum (the muscular wall separating the right and left side of the heart). If the hole is large, blood from the left side of the heart flows back into the right side of the heart and gets pumped back to the lungs again.

In general, most women with a congenital heart defect, especially those who have had corrective surgery, can safely become pregnant. However, the type of heart defect, severity of symptoms, presence of pulmonary hypertension or other cardiac or lung disease, and any prior heart surgeries may affect the outcome of the pregnancy. In some women who have a congenital heart defect and who also have pulmonary hypertension, pregnancy is not recommended, as there's a high risk of maternal death.

Over time, symptoms of heart failure can occur or worsen in women with a congenital heart defect, increasing the mother's risk of long-term complications.

There is a greater risk that the baby will develop a heart condition if either parent has a congenital heart defect. Your cardiologist may recommend a fetal echocardiogram to check the fetus's heart for possible defects. This test is usually done in the eighteenth week of pregnancy.

If you have been diagnosed with a congenital heart defect, a cardiologist should evaluate your heart condition before you plan a pregnancy. The cardiologist can provide you with guidance on the possible risks of pregnancy and can work with your health care team to monitor your health and your baby's health during pregnancy.

Valve Disease and Pregnancy

Aortic valve stenosis means the aortic valve (the valve between the left ventricle and the aorta) is narrowed or stiff. If the narrowing is severe, the heart has to work harder to pump the increased blood volume out of the narrowed valve. This, in turn, can cause the left ventricle (the major pumping chamber of the heart) to enlarge (hypertrophy). Over time, symptoms of heart failure can occur or worsen, increasing the mother's risk of long-term complications.

One common cause of aortic valve stenosis is bicuspid aortic valve disease, a congenital heart condition in which there are only two leaflets or cusps, instead of the normal three leaflets. Without the third leaflet, the valve can become narrowed or stiff.

Women with bicuspid aortic valve disease or any type of aortic valve stenosis need to be evaluated by a cardiologist before planning a pregnancy. In some cases, surgery to correct the valve may be recommended before pregnancy.

Mitral valve stenosis means the mitral valve (the valve between the left atrium and left ventricle) is narrowed. This is often caused by rheumatic fever.

The increased blood volume and increased heart rate that occurs with pregnancy can worsen symptoms of mitral stenosis. The right atrium can enlarge in size, causing a rapid irregular heart rhythm called atrial fibrillation. In addition, heart failure symptoms can occur (shortness of breath, irregular heartbeat, fatigue, and swelling or edema). This can increase the risk to the mother. Medications may be used during surgery, and in some cases, percutaneous valvuloplasty may be required during pregnancy to correct the narrowed valve. Patients with mitral stenosis need to have their valve evaluated prior to becoming pregnant. In some cases, surgery to correct the valve will be recommended before pregnancy.

Mitral valve prolapse is a common condition, often not causing symptoms or requiring any treatment. Most patients with mitral valve prolapse tolerate pregnancy. If the prolapse causes a severe leak, treatment may be needed prior to pregnancy. It is always best to follow your doctor's recommendations if you have mitral valve prolapse.

Pregnancy in Women with Prosthetic (Artificial) Valves

Women who have artificial heart valves may experience complications during pregnancy because:

1. Women who have an artificial heart valve need to take lifelong anticoagulant medication, and certain anticoagulant medications can be harmful to the fetus. There is controversy regarding the best anticoagulant regimen.

2. During pregnancy, the risk of blood clots increases.

Use of warfarin, heparin, aspirin, and combinations of these have been suggested and compared. The most recent recommendations from the European Heart Association suggest the use of heparin during first trimester followed by warfarin up to the thirty-sixth week of pregnancy, with subsequent replacement by heparin until delivery or oral anticoagulation throughout pregnancy, until the thirty-sixth week, followed by heparin until delivery.

Warfarin doses are less harmful if the dose is kept to less than 5 mg. In addition, other specialists have recommended the addition of low-dose aspirin for women at high risk.

If you have a prosthetic valve and are taking an anticoagulant medication, it is very important to be evaluated by a cardiologist before planning a pregnancy so you can discuss your potential risks and determine the best anticoagulant therapy.

In addition, ask your doctor what precautions you should continue to follow to prevent endocarditis.

Arrhythmias and Pregnancy

Abnormal heartbeats (arrhythmias) during pregnancy are common. They may develop for the first time during pregnancy in a woman with a normal heart, or arrhythmias may be the result of a previously unknown heart condition. Most of the time, there are no symptoms of arrhythmias and no treatment is required. If symptoms develop, your doctor may order additional tests to determine the cause of the arrhythmias.

Aorta Disease and Pregnancy

Women who have conditions affecting their aorta, such as aortic aneurysm, dilated aorta, or connective tissue disorders such as Marfan syndrome are at increased risk during pregnancy.

Increased pressures in the aorta during pregnancy and bearing down during labor and delivery can increase risk for aorta dissection or rupture, which can be life threatening.

It is very important for women who have aorta disease to be evaluated by a cardiologist before planning a pregnancy. A thorough evaluation of the mother's condition will provide the physician with information about the potential risks of pregnancy. It is also important to note that some conditions, such as Marfan syndrome, are genetic and can be passed down to children, so genetic counseling may be recommended.

Cardiovascular Disorders that May Develop during Pregnancy

Peripartum Cardiomyopathy

Peripartum cardiomyopathy is the rare development of heart failure within the last month of pregnancy or within five months after delivery. The cause of peripartum cardiomyopathy remains unknown.

Women with peripartum cardiomyopathy have symptoms of heart failure. After pregnancy, the heart often returns to its normal size and function, although some women continue to have poor left ventricular function and symptoms. Women with peripartum cardiomyopathy have an increased risk for complications during subsequent pregnancies.

Hypertension (High Blood Pressure)

About 6 to 8 percent of women develop high blood pressure, also called hypertension, during pregnancy. This is called pregnancy-induced hypertension (PIH) and is related to preeclampsia, toxemia, or toxemia of pregnancy. PIH is a complication characterized by high blood pressure, swelling due to fluid retention, and protein in the urine. PIH can be harmful to the mother and the baby.

Heart Murmur

Sometimes, a heart murmur or abnormal "swishing" sound, can develop as a result of the increase in blood volume that occurs during pregnancy. In most cases, the murmur is harmless but in rare cases, it could mean there's a problem with a heart valve. Your doctor can evaluate your condition and determine the cause of the murmur.

After You Become Pregnant

Congratulations on your pregnancy! During pregnancy, it's important to:

- continue following a heart-healthy diet;
- exercise regularly, as recommended by your cardiologist;
- quit smoking!

In addition to keeping your follow-up appointments with your obstetric provider throughout pregnancy, schedule regular follow-up visits with your cardiologist and follow your cardiologist's recommendations carefully. Your cardiologist can evaluate your heart condition throughout your pregnancy so symptoms and/or potential complications can be detected and treated early. This will help ensure a safe outcome for you and your baby.

Some conditions may require a team approach with the patient, obstetrician, cardiologist, anesthesiologist, and pediatrician. Depending on the woman's heart condition, special arrangements may need to be made for labor and delivery.

Section 32.5

Menopause and Heart Disease

Heart disease risk rises for everyone as they age, but for women symptoms can become more evident after the onset of menopause.

Menopause does not cause cardiovascular diseases. However, certain risk factors increase around the time of menopause, and a high-fat diet, smoking, or other unhealthy habits begun earlier in life can also take a toll, said Dr. Nieca Goldberg, a cardiologist and an American Heart Association volunteer.

"Menopause isn't a disease. It's a natural phase of a woman's life cycle," Dr. Goldberg said. "It's important for women, as they approach menopause, to really take stock of their health."

On average, the onset of menopause, when menstrual periods permanently stop, occurs at age fifty-four, said Dr. Goldberg, medical director of the Joan H. Tisch Center for Women's Health at New York University Langone Medical Center.

About thirty-five thousand American women under fifty have a heart attack each year, Dr. Goldberg said. An overall increase in heart attacks among women is seen about ten years after menopause. Heart disease is the leading killer of women.

Estrogen Levels May Play a Role

A decline in the natural hormone estrogen may be a factor in heart disease increase among postmenopausal women. Estrogen is believed to have a positive effect on the inner layer of artery wall, helping to keep blood vessels flexible. That means they can relax and expand to accommodate blood flow.

Despite the benefits of estrogen, the American Heart Association recommends against using postmenopausal hormone therapy to reduce the risk of coronary heart disease or stroke because some studies have shown it appears to not reduce the risk.

Estrogen decline isn't the only reason women face a higher cardiovascular disease risk after reaching menopause, Dr. Goldberg said.

"We're trying to figure the rest of it out," she said.

Assorted changes in the body occur with menopause. Blood pressure starts to go up. Low-density lipoprotein (LDL) cholesterol, or "bad" cholesterol, tends to increase while high-density lipoprotein (HDL), or "good" cholesterol declines or remains the same. Triglycerides, certain types of fats in the blood, also increase.

Strive for Heart Health

If you've followed a healthy lifestyle and continue doing so at menopause, your risk for heart disease and stroke is lower. Family history also contributes to your risk.

Women should take care of their heart through regular exercise and good nutrition and by eliminating unhealthy habits like smoking, which may contribute to early menopause, increase the risk of blood clots, decrease the flexibility of arteries, and lower the levels of HDL cholesterol, Dr. Goldberg said.

The American Heart Association recommends at least 4.5 cups per day of fruits and vegetables, at least six to eight servings per day of fiber-rich whole grains based on a two-thousand-calorie diet, and a variety of nutritious foods each week such as fatty fish, unsalted nuts, and legumes.

Women should aim for a 150 minutes of physical activity each week to help prevent heart disease, and an hour daily for a weight loss program, depending on individual needs. Walking, cycling, dancing, or swimming—activities that use larger muscles at low resistance—are good aerobic exercises, said Dr. Goldberg. And, she advised, don't worry about how you look while exercising or whether you have fashionable workout clothes.

"You have to get over that," she said, adding: "Do the activity that works for you."

Chapter 33

Cardiovascular Disease in Minority Populations

Chapter Contents

Section 33.1

Cardiovascular Disease among U.S. Racial and Ethnic Minorities: Some Statistics

"Heart Disease Data/Statistics," U.S. Department of Health and Human Services, Office of Minority Health, July 9, 2012.

Heart disease is the leading killer across most racial and ethnic minority communities in the United States, accounting for 25 percent of all deaths in 2008.

African American men and women are 30 percent more likely to die from heart disease than non-Hispanic white males. This occurs despite the fact that 6 percent of African Americans have heart disease. Some 34 percent of African Americans have hypertension compared to 24 percent of whites, in 2009.

Mexican Americans, who make up the largest share of the U.S. Hispanic population, suffer in greater percentages than whites from overweight and obesity, two of the leading risk factors for heart disease. Premature death was higher for Hispanics (23.5 percent) than non-Hispanics (16.5 percent). In 2008, in the Asian and Pacific Islander community, 33 percent of deaths are caused by heart disease. In 2001, the number of premature deaths (before age sixty-five) from heart disease was greatest among American Indians or Alaska Natives (36 percent) and lowest among whites.

Quick Facts

- African Americans are 1.4 times as likely as non-Hispanic whites to have high blood pressure.

- American Indian/Alaska Native adults are 1.3 times as likely as white adults to have high blood pressure.

- Overall, Asian American adults are less likely than white adults to have heart disease and they are less likely to die from heart disease.

- Mexican American women are less likely than non-Hispanic white women to have high blood pressure.

Section 33.2

African Americans and Cardiovascular Disease

Heart disease is the number one killer for all Americans, and stroke is the fourth-leading cause of death. As frightening as those statistics are the risks of getting those diseases are even higher for African Americans.

The good news is, African Americans can improve their odds of preventing and beating these diseases by understanding the risks and taking simple steps to address them.

"Get checked, then work with your medical professional on your specific risk factors and the things that you need to do to take care of your personal health," said Winston Gandy, M.D., a cardiologist and chief medical marketing officer with the Piedmont Heart Institute in Atlanta and a volunteer with the American Heart Association.

High blood pressure, obesity, and diabetes are the most common conditions that increase the risk of heart disease and stroke. Here's how they affect African Americans and some tips to lower your risk.

High Blood Pressure

The prevalence of high blood pressure in African Americans is the highest in the world. Also known as hypertension, high blood pressure (HBP) increases your risk of heart disease and stroke, and it can cause permanent damage to the heart before you even notice any symptoms, that's why it is often referred to as the "silent killer." Not only is HBP more severe in blacks than whites, but it also develops earlier in life.

Research suggests African Americans may carry a gene that makes them more salt sensitive, increasing the risk of high blood pressure. Your health care provider can help you find the right medication, and lifestyle changes can also have a big impact.

"You can't do anything about your family history, but you can control your blood pressure," Dr. Gandy said.

355

If you know your blood pressure is high, keeping track of changes is important. Check it regularly, and notify your doctor of changes in case treatment needs to be adjusted, Dr. Gandy said. Even if you don't have high blood pressure, he recommends checking it every two years.

"The number one thing you can do is check your blood pressure regularly," he said.

Obesity

African Americans are disproportionately affected by obesity. Among non-Hispanic blacks age twenty and older, 63 percent of men and 77 percent of women are overweight or obese.

If you're carrying extra weight, Dr. Gandy suggests focusing on the quality of your diet throughout the day, not just during mealtime.

"You can add hundreds of calories to your diet just on snacking," he said.

Dr. Gandy knows all too well how challenging it can be to lose weight. After years of prescribing diet changes for his patients, he decided it was time to follow his own advice by walking at least thirty minutes a day and eliminating sugary drinks and desserts. The hard work paid off. Dr. Gandy lost twenty-five pounds in six months and feels much better.

He also suggests limiting red meat in favor of lean meats such as chicken or fish, and watching portions on carbohydrate-heavy foods, such as pasta and rice.

"Make vegetables the main part of the meal and fill up with those rather than other foods," he said.

Dr. Gandy cautioned that even things that are healthy can pack in calories.

"If you're thirsty, drink water, not juice," Dr. Gandy said.

Diabetes

African Americans are nearly twice as likely to have diabetes as non-Hispanic whites. In fact, about 15 percent of all African Americans age twenty and older have the disease.

Diabetes is treatable and preventable, but many people don't recognize early warning signs. Or, they avoid seeking treatment out of fear of complications.

Dr. Gandy said many people associate the disease with older relatives who were diagnosed too late and suffered preventable complications such as blindness, amputations, or renal failure.

For diabetes and other heart disease risks, regular exercise also plays a key role—both in strengthening the cardiovascular system and burning extra calories.

Aim for at least thirty minutes of walking a day, Dr. Gandy said. "That's enough to get the heart rate up," he said. "There's no need to do a marathon."

Section 33.3

Cardiovascular Disease in the Hispanic Population

"Hispanics and Heart Disease, Stroke," reprinted with permission from www.heart.org. © 2013 American Heart Association, Inc. All rights reserved.

Heart disease is the number one killer for all Americans and stroke is the fourth leading cause of death. Hispanics and Latinos, however, face even higher risks of cardiovascular diseases because of high blood pressure, obesity, and diabetes.

There is good news in the fact that a few simple lifestyle changes can reduce the chances of getting these diseases. Yet at the same time, Hispanics and Latinos face hurdles when it comes to making those changes and accessing health care, including language barriers, lack of transportation, and lack of health insurance.

Those factors can make early diagnoses and management of risks difficult, said Martha L. Daviglus, M.D., Ph.D., a cardiovascular epidemiologist at Northwestern University and University of Illinois and an American Heart Association volunteer.

"Hispanics are more likely to delay care, drop out of treatment when symptoms disappear, and avoid visits to the doctor," Dr. Daviglus said.

Here are some of the primary conditions affecting Hispanics and what you can do to lower your risk for heart disease and stroke.

High Blood Pressure

Hypertension, the medical term for high blood pressure, is a major risk factor for heart disease and stroke among Hispanics. Among Hispanics who experienced a stroke, 72 percent had high blood pressure, compared to 66 percent in non-Hispanic whites.

Checking your blood pressure regularly is an important first step for understanding your risks. If it's high, work with your doctor to create a treatment plan. If it's normal, be sure to keep checking it a couple times a year.

You can also lower your risk by maintaining a healthy weight and eating a healthy diet that focuses on fruit and vegetables and avoids excessive salt, Dr. Daviglus said.

"If you do these things and are still unable to control your blood pressure, you will need to consult your physician and follow advice regarding medications to help lower blood pressure," Dr. Daviglus said.

Obesity Is More Prevalent

Carrying extra weight is also a key risk factor for Hispanics. Seventy-five percent of Mexican-American men and 72 percent of women age twenty and older are overweight or obese.

That's partly because of cultural influences, Dr. Daviglus said, pointing to popular fatty foods such as refried beans and sour cream.

But environmental factors also play an important role. Both parents work in many Hispanic families, which means it can be hard to find time to prepare healthy meals, Dr. Daviglus said.

"Any family with two working parents may find that five dollars can get several hamburgers, but fruits and veggies are more expensive and take more time to prepare," she said. "It's an issue of time and money."

Watching portion size, even for seemingly healthy foods, is important as well.

Getting plenty of exercise is also important. The National Health and Nutrition Examination Survey reported that 65 percent of Mexican-American men and 74 percent of Mexican-American women did not participate in leisure-time physical activity.

Dr. Daviglus said many Hispanics find it difficult to exercise because they work multiple jobs, or they live in areas lacking in safe walking areas or health clubs. In such cases you have to try to be creative to squeeze in thirty minutes of daily physical activity.

"If you can't walk outside in your neighborhood, perhaps the area where you work is a safer choice," she said. "Perhaps there is a nearby park with an indoor or outdoor track that can provide a secure area for walking."

Diabetes Is Growing

An estimated 30 percent of adult Hispanics have diabetes, but as many as half don't realize it. Untreated, diabetes can lead to serious complications, including cardiovascular disease and renal failure.

The prevalence of diagnosed diabetes in Mexican-Americans and Puerto Ricans between the ages of twenty-four and seventy-four was 2.4 times greater than in non-Hispanic whites.

"We're seeing diabetes even in children and in much higher proportion than other communities," Dr. Daviglus said. A family history of diabetes can be an important red flag signaling increased risks, but many of the risks for type 2 diabetes can be lowered with lifestyle changes and proper medical care.

"Make every effort to make healthy lifestyle changes," Dr. Daviglus said. "Family history is important, but even if your parents or other family has diabetes, you can eat right and exercise and not get it."

Section 33.4

Things to Know about Cardiovascular Disease in Asian Americans

"Top Ten Things to Know: Cardiovascular Disease in Asian Americans," reprinted with permission from www.heart.org. © 2013 American Heart Association, Inc. All rights reserved.

1. Asian Americans are the fastest growing racial/ethnic group in the United States, representing 25 percent of all foreign-born people.

2. Asian Americans are projected to reach nearly thirty-four million by 2050.

3. Six subgroups of Asian Americans make up 90 percent of the Asian American population; the three largest Asian subgroups are Asian Indian, Chinese, and Filipino.

4. Major federal surveys have only recently started to classify Asian Americans into six subgroups and have added an additional category for a total of seven: Asian Indian, Chinese, Filipino, Korean, Japanese, Vietnamese, and Other Asian.

5. Although few studies of cardiovascular disease (CVD) have examined Asian American subgroups separately, limited data

on coronary artery disease (CAD) in Asian Americans strongly suggest that some subgroups are at increased risk.

6. Studies that have evaluated specific subgroups show higher rates of CAD in Asian Indians, higher rates of hemorrhagic stroke among Japanese and Chinese Americans, and more intracerebral hemorrhage in Filipino Americans.

7. Risk factors for Asian Americans differ from those for Caucasians; for example, body mass index (BMI) is normal at less than 25 for Caucasians, but among Asians normal BMI is less than 23.

8. Adoption of Western culture may result in unhealthy dietary and physical activity practices, which has been shown both in Asia and in the United States.

Section 33.5

Cardiovascular Disease among American Indians and Alaska Natives

Excerpted from "American Indian and Alaska Native Heart Disease and Stroke Fact Sheet," Centers for Disease Control and Prevention, January 17, 2012.

The American Indian and Alaska Native Population

- There are approximately 4.5 million American Indians and Alaska Natives in the United States, 1.5 percent of the population, including those of more than one race.

- The median age of American Indians and Alaska Natives is 30.7 years, which is younger than the 36.2 years of the total U.S. population.

- California has the largest population of American Indians and Alaska Natives (696,600), followed by Oklahoma (401,100), and Arizona (334,700). Alaska has the highest proportion of American Indians and Alaska Natives in its populations (20 percent), followed by Oklahoma and New Mexico (11 percent each). Los

Angeles County is the county with the most American Indians and Alaska Natives (154,000).

- A language other than English is spoken at home by 25 percent of American Indians and Alaska Natives aged five years and older.

- A high school diploma is held by 76 percent of American Indians and Alaska Natives over age twenty-five; 14 percent have a bachelor's degree or higher. The poverty rate of people who report American Indian and Alaska Native race only is 25 percent.

- Approximately 177,000 American Indians and Alaska Natives are veterans.

American Indian and Alaska Native Heart Disease and Stroke Facts

- Heart Disease is the first and stroke the sixth leading cause of death among American Indians and Alaska Natives.

- The heart disease death rate was 20 percent greater and the stroke death rate 14 percent greater among American Indians and Alaska Natives (1996–1998) than among all U.S. races (1997) after adjusting for misreporting of American Indian and Alaska Native race on state death certificates.

- The highest heart disease death rates are located primarily in South Dakota and North Dakota, Wisconsin, and Michigan.

- Counties with the highest stroke death rates are primarily in Alaska, Washington, Idaho, Montana, Wyoming, South Dakota, Wisconsin, and Minnesota.

- American Indians and Alaska Natives die from heart diseases at younger ages than other racial and ethnic groups in the United States. Thirty-six percent of those who die of heart disease die before age sixty-five.

- Diabetes is an extremely important risk factor for cardiovascular disease among American Indians.

- Cigarette smoking, a risk factor for heart disease and stroke, is highest in the Northern Plains (44.1 percent) and Alaska (39.0 percent) and lowest in the Southwest (21.2 percent) among American Indians and Alaska Natives.

Part Five

Diagnosing Cardiovascular Disorders

Chapter 34

Recognizing Signs and Symptoms of Heart Disease

What Are the Signs and Symptoms of Heart Disease

The signs and symptoms of coronary heart disease (CHD) may differ between women and men. Some women who have CHD have no signs or symptoms. This is called silent CHD.

Silent CHD may not be diagnosed until a woman has signs and symptoms of a heart attack, heart failure, or an arrhythmia (irregular heartbeat).

Other women who have CHD will have signs and symptoms of the disease.

A common symptom of CHD is angina. Angina is chest pain or discomfort that occurs when your heart muscle doesn't get enough oxygen-rich blood.

In men, angina often feels like pressure or squeezing in the chest. This feeling may extend to the arms. Women can also have these angina symptoms. But women also tend to describe a sharp, burning chest pain. Women are more likely to have pain in the neck, jaw, throat, abdomen, or back.

In men, angina tends to worsen with physical activity and go away with rest. Women are more likely than men to have angina while they're resting or sleeping.

Reprinted from "What Are the Signs and Symptoms of Heart Disease" and "How Is Heart Disease Diagnosed," National Heart, Lung, and Blood Institute, National Institutes of Health, September 26, 2011.

In women who have coronary microvascular disease, angina often occurs during routine daily activities, such as shopping or cooking, rather than while exercising. Mental stress also is more likely to trigger angina pain in women than in men.

The severity of angina varies. The pain may get worse or occur more often as the buildup of plaque continues to narrow the coronary (heart) arteries.

Signs and Symptoms of Coronary Heart Disease Complications

Heart attack: The most common heart attack symptom in men and women is chest pain or discomfort. However, only half of women who have heart attacks have chest pain.

Women are more likely than men to report back or neck pain, indigestion, heartburn, nausea (feeling sick to the stomach), vomiting, extreme fatigue (tiredness), or problems breathing.

Heart attacks also can cause upper body discomfort in one or both arms, the back, neck, jaw, or upper part of the stomach. Other heart attack symptoms are light-headedness and dizziness, which occur more often in women than men.

Men are more likely than women to break out in a cold sweat and to report pain in the left arm during a heart attack.

Heart failure: Heart failure is a condition in which your heart can't pump enough blood to meet your body's needs. Heart failure doesn't mean that your heart has stopped or is about to stop working. It means that your heart can't cope with the demands of everyday activities.

Heart failure causes shortness of breath and fatigue that tends to increase with physical exertion. Heart failure also can cause swelling in the feet, ankles, legs, abdomen, and veins in the neck.

Arrhythmia: An arrhythmia is a problem with the rate or rhythm of the heartbeat. During an arrhythmia, the heart can beat too fast, too slow, or with an irregular rhythm.

Some people describe arrhythmias as fluttering or thumping feelings or skipped beats in their chests. These feelings are called palpitations.

Some arrhythmias can cause your heart to suddenly stop beating. This condition is called sudden cardiac arrest (SCA).

SCA causes loss of consciousness and death if it's not treated right away.

Signs and Symptoms of Broken Heart Syndrome

The most common signs and symptoms of broken heart syndrome are chest pain and shortness of breath. In this disorder, these symptoms tend to occur suddenly in people who have no history of heart disease.

Arrhythmias or cardiogenic shock also may occur. Cardiogenic shock is a condition in which a suddenly weakened heart isn't able to pump enough blood to meet the body's needs.

Some of the signs and symptoms of broken heart syndrome differ from those of heart attack. For example, in people who have broken heart syndrome the following is true:

- Symptoms occur suddenly after having extreme emotional or physical stress.

- Electrocardiogram (EKG) results don't look the same as the EKG results for a person having a heart attack. (An EKG is a test that records the heart's electrical activity.)

- Blood tests show no signs or mild signs of heart damage.

- Tests show no signs of blockages in the coronary arteries.

- Tests show ballooning and unusual movement of the lower left heart chamber (left ventricle).

- Recovery time is quick, usually within days or weeks (compared with the recovery time of a month or more for a heart attack).

How Is Heart Disease Diagnosed?

Your doctor will diagnose coronary heart disease (CHD) based on your medical and family histories, your risk factors, a physical exam, and the results from tests and procedures.

No single test can diagnose CHD. If your doctor thinks you have CHD, he or she may recommend one or more of the following tests.

Electrocardiogram (EKG)

An EKG is a simple, painless test that detects and records the heart's electrical activity. The test shows how fast the heart is beating and its rhythm (steady or irregular). An EKG also records the strength and timing of electrical signals as they pass through the heart.

An EKG can show signs of heart damage due to CHD and signs of a previous or current heart attack.

367

Stress Testing

During stress testing, you exercise to make your heart work hard and beat fast while heart tests are done. If you can't exercise, you may be given medicines to increase your heart rate.

When your heart is working hard and beating fast, it needs more blood and oxygen. Plaque-narrowed coronary (heart) arteries can't supply enough oxygen-rich blood to meet your heart's needs.

A stress test can show possible signs and symptoms of CHD, such as the following:

- Abnormal changes in your heart rate or blood pressure

- Shortness of breath or chest pain

- Abnormal changes in your heart rhythm or your heart's electrical activity

If you can't exercise for as long as what is considered normal for someone your age, your heart may not be getting enough oxygen-rich blood. However, other factors also can prevent you from exercising long enough (for example, lung diseases, anemia, or poor general fitness).

As part of some stress tests, pictures are taken of your heart while you exercise and while you rest. These imaging stress tests can show how well blood is flowing in your heart and how well your heart pumps blood when it beats.

Echocardiography

Echocardiography (echo) uses sound waves to create a moving picture of your heart. The test provides information about the size and shape of your heart and how well your heart chambers and valves are working.

Echo also can show areas of poor blood flow to the heart, areas of heart muscle that aren't contracting normally, and previous injury to the heart muscle caused by poor blood flow.

Chest X-Ray

A chest x-ray creates pictures of the organs and structures inside your chest, such as your heart, lungs, and blood vessels.

A chest x-ray can reveal signs of heart failure, as well as lung disorders and other causes of symptoms not related to CHD.

Blood Tests

Blood tests check the levels of certain fats, cholesterol, sugar, and proteins in your blood. Abnormal levels may be a sign that you're at risk for CHD. Blood tests also help detect anemia, a risk factor for CHD.

During a heart attack, heart muscle cells die and release proteins into the bloodstream. Blood tests can measure the amount of these proteins in the bloodstream. High levels of these proteins are a sign of a recent heart attack.

Electron-Beam Computed Tomography

Electron-beam computed tomography (EBCT) is a test that looks for specks of calcium (called calcifications) in the walls of the coronary arteries. Calcifications are an early sign of CHD.

The test can show whether you're at increased risk for a heart attack or other heart problems before other signs and symptoms occur.

EBCT isn't routinely used to diagnose CHD because its accuracy isn't yet known.

Coronary Angiography and Cardiac Catheterization

Your doctor may recommend coronary angiography if other tests or factors suggest you have CHD. This test uses dye and special x-rays to look inside your coronary arteries.

To get the dye into your coronary arteries, your doctor will use a procedure called cardiac catheterization.

A thin, flexible tube called a catheter is put into a blood vessel in your arm, groin (upper thigh), or neck. The tube is threaded into your coronary arteries, and the dye is released into your bloodstream.

Special x-rays are taken while the dye is flowing through your coronary arteries. The dye lets your doctor study the flow of blood through your heart and blood vessels.

Coronary angiography detects blockages in the large coronary arteries. However, the test doesn't detect coronary microvascular disease (MVD). This is because coronary MVD doesn't cause blockages in the large coronary arteries.

Even if the results of your coronary angiography are normal, you may still have chest pain or other CHD symptoms. If so, talk with your doctor about whether you might have coronary MVD.

Your doctor may ask you to fill out a questionnaire called the Duke Activity Status Index. This questionnaire measures how easily you can do routine tasks. It gives your doctor information about how well blood is flowing through your coronary arteries.

Your doctor also may recommend other tests that measure blood flow in the heart, such as a cardiac magnetic resonance imaging (MRI) stress test.

Cardiac MRI uses radio waves, magnets, and a computer to create pictures of your heart as it beats. The test produces both still and moving pictures of your heart and major blood vessels.

Other tests done during cardiac catheterization can check blood flow in the heart's small arteries and the thickness of the artery walls.

Tests Used to Diagnose Broken Heart Syndrome

If your doctor thinks you have broken heart syndrome, he or she may recommend coronary angiography. Other tests are also used to diagnose this disorder, including blood tests, EKG, echo, and cardiac MRI.

Chapter 35

Blood Tests Used to Diagnose Cardiovascular Disorders

Chapter Contents

Section 35.1

Blood Tests Basics

Excerpted from "What Are Blood Tests?" National Heart, Lung, and
Blood Institute, National Institutes of Health, January 6, 2012.

What Are Blood Tests?

Blood tests help doctors check for certain diseases and conditions.
They also help check the function of your organs and show how well
treatments are working.

Specifically, blood tests can help doctors do the following things:

- Evaluate how well organs—such as the kidneys, liver, thyroid,
  and heart—are working

- Diagnose diseases and conditions such as cancer, human immunodeficiency virus (HIV)/acquired immunodeficiency syndrome
  (AIDS), diabetes, anemia, and coronary heart disease

- Find out whether you have risk factors for heart disease

- Check whether medicines you're taking are working

- Assess how well your blood is clotting

Types of Blood Tests

Some of the most common blood tests are as follows:

- A complete blood count (CBC)

- Blood chemistry tests

- Blood enzyme tests

- Blood tests to assess heart disease risk

- Blood clotting tests

Complete Blood Count

The CBC is one of the most common blood tests. It's often done as
part of a routine checkup.

The CBC can help detect blood diseases and disorders, such as anemia, infections, clotting problems, blood cancers, and immune system disorders. This test measures many parts of your blood, as discussed in the following paragraphs.

Red blood cells: Red blood cells carry oxygen from your lungs to the rest of your body. Abnormal red blood cell levels might be a sign of anemia, dehydration (too little fluid in the body), bleeding, or another disorder.

White blood cells: White blood cells are part of your immune system, which fights infections and diseases. Abnormal white blood cell levels might be a sign of infection, blood cancer, or an immune system disorder.

A CBC measures the overall number of white blood cells in your blood. A test called a CBC with differential can measure the amounts of different types of white blood cells in your blood.

Platelets: Platelets are blood cell fragments that help your blood clot. They stick together to seal cuts or breaks on blood vessel walls and stop bleeding.

Abnormal platelet levels might be a sign of a bleeding disorder (not enough clotting) or a thrombotic disorder (too much clotting).

Hemoglobin: Hemoglobin is an iron-rich protein in red blood cells that carries oxygen. Abnormal hemoglobin levels might be a sign of anemia, sickle cell anemia, thalassemia, or other blood disorders.

If you have diabetes, excess glucose (sugar) in your blood can attach to hemoglobin and raise the level of hemoglobin A1c.

Hematocrit: Hematocrit is a measure of how much space red blood cells take up in your blood. A high hematocrit level might mean you're dehydrated. A low hematocrit level might mean you have anemia. Abnormal hematocrit levels also might be a sign of a blood or bone marrow disorder.

Mean corpuscular volume: Mean corpuscular volume (MCV) is a measure of the average size of your red blood cells. Abnormal MCV levels might be a sign of anemia or thalassemia.

Blood Chemistry Tests/Basic Metabolic Panel

The basic metabolic panel (BMP) is a group of tests that measures different chemicals in the blood. These tests usually are done on the fluid (plasma) part of blood.

The BMP can give doctors information about your muscles (including the heart), bones, and organs (such as the kidneys and liver).

The BMP includes blood glucose, calcium, electrolyte, and kidney function tests. Some of these tests require you to fast (not eat any food) before the test, and others don't. Your doctor will tell you how to prepare for the test(s) you're having.

Blood glucose: Glucose is a type of sugar that the body uses for energy. Abnormal glucose levels in your blood might be a sign of diabetes.

For some blood glucose tests, you have to fast before your blood is drawn. Other blood glucose tests are done after a meal or at any time with no preparation.

Calcium: Calcium is an important mineral in the body. Abnormal calcium levels in the blood might suggest kidney problems, bone disease, thyroid disease, cancer, malnutrition, or another disorder.

Electrolytes: Electrolytes are minerals that help maintain fluid levels and acid-base balance in the body. They include sodium, potassium, bicarbonate, and chloride.

Abnormal electrolyte levels might be a sign of dehydration, kidney disease, liver disease, heart failure, high blood pressure, or other disorders.

Kidney function: Blood tests for kidney function measure levels of blood urea nitrogen (BUN) and creatinine. Both of these are waste products that the kidneys filter out of the body. Abnormal BUN and creatinine levels might suggest a kidney disease or disorder.

Blood Enzyme Tests

Enzymes help control chemical reactions in your body. There are many blood enzyme tests. This section focuses on blood enzyme tests used to help diagnose a heart attack. These tests include troponin and creatine kinase (CK) tests.

Troponin: Troponin is a protein that helps your muscles contract. When muscle or heart cells are injured, troponin leaks out, and its levels in your blood rise.

For example, blood levels of troponin rise when you have a heart attack. For this reason, doctors often order troponin tests when patients have chest pain or other heart attack signs and symptoms.

Creatine kinase: A blood product called CK-MB is released when the heart muscle is damaged. High levels of CK-MB in the blood can mean that you've had a heart attack.

Blood Tests to Assess Heart Disease Risk

A lipoprotein panel is a blood test that can help show whether you're at risk for coronary heart disease (CHD). This test looks at substances in your blood that carry cholesterol.

A lipoprotein panel gives information about the following things:

- Your total cholesterol.

- Your low-density lipoprotein (LDL, or "bad") cholesterol. This is the main source of cholesterol buildup and blockages in the arteries.

- Your high-density lipoprotein (HDL, or "good") cholesterol. This type of cholesterol helps decrease blockages in the arteries.

- Triglycerides. Triglycerides are a type of fat in your blood.

A lipoprotein panel measures the levels of LDL and HDL cholesterol and triglycerides in your blood. Abnormal cholesterol or triglyceride levels might be signs of increased risk of CHD.

Most people will need to fast for nine to twelve hours before a lipoprotein panel.

Blood Clotting Tests

Blood clotting tests sometimes are called a coagulation panel. These tests check proteins in your blood that affect the blood clotting process. Abnormal test results might suggest that you're at risk of bleeding or developing clots in your blood vessels.

Your doctor may recommend these tests if he or she thinks you have a disorder or disease related to blood clotting.

Blood clotting tests also are used to monitor people who are taking medicines to lower the risk of blood clots. Warfarin and heparin are two examples of such medicines.

What to Expect with Blood Tests

What to Expect Before Blood Tests

Many blood tests don't require any special preparation and take only a few minutes.

Other blood tests require fasting (not eating any food) for eight to twelve hours before the test. Your doctor will tell you how to prepare for your blood test(s).

What to Expect During Blood Tests

Blood usually is drawn from a vein in your arm or other part of your body using a needle. It also can be drawn using a finger prick.

The person who draws your blood might tie a band around the upper part of your arm or ask you to make a fist. Doing this can make the veins in your arm stick out more, which makes it easier to insert the needle.

The needle that goes into your vein is attached to a small test tube. The person who draws your blood removes the tube when it's full, and the tube seals on its own. The needle is then removed from your vein.

If you're getting a few blood tests, more than one test tube might be attached to the needle before it's withdrawn.

Some people get nervous about blood tests because they're afraid of needles. Others don't want to see blood leaving their bodies.

If you're nervous or scared, it can help to look away or talk to someone to distract yourself. You might feel a slight sting when the needle goes in or comes out.

Drawing blood usually takes only a few minutes.

What to Expect After Blood Tests

When the needle is withdrawn, you'll be asked to apply gentle pressure with a piece of gauze or bandage to the site. This stops bleeding and helps prevent swelling and bruising.

Most of the time, you can remove the pressure after a minute or two. You may want to keep a bandage on for a few hours.

Usually, you don't need to do anything else after a blood test. Results can take anywhere from a few minutes to a few weeks to come back. Your doctor will get the results. It's important that you follow up with your doctor to discuss your test results.

What Are the Risks of Blood Tests?

The main risks of blood tests are discomfort and bruising at the site where the needle is inserted. These issues usually are minor and go away shortly after the tests are done.

What Do Blood Tests Show?

Blood tests show whether the levels of different substances in your blood fall within a normal range.

For many blood substances, the normal range is the range of levels seen in 95 percent of healthy people in a certain group. For many tests, normal ranges vary depending on your age, gender, race, and other factors.

Your blood test results may fall outside the normal range for many reasons. Abnormal results might be a sign of a disorder or disease. Other factors—such as diet, menstrual cycle, physical activity level, alcohol intake, and medicines (both prescription and over the counter)—also can cause abnormal results.

Your doctor should discuss any unusual or abnormal blood test results with you. These results may or may not suggest a health problem.

Many diseases and medical problems can't be diagnosed with blood tests alone. However, blood tests can help you and your doctor learn more about your health. Blood tests also can help find potential problems early, when treatments or lifestyle changes may work best.

Section 35.2

Cardiac Biomarker Tests

What Are Cardiac Biomarkers?

Cardiac biomarkers are substances that are released into the blood when the heart is damaged or stressed. Measurement of these biomarkers is used to help diagnose, risk stratify, monitor, and manage people with suspected acute coronary syndrome (ACS) and cardiac ischemia. The symptoms of ACS and cardiac ischemia can vary greatly but frequently include chest pain, pressure, nausea, and/or shortness of breath. These symptoms are associated with heart attacks and angina, but they may also be seen with non-heart-related conditions. Increases in one or more cardiac biomarkers can identify people with ACS or cardiac ischemia, allowing rapid and accurate diagnosis and appropriate treatment of their condition.

ACS is caused by rupture of a plaque that results from atherosclerosis. Plaque rupture causes blood clot (thrombus) formation in coronary arteries, which results in a sudden decrease in the amount of blood and oxygen reaching the heart. Cardiac ischemia is caused when the supply of blood reaching heart tissue is not enough to meet the heart's needs. The root causes of both ACS and cardiac ischemia are usually atherosclerosis and buildup of plaque, resulting in severe narrowing of the coronary arteries or a sudden blockage of blood flow through these arteries. Angina is caused by a decrease in the supply of blood to the heart. When blood flow to the heart is blocked or significantly reduced for a longer period of time (usually for more than thirty to sixty minutes), it can cause heart cells to die and is called an acute myocardial infarction (AMI or heart attack). This leads to death of the affected portion of heart muscle with permanent damage and scarring of the heart and sometimes can cause sudden death to the person.

Cardiac biomarker tests are ordered to help detect the presence of ACS and cardiac ischemia and to evaluate their severity as soon as possible so that appropriate therapy can be initiated. It is important to distinguish heart attacks from angina, heart failure, or other conditions that may have similar signs and symptoms because the treatments and monitoring requirements are different. For heart attacks, prompt medical intervention is crucial to minimize heart damage and future complications. Cardiac biomarker tests must be available to the doctor twenty-four hours a day, seven days a week with a rapid turnaround-time. Some of the tests may be performed at the point of care (POC)—in the emergency room or at the person's bedside. Serial testing of one or more cardiac biomarkers is necessary to ensure that a rise in blood levels is not missed and to estimate the severity of a heart attack.

Only a few cardiac biomarker tests are routinely used by physicians. The current biomarker test of choice for detecting heart damage is troponin. Other cardiac biomarkers are less specific for the heart and may be elevated in skeletal muscle injury, liver disease, or kidney disease. Many other potential cardiac biomarkers are being researched, but their clinical utility has yet to be established.

Laboratory Tests

Current cardiac biomarker tests used to help diagnose, evaluate, and monitor individuals suspected of having acute coronary syndrome (ACS) include:

- troponin I or T;
- creatine kinase (CK);

- CK-MB.

Other biomarker tests that may be used:

- myoglobin;
- B-type natriuretic peptide (BNP, or N-terminal pro b-type natriuretic peptide [NT-proBNP])—although usually used to recognize heart failure, an increased level in people with ACS indicates an increased risk of recurrent events;
- high-sensitivity C-reactive protein (hs-CRP).

Phased out biomarkers—the tests below are not specific for damage to the heart and are no longer recommended for evaluating people with suspected ACS:

- Aspartate aminotransferase (AST)
- Lactate dehydrogenase (LDH)

More general tests frequently ordered along with cardiac biomarkers include:

- blood gases;
- comprehensive metabolic panel (CMP);
- basic metabolic panel (BMP);
- electrolytes;
- complete blood count (CBC).

Nonlaboratory Tests

These tests allow doctors to look at the size, shape, and function of the heart as it is beating. They can be used to detect changes to the rhythm of the heart as well as to detect and evaluate damaged tissues and blocked arteries:

- Electrocardiogram (EKG, ECG)
- Nuclear scan
- Coronary angiography (or arteriography)
- Echocardiogram (Cardiac echo, transthoracic echocardiography [TTE])
- Stress testing

- Chest x-ray

Summary Tables

Tables 35.1 and 35.2 summarize currently used cardiac biomarkers.

Table 35.1. Cardiac Biomarker Tests

Marker	What It Is	Tissue Source	Reason for Increase	Time to Increase	Time Back to Normal	When/How Used
Cardiac Troponin	Regulatory protein complex; two cardiac-specific isoforms: T and I	Heart	Injury to heart	2 to 8 hours	Remains elevated for 7 to 14 days	Diagnose heart attack, risk stratification, assist in deciding management, assess degree of damage
CK	Enzyme; total of three different isoenzymes	Heart, brain, and skeletal muscle	Injury to skeletal muscle and/or heart cells	4 to 6 hours after injury, peaks in 18 to 24 hours	48 to 72 hours, unless due to continuing injury	Frequently performed in combination with CK-MB
CK-MB	Heart-related isoenzymes of CK	Heart primarily, but also in skeletal muscle	Injury to heart and/or muscle cells	4 to 6 hours after heart attack, peaks in 12 to 20 hours	24 to 48 hours, unless new or continuing damage	Less specific than troponin, may be ordered when troponin is not available
Myoglobin	Oxygen-storing protein	Heart and other muscle cells	Injury to muscle and/or heart cells	2 to 3 hours after injury, peaks in 8 to 12 hours	Within one day after injury	Used less frequently; sometimes performed with troponin to provide early diagnosis

Table 35.2. Biomarker Tests Used for Prognosis

Biomarker	What It Is	Reason for Increase	When/How Used
hs-CRP	Protein	Inflammation	May help determine risk of future cardiac events in those patients who have had a heart attack
BNP and NT-proBNP	Heart hormone	Heart failure; increased risk of another heart attack	Usually used to recognize heart failure, but an increased level in people with ACS indicates an increased risk of recurrent events

Cardiac biomarker tests: Tests [listed in Table 35.1] are used to help diagnose, evaluate, and monitor people suspected of having acute coronary syndrome (ACS).

Biomarker tests used for prognosis: Tests [listed in Table 35.2] may be used to evaluate risk of future cardiac events.

Section 35.3

C-Reactive Protein Test

"C-Reactive Protein (CRP) Test," reprinted with permission from www.SecondsCount.org. Copyright © 2013 Society for Cardiovascular Angiography and Interventions. All rights reserved.

A high-sensitivity C-reactive protein (HS-CRP) test measures levels of CRP in the bloodstream. CRP is a protein that is released when inflammation is present in the body. Inflammation of the arteries is a risk factor for cardiovascular disease, and CRP may be a predictor of risk for heart attack, stroke, or other cardiovascular problems. An elevated CRP may confer additional predictive value to your other cardiac risk factors.

A high-sensitivity CRP test is better at assessing heart disease than a general CRP test. In either case, inflammation elsewhere in the body can be due to an infection or other illness. Results from an HS-CRP test should be considered in conjunction with symptom evaluation and the results of other tests.

How does it work?

Your blood will be drawn and sent to a lab for analysis. The amount of C-reactive protein in your blood will be measured. The test results will be communicated back to your physician.

How is it performed?

A CRP test is like any other blood test. Having blood drawn typically only takes a few minutes. You will be asked to roll up your shirt

381

sleeve (if necessary) and the medical professional who will be drawing the blood will swab the area where the needle will be inserted with an alcohol wipe. A rubber tube may be tied around the upper part of your arm, or you may be asked to make a fist, to make the veins stand out more and easier to access.

A needle attached to a small test tube will be inserted into your vein and blood will begin to flow into the tube. When a sample that is appropriate for the test has been gathered, the needle will be removed, and you may be asked to press on a piece of gauze placed over the insertion site. This pressure will help stop any bleeding from the tiny puncture site. A bandage will then be placed over the site where the needle was inserted.

Your blood sample will then be sent to lab technicians for analysis. You will receive information when you have the blood test as to when you can expect results.

Is it safe?

Having blood drawn by a qualified medical professional is very safe. You will experience momentary pain when the needle is inserted, and you may experience bruising at the needle insertion site after the test is complete. If you have an allergy to latex or to any adhesives, let the person who is drawing the blood know, so he or she can make any necessary adjustments.

Questions to Ask Your Doctor about C-reactive Protein Tests

The following questions can help you talk to your physician about a C-reactive protein test. Write down these questions and take them with you to your appointment. Taking notes can help you remember your physician's response when you get home.

Questions to ask:

- Am I at high risk for heart disease?

- What will the CRP test results tell us about my cardiovascular health?

- How accurate is a CRP test?

- What comes next if the test finds inflammation?

Section 35.4

Homocysteine Test

Reprinted from "Homocysteine Test." The information in this chapter is from the U.S. Department of Health and Human Services, Office on Women's Health, 2013. For additional information, visit www.womenshealth.gov or www.hearthealthywomen.org.

What is homocysteine?

Homocysteine is a chemical found in the blood that is produced when the amino acid methionine (a building block for proteins) is broken down. High levels are linked to an increased risk of heart disease.

Who might have a homocysteine test?

Homocystcine testing may be useful if you or a family member have heart or blood vessel disease, but do not have any of the well-established risk factors such as smoking, high blood cholesterol, high blood pressure, obesity, or diabetes.

What does the homocysteine test entail?

Homocysteine is measured through a routine blood test. It is not widely available, costs about $100.00, and is not currently covered by insurance. More rarely, your health care provider may order a methionine-load test, which measures homocysteine before and after you swallow 100 mg/kg of methionine (dissolved in orange juice). This test can diagnose homocysteine abnormalities in people at high risk for heart disease who have normal homocysteine levels when tested with the routine blood test.

What do the results of a homocysteine test mean?

If you have high homocysteine levels, you have a higher risk of heart attack, stroke, and developing blood clots in the arteries and veins in the legs. However, there is no treatment plan for high homocysteine levels, since it has not been shown that lowering homocysteine cuts down your heart disease risk.[1]

Table 35.3. Homocysteine Blood Levels[1]

Fasting Plasma Homocysteine Level (micromoles per liter of blood)	
Normal	5–15
Moderately high	16–30
Intermediately high	31–100
Severely high	>100

Reference

1. Malinow MR, Bostom AG, Krauss RM. Homocyst(e)ine, diet, and cardiovascular diseases: a statement for healthcare professionals from the Nutrition Committee, American Heart Association. *Circulation*. Jan 5–12 1999; 99(1):178–82.

Section 35. 5

Troponin Test

The Test Sample

What Is Being Tested?

The troponins are a family of proteins found in skeletal and heart muscle (cardiac) fibers. There are three different types: troponin C (TnC), troponin T (TnT), and troponin I (TnI). Together, these three proteins regulate muscular contraction.

Cardiac-specific troponins I and T (cTnI and cTnT) are troponins that are found only in the heart. They are normally present in very small to undetectable quantities in the blood. When there is damage to heart muscle cells, cardiac-specific troponins I and T are released into circulation. The more damage there is, the greater their concentration in the blood. The troponin test measures the amount of cardiac-specific troponin I or T in the blood and is used to help determine if an individual has suffered a heart attack.

When a person has a heart attack, levels of cardiac-specific troponins I and T can become elevated in the blood within three or four hours after injury and may remain elevated for ten to fourteen days.

How Is the Sample Collected for Testing?

A blood sample is taken by needle from a vein in the arm.

Is Any Test Preparation Needed to Ensure the Quality of the Sample?

No test preparation is needed.

The Test

How Is It Used?

Troponin tests are primarily ordered to evaluate people who have chest pain to see if they have had a heart attack or other damage to their heart. Either a cardiac-specific troponin I or troponin T test can be performed; usually a laboratory will offer one test or the other. Troponin tests are sometimes ordered along with other cardiac biomarkers, such as CK-MB or myoglobin. However, troponins are the preferred tests for a suspected heart attack because they are more specific for heart injury than other tests (which may become positive in skeletal muscle injury) and remain elevated for a longer period of time.

The troponin test is used to help diagnose a heart attack, to detect and evaluate mild to severe heart injury, and to distinguish chest pain that may be due to other causes. In those who experience heart-related chest pain, discomfort, or other symptoms and do not seek medical attention for a day or more, the troponin test will still be positive if the symptoms are due to heart damage.

When Is It Ordered?

A cardiac-specific troponin I or T test will usually be ordered when a person with a suspected heart attack first comes into the emergency room, followed by a series of troponin tests performed over several hours. It is sometimes ordered along with other tests such as CK, CK-MB, or myoglobin.

In people with stable angina, a troponin test may be ordered when:

- symptoms worsen;
- symptoms occur when a person is at rest;
- symptoms are no longer eased with treatment.

These are all signs that the angina is becoming unstable, which increases the risk of a heart attack or other serious heart problem in the near future.

What Does the Test Result Mean?

Because troponin is specific to the heart, even slight elevations may indicate some degree of damage to the heart. When a person has significantly elevated troponin levels and, in particular, a rise or fall in the results from a series of tests done over several hours, then it is likely that the person has had a heart attack or some other form of damage to the heart.

When someone with chest pain and/or known stable angina has normal troponin values in a series of measurements over several hours, then it is unlikely that their heart has been injured.

Troponin values can remain high for one to two weeks after a heart attack. The test is not affected by damage to other muscles, so injections, accidents, and drugs that can damage muscle do not affect cardiac troponin levels. Troponin may rise following strenuous exercise, although in the absence of signs and symptoms of heart disease, it is usually of no medical significance.

Is There Anything Else I Should Know?

Increased troponin concentrations should not be used by themselves to diagnose or rule out a heart attack. A physical exam, clinical history, and ECG are also important, as is whether the troponin levels from a series of tests are stably elevated or show a rise or fall over several hours. Very rarely, people who have a heart attack will have normal troponin concentrations, and some people with increased troponin concentrations have no apparent heart injury. Troponin levels may also be elevated with acute or chronic conditions such as myocarditis (heart inflammation), congestive heart failure, severe infections, kidney disease, and certain chronic inflammatory conditions of muscles and skin.

Chapter 36

Electrocardiogram (EKG)

What Is an Electrocardiogram?

An electrocardiogram, also called an EKG or ECG, is a simple, painless test that records the heart's electrical activity. To understand this test, it helps to understand how the heart works.

With each heartbeat, an electrical signal spreads from the top of the heart to the bottom. As it travels, the signal causes the heart to contract and pump blood. The process repeats with each new heartbeat.

The heart's electrical signals set the rhythm of the heartbeat.

An EKG shows the following things:

- How fast your heart is beating

- Whether the rhythm of your heartbeat is steady or irregular

- The strength and timing of electrical signals as they pass through each part of your heart

Doctors use EKGs to detect and study many heart problems, such as heart attacks, arrhythmias, and heart failure. The test's results also can suggest other disorders that affect heart function.

Other Names for an Electrocardiogram

An electrocardiogram also is called an EKG or ECG. Sometimes the test is called a twelve-lead EKG or twelve-lead ECG. This is because

"What Is an Electrocardiogram?" National Heart, Lung, and Blood Institute, National Institutes of Health, October 1, 2010.

the heart's electrical activity most often is recorded from twelve different places on the body at the same time.

Who Needs an Electrocardiogram?

Your doctor may recommend an electrocardiogram (EKG) if you have signs or symptoms that suggest a heart problem. Examples of such signs and symptoms include the following:

- Chest pain

- Heart pounding, racing, or fluttering, or the sense that your heart is beating unevenly

- Breathing problems

- Tiredness and weakness

- Unusual heart sounds when your doctor listens to your heartbeat

You may need to have more than one EKG so your doctor can diagnose certain heart conditions.

An EKG also may be done as part of a routine health exam. The test can screen for early heart disease that has no symptoms. Your doctor is more likely to look for early heart disease if your mother, father, brother, or sister had heart disease—especially early in life.

You may have an EKG so your doctor can check how well heart medicine or a medical device, such as a pacemaker, is working. The test also may be used for routine screening before major surgery.

Your doctor also may use EKG results to help plan your treatment for a heart condition.

What to Expect Before an Electrocardiogram

You don't need to take any special steps before having an electrocardiogram (EKG). However, tell your doctor or his or her staff about the medicines you're taking. Some medicines can affect EKG results.

What to Expect During an Electrocardiogram

An electrocardiogram (EKG) is painless and harmless. A nurse or technician will attach soft, sticky patches called electrodes to the skin of your chest, arms, and legs. The patches are about the size of a quarter.

Often, twelve patches are attached to your body. This helps detect your heart's electrical activity from many areas at the same time. The nurse may have to shave areas of your skin to help the patches stick.

After the patches are placed on your skin, you'll lie still on a table while the patches detect your heart's electrical signals. A machine will record these signals on graph paper or display them on a screen.

The entire test will take about ten minutes.

Special Types of Electrocardiogram

The standard EKG described above, called a resting twelve-lead EKG, only records seconds of heart activity at a time. It will show a heart problem only if the problem occurs during the test.

Many heart problems are present all the time, and a resting twelve-lead EKG will detect them. But some heart problems, like those related to an irregular heartbeat, can come and go. They may occur for only a few minutes a day or only while you exercise.

Doctors use special EKGs, such as stress tests and Holter and event monitors, to help diagnose these kinds of problems.

Stress test: Some heart problems are easier to diagnose when your heart is working hard and beating fast. During stress testing, you exercise to make your heart work hard and beat fast while an EKG is done. If you can't exercise, you'll be given medicine to make your heart work hard and beat fast.

Holter and event monitors: Holter and event monitors are small, portable devices. They record your heart's electrical activity while you do your normal daily activities. A Holter monitor records your heart's electrical activity for a full twenty-four- or forty-eight-hour period.

An event monitor records your heart's electrical activity only at certain times while you're wearing it. For many event monitors, you push a button to start the monitor when you feel symptoms. Other event monitors start automatically when they sense abnormal heart rhythms.

What to Expect After an Electrocardiogram

After an electrocardiogram (EKG), the nurse or technician will remove the electrodes (soft patches) from your skin. You may develop a rash or redness where the EKG patches were attached. This mild rash often goes away without treatment.

You usually can go back to your normal daily routine after an EKG.

What Does an Electrocardiogram Show?

Many heart problems change the heart's electrical activity in distinct ways. An electrocardiogram (EKG) can help detect these heart problems.

EKG recordings can help doctors diagnose heart attacks that are in progress or have happened in the past. This is especially true if doctors can compare a current EKG recording to an older one.

An EKG also can show the following things:

- Lack of blood flow to the heart muscle (coronary heart disease)

- A heartbeat that's too fast, too slow, or irregular (arrhythmia)

- A heart that doesn't pump forcefully enough (heart failure)

- Heart muscle that's too thick or parts of the heart that are too big (cardiomyopathy)

- Birth defects in the heart (congenital heart defects)

- Problems with the heart valves (heart valve disease)

- Inflammation of the sac that surrounds the heart (pericarditis)

An EKG can reveal whether the heartbeat starts in the correct place in the heart. The test also shows how long it takes for electrical signals to travel through the heart. Delays in signal travel time may suggest heart block or long QT syndrome.

What Are the Risks of an Electrocardiogram?

An electrocardiogram (EKG) has no serious risks. It's a harmless, painless test that detects the heart's electrical activity. EKGs don't give off electrical charges, such as shocks.

You may develop a mild rash where the electrodes (soft patches) were attached. This rash often goes away without treatment.

Chapter 37

Echocardiography

What Is Echocardiography?

Echocardiography, or echo, is a painless test that uses sound waves to create moving pictures of your heart. The pictures show the size and shape of your heart. They also show how well your heart's chambers and valves are working.

Echo also can pinpoint areas of heart muscle that aren't contracting well because of poor blood flow or injury from a previous heart attack. A type of echo called Doppler ultrasound shows how well blood flows through your heart's chambers and valves.

Echo can detect possible blood clots inside the heart, fluid buildup in the pericardium (the sac around the heart), and problems with the aorta. The aorta is the main artery that carries oxygen-rich blood from your heart to your body.

Doctors also use echo to detect heart problems in infants and children.

Who Needs Echocardiography?

Your doctor may recommend echocardiography (echo) if you have signs or symptoms of heart problems.

Excerpted from "What Is Echocardiography?" National Heart, Lung, and Blood Institute, National Institutes of Health, October 31, 2011.

For example, shortness of breath and swelling in the legs are possible signs of heart failure. Heart failure is a condition in which your heart can't pump enough oxygen-rich blood to meet your body's needs. Echo can show how well your heart is pumping blood.

Echo also can help your doctor find the cause of abnormal heart sounds, such as heart murmurs. Heart murmurs are extra or unusual sounds heard during the heartbeat. Some heart murmurs are harmless, while others are signs of heart problems.

Your doctor also may use echo to learn about the following things:

- **The size of your heart:** An enlarged heart might be the result of high blood pressure, leaky heart valves, or heart failure. Echo also can detect increased thickness of the ventricles (the heart's lower chambers). Increased thickness may be due to high blood pressure, heart valve disease, or congenital heart defects.

- **Heart muscles that are weak and aren't pumping well:** Damage from a heart attack may cause weak areas of heart muscle. Weakening also might mean that the area isn't getting enough blood supply, a sign of coronary heart disease.

- **Heart valve problems:** Echo can show whether any of your heart valves don't open normally or close tightly.

- **Problems with your heart's structure:** Echo can detect congenital heart defects, such as holes in the heart. Congenital heart defects are structural problems present at birth. Infants and children may have echo to detect these heart defects.

- **Blood clots or tumors:** If you've had a stroke, you may have echo to check for blood clots or tumors that could have caused the stroke.

Your doctor also might recommend echo to see how well your heart responds to certain heart treatments, such as those used for heart failure.

Types of Echocardiography

There are several types of echocardiography (echo)—all use sound waves to create moving pictures of your heart. This is the same technology that allows doctors to see an unborn baby inside a pregnant woman.

Unlike x-rays and some other tests, echo doesn't involve radiation.

Transthoracic Echocardiography

Transthoracic echo is the most common type of echocardiogram test. It's painless and noninvasive. "Noninvasive" means that no surgery is done and no instruments are inserted into your body.

This type of echo involves placing a device called a transducer on your chest. The device sends special sound waves, called ultrasound, through your chest wall to your heart. The human ear can't hear ultrasound waves.

As the ultrasound waves bounce off the structures of your heart, a computer in the echo machine converts them into pictures on a screen.

Stress Echocardiography

Stress echo is done as part of a stress test. During a stress test, you exercise or take medicine (given by your doctor) to make your heart work hard and beat fast. A technician will use echo to create pictures of your heart before you exercise and as soon as you finish.

Some heart problems, such as coronary heart disease, are easier to diagnose when the heart is working hard and beating fast.

Transesophageal Echocardiography

Your doctor may have a hard time seeing the aorta and other parts of your heart using a standard transthoracic echo. Thus, he or she may recommend transesophageal echo, or TEE.

During this test, the transducer is attached to the end of a flexible tube. The tube is guided down your throat and into your esophagus (the passage leading from your mouth to your stomach). This allows your doctor to get more detailed pictures of your heart.

Fetal Echocardiography

Fetal echo is used to look at an unborn baby's heart. A doctor may recommend this test to check a baby for heart problems. When recommended, the test is commonly done at about eighteen to twenty-two weeks of pregnancy. For this test, the transducer is moved over the pregnant woman's belly.

Three-Dimensional Echocardiography

A three-dimensional (3D) echo creates 3D images of your heart. These detailed images show how your heart looks and works.

During transthoracic echo or TEE, 3D images can be taken as part of the process used to do these types of echo.

Doctors may use 3D echo to diagnose heart problems in children. They also may use 3D echo for planning and overseeing heart valve surgery.

Researchers continue to study new ways to use 3D echo.

Other Names for Echocardiography

- Echo

- Surface echo

- Ultrasound of the heart

What to Expect Before Echocardiography

Echocardiography (echo) is done in a doctor's office or a hospital. No special preparations are needed for most types of echo. You usually can eat, drink, and take any medicines as you normally would.

The exception is if you're having a transesophageal echo. This test usually requires that you don't eat or drink for eight hours prior to the test.

If you're having a stress echo, you may need to take steps to prepare for the stress test. Your doctor will let you know what steps you need to take.

What to Expect During Echocardiography

Echocardiography (echo) is painless; the test usually takes less than an hour to do. For some types of echo, your doctor will need to inject saline or a special dye into one of your veins. The substance makes your heart show up more clearly on the echo pictures.

The dye used for echo is different from the dye used during angiography (a test used to examine the body's blood vessels).

For most types of echo, you will remove your clothing from the waist up. Women will be given a gown to wear during the test. You'll lie on your back or left side on an exam table or stretcher.

Soft, sticky patches called electrodes will be attached to your chest to allow an EKG (electrocardiogram) to be done. An EKG is a test that records the heart's electrical activity.

A doctor or sonographer (a person specially trained to do ultrasounds) will apply gel to your chest. The gel helps the sound waves reach your heart. A wand-like device called a transducer will then be moved around on your chest.

The transducer transmits ultrasound waves into your chest. A computer will convert echoes from the sound waves into pictures of your heart on a screen. During the test, the lights in the room will be dimmed so the computer screen is easier to see.

The sonographer will record pictures of various parts of your heart. He or she will put the recordings on a computer disc for a cardiologist (heart specialist) to review.

During the test, you may be asked to change positions or hold your breath for a short time. This allows the sonographer to get better pictures of your heart.

At times, the sonographer may apply a bit of pressure to your chest with the transducer. You may find this pressure a little uncomfortable, but it helps get the best picture of your heart. You should let the sonographer know if you feel too uncomfortable.

The process described above is similar to the process for fetal echo. For that test, however, the transducer is placed over the pregnant woman's belly at the location of the baby's heart.

Transesophageal Echocardiography

Transesophageal echo (TEE) is used if your doctor needs a more detailed view of your heart. For example, your doctor may use TEE to look for blood clots in your heart. A doctor, not a sonographer, will perform this type of echo.

TEE uses the same technology as transthoracic echo, but the transducer is attached to the end of a flexible tube.

Your doctor will guide the tube down your throat and into your esophagus (the passage leading from your mouth to your stomach). From this angle, your doctor can get a more detailed image of the heart and major blood vessels leading to and from the heart.

For TEE, you'll likely be given medicine to help you relax during the test. The medicine will be injected into one of your veins.

Your blood pressure, the oxygen content of your blood, and other vital signs will be checked during the test. You'll be given oxygen through a tube in your nose. If you wear dentures or partials, you'll have to remove them.

The back of your mouth will be numbed with gel or spray. Your doctor will gently place the tube with the transducer in your throat and guide it down until it's in place behind your heart.

The pictures of your heart are then recorded as your doctor moves the transducer around in your esophagus and stomach. You shouldn't feel any discomfort as this happens.

Although the imaging usually takes less than an hour, you may be watched for a few hours at the doctor's office or hospital after the test.

Stress Echocardiography

Stress echo is a transthoracic echo combined with either an exercise or pharmacological stress test.

For an exercise stress test, you'll walk or run on a treadmill or pedal a stationary bike to make your heart work hard and beat fast. For a pharmacological stress test, you'll be given medicine to increase your heart rate.

A technician will take pictures of your heart using echo before you exercise and as soon as you finish.

What You May See and Hear During Echocardiography

As the doctor or sonographer moves the transducer around, you will see different views of your heart on the screen of the echo machine. The structures of your heart will appear as white objects, while any fluid or blood will appear black on the screen.

Doppler ultrasound often is used during echo tests. Doppler ultrasound is a special ultrasound that shows how blood is flowing through the blood vessels.

This test allows the sonographer to see blood flowing at different speeds and in different directions. The speed and direction of blood flow appear as different colors moving within the black and white images.

The human ear is unable to hear the sound waves used in echo. If you have a Doppler ultrasound, you may be able to hear "whooshing" sounds. Your doctor can use these sounds to learn about blood flow through your heart.

What to Expect after Echocardiography

You usually can go back to your normal activities right after having echocardiography (echo).

If you have a transesophageal echo (TEE), you may be watched for a few hours at the doctor's office or hospital after the test. Your throat might be sore for a few hours after the test.

You also may not be able to drive for a short time after having TEE. Your doctor will let you know whether you need to arrange for a ride home.

What Does Echocardiography Show?

Echocardiography (echo) shows the size, structure, and movement of various parts of your heart. These parts include the heart valves, the septum (the wall separating the right and left heart chambers), and the walls of the heart chambers. Doppler ultrasound shows the movement of blood through your heart.

Your doctor may use echo to do the following things:

- Diagnose heart problems

- Guide or determine next steps for treatment

- Monitor changes and improvement

- Determine the need for more tests

Echo can detect many heart problems. Some might be minor and pose no risk to you. Others can be signs of serious heart disease or other heart conditions. Your doctor may use echo to learn about the following things:

- **The size of your heart:** An enlarged heart might be the result of high blood pressure, leaky heart valves, or heart failure. Echo also can detect increased thickness of the ventricles (the heart's lower chambers). Increased thickness may be due to high blood pressure, heart valve disease, or congenital heart defects.

- **Heart muscles that are weak and aren't pumping well:** Damage from a heart attack may cause weak areas of heart muscle. Weakening also might mean that the area isn't getting enough blood supply, a sign of coronary heart disease.

- **Heart valve problems:** Echo can show whether any of your heart valves don't open normally or close tightly.

- **Problems with your heart's structure:** Echo can detect congenital heart defects, such as holes in the heart. Congenital heart defects are structural problems present at birth. Infants and children may have echo to detect these heart defects.

- **Blood clots or tumors:** If you've had a stroke, you may have echo to check for blood clots or tumors that could have caused the stroke.

What Are the Risks of Echocardiography?

Transthoracic and fetal echocardiography (echo) have no risks. These tests are safe for adults, children, and infants.

If you have a transesophageal echo (TEE), some risks are associated with the medicine given to help you relax. For example, you may have a bad reaction to the medicine, problems breathing, and nausea (feeling sick to your stomach).

Your throat also might be sore for a few hours after the test. Rarely, the tube used during TEE causes minor throat injuries.

Stress echo has some risks, but they're related to the exercise or medicine used to raise your heart rate, not the echo. Serious complications from stress tests are very uncommon.

Chapter 38

Carotid Ultrasound

What Is Carotid Ultrasound?

Carotid ultrasound is a painless and harmless test that uses high-frequency sound waves to create pictures of the insides of your carotid arteries.

You have two common carotid arteries, one on each side of your neck. They each divide into internal and external carotid arteries.

The internal carotid arteries supply oxygen-rich blood to your brain. The external carotid arteries supply oxygen-rich blood to your face, scalp, and neck.

Other Names for Carotid Ultrasound

- Doppler ultrasound
- Carotid duplex ultrasound

Who Needs Carotid Ultrasound?

A carotid ultrasound shows whether you have plaque buildup in your carotid arteries. Over time, plaque can harden or rupture (break open). This can reduce or block the flow of oxygen-rich blood to your brain and cause a stroke.

Excerpted from "What Is Carotid Ultrasound?" National Heart, Lung, and Blood Institute, National Institutes of Health, February 3, 2012.

Your doctor may recommend a carotid ultrasound if you:

- Had a stroke or mini-stroke recently. During a mini-stroke, you may have some or all of the symptoms of a stroke. However, the symptoms usually go away on their own within twenty-four hours.

- Have an abnormal sound called a carotid bruit in one of your carotid arteries. Your doctor can hear a carotid bruit using a stethoscope. A bruit might suggest a partial blockage in your carotid artery, which could lead to a stroke.

Your doctor also may recommend a carotid ultrasound if he or she thinks you have either of the following:

- Blood clots in one of your carotid arteries.

- A split between the layers of your carotid artery wall. The split can weaken the wall or reduce blood flow to your brain.

A carotid ultrasound also might be done to see whether carotid artery surgery, also called carotid endarterectomy, has restored normal blood flow through a carotid artery.

If you have a procedure called carotid stenting, your doctor might use carotid ultrasound afterward to check the position of the stent in your carotid artery. (The stent, a small mesh tube, supports the inner artery wall.)

Carotid ultrasound sometimes is used as a preventive screening test in people at increased risk of stroke, such as those who have high blood pressure and diabetes.

What to Expect Before Carotid Ultrasound

Carotid ultrasound is a painless test. Typically, there is little to do in advance of the test. Your doctor will tell you how to prepare for your carotid ultrasound.

What to Expect During Carotid Ultrasound

Carotid ultrasound usually is done in a doctor's office or hospital. The test is painless and often doesn't take more than thirty minutes.

The ultrasound machine includes a computer, a screen, and a transducer. The transducer is a hand-held device that sends and receives ultrasound waves.

You will lie on your back on an exam table for the test. Your technician or doctor will put gel on your neck where your carotid arteries are located. The gel helps the ultrasound waves reach the arteries.

Your technician or doctor will put the transducer against different spots on your neck and move it back and forth. The transducer gives off ultrasound waves and detects their echoes as they bounce off the artery walls and blood cells. Ultrasound waves can't be heard by the human ear.

The computer uses the echoes to create and record pictures of the insides of the carotid arteries. These pictures usually appear in black and white. The screen displays these live images for your doctor to review.

Your carotid ultrasound test might include a Doppler ultrasound. Doppler ultrasound is a special test that shows the movement of blood through your arteries. Blood flow through the arteries usually appears in color on the ultrasound pictures.

What to Expect After Carotid Ultrasound

You usually can return to your normal activities as soon as the carotid ultrasound is over. Your doctor will likely be able to tell you the results of the carotid ultrasound when it occurs or soon afterward.

What Does a Carotid Ultrasound Show?

A carotid ultrasound can show whether plaque buildup has narrowed one or both of your carotid arteries. If so, you might be at risk of having a stroke. The risk depends on the extent of the blockage and how much it has reduced blood flow to your brain.

To lower your risk of stroke, your doctor may recommend medical or surgical treatments to reduce or remove plaque from your carotid arteries.

What Are the Risks of Carotid Ultrasound?

Carotid ultrasound has no risks because the test uses harmless sound waves. They are the same type of sound waves that doctors use to record pictures of fetuses in pregnant women.

Chapter 39

Holter and Event Monitors

What Are Holter and Event Monitors?

Holter and event monitors are medical devices that record the heart's electrical activity. Doctors most often use these monitors to diagnose arrhythmias.

Arrhythmias are problems with the rate or rhythm of the heartbeat. During an arrhythmia, the heart can beat too fast, too slow, or with an irregular rhythm.

Holter and event monitors also are used to detect silent myocardial ischemia. In this condition, not enough oxygen-rich blood reaches the heart muscle. "Silent" means that no symptoms occur.

The monitors also can check whether treatments for an arrhythmia or silent myocardial ischemia are working.

This chapter focuses on using Holter and event monitors to diagnose problems with the heart's rate or rhythm.

Overview

Holter and event monitors are similar to an electrocardiogram (EKG). An EKG is a simple test that detects and records the heart's electrical activity. It's a common test for diagnosing heart rhythm problems.

Excerpted from "What Are Holter and Event Monitors?" National Heart, Lung, and Blood Institute, National Institutes of Health, March 16, 2012.

However, a standard EKG records the heartbeat for a only few seconds. It won't detect heart rhythm problems that don't occur during the test.

Holter and event monitors are small, portable devices. You can wear one while you do your normal daily activities. This allows the monitor to record your heart for a longer time than an EKG.

Some people have heart rhythm problems that occur only during certain activities, such as sleeping or physical exertion. Using a Holter or event monitor increases the chance of recording these problems.

Although similar, Holter and event monitors aren't the same. A Holter monitor records your heart's electrical activity the entire time you're wearing it. An event monitor records your heart's electrical activity only at certain times while you're wearing it.

Types of Holter and Event Monitors

Holter Monitors

Holter monitors sometimes are called continuous EKGs (electrocardiograms). This is because Holter monitors record your heart rhythm continuously for twenty-four to forty-eight hours.

A Holter monitor is about the size of a large deck of cards. You can clip it to a belt or carry it in a pocket. Wires connect the device to sensors (called electrodes) that are stuck to your chest using sticky patches. These sensors detect your heart's electrical signals, and the monitor records your heart rhythm.

Wireless Holter Monitors

Wireless Holter monitors have a longer recording time than standard Holter monitors. Wireless monitors record your heart's electrical activity for a preset amount of time.

These monitors use wireless cellular technology to send the recorded data to your doctor's office or a company that checks the data. The device sends the data automatically at certain times. Wireless monitors still have wires that connect the device to the sensors on your chest.

You can use a wireless Holter monitor for days or even weeks, until signs or symptoms of a heart rhythm problem occur. These monitors usually are used to detect heart rhythm problems that don't occur often.

Although wireless Holter monitors work for longer periods, they have a down side. You must remember to write down the time of symptoms so your doctor can match it to the heart rhythm recording. Also, the batteries in the wireless monitor must be changed every one to two days.

Event Monitors

Event monitors are similar to Holter monitors. You wear one while you do your normal daily activities. Most event monitors have wires that connect the device to sensors. The sensors are stuck to your chest using sticky patches.

Unlike Holter monitors, event monitors don't continuously record your heart's electrical activity. They record only during symptoms. For many event monitors, you need to start the device when you feel symptoms. Some event monitors start automatically if they detect abnormal heart rhythms.

Event monitors tend to be smaller than Holter monitors because they don't need to store as much data.

Different types of event monitors work in slightly different ways. Your doctor will explain how to use the monitor before you start wearing it.

Postevent Recorders

Postevent recorders are among the smallest event monitors. You can wear a postevent recorder like a wristwatch or carry it in your pocket. The pocket version is about the size of a thick credit card. These monitors don't have wires that connect the device to chest sensors.

To start the recorder when you feel a symptom, you hold it to your chest. To start the wristwatch version, you touch a button on the side of the watch.

A postevent recorder records only what happens after you start it. It may miss a heart rhythm problem that occurs before and during the onset of symptoms. Also, it might be hard to start the monitor when a symptom is in progress.

In some cases, the missing data could have helped your doctor diagnose the heart rhythm problem.

Presymptom Memory Loop Recorders

Presymptom memory loop recorders are the size of a small cell phone. They're also called continuous loop event recorders.

You can clip this event monitor to your belt or carry it in your pocket. Wires connect the device to sensors on your chest.

These recorders are always recording and erasing data. When you feel a symptom, you push a button on the device. The normal erase process stops. The recording will show a few minutes of data from before, during, and after the symptom. This may make it possible for your doctor to see very brief changes in your heart rhythm.

Autodetect Recorders

Autodetect recorders are about the size of the palm of your hand. Wires connect the device to sensors on your chest.

You don't need to start an autodetect recorder during symptoms. These recorders detect abnormal heart rhythms and automatically record and send the data to your doctor's office.

Implantable Loop Recorders

You may need an implantable loop recorder if other event monitors can't provide enough data. Implantable loop recorders are about the size of a pack of gum. This type of event monitor is inserted under the skin on your chest. No wires or chest sensors are used.

Your doctor can program the device to record when you start it during symptoms or automatically if it detects an abnormal heart rhythm. Devices may differ, so your doctor will tell you how to use your recorder. Sometimes a special card is held close to the recorder to start it.

Who Needs a Holter or Event Monitor?

Your doctor may recommend a Holter or event monitor if he or she thinks you have an arrhythmia. An arrhythmia is a problem with the rate or rhythm of the heartbeat.

Holter and event monitors most often are used to detect arrhythmias in people who have the following symptoms:

- **Issues with fainting or feeling dizzy:** A monitor might be used if causes other than a heart rhythm problem have been ruled out.

- **Palpitations that recur with no known cause:** Palpitations are feelings that your heart is skipping a beat, fluttering, or beating too hard or fast. You may have these feelings in your chest, throat, or neck.

People who are being treated for heart rhythm problems also may need to use Holter or event monitors. The monitors can show how well their treatments are working.

Heart rhythm problems may occur only during certain activities, such sleeping or physical exertion. Holter and event monitors record your heart rhythm while you do your normal daily routine. This allows your doctor to see how your heart responds to various activities.

What to Expect Before Using a Holter or Event Monitor

Your doctor will do a physical exam before giving you a Holter or event monitor. He or she may do the following things:

- Check your pulse to find out how fast your heart is beating (your heart rate) and whether your heart rhythm is steady or irregular.

- Measure your blood pressure.

- Check for swelling in your legs or feet. Swelling could be a sign of an enlarged heart or heart failure, which may cause an arrhythmia. An arrhythmia is a problem with the rate or rhythm of the heartbeat.

- Look for signs of other diseases that might cause heart rhythm problems, such as thyroid disease.

You may have an EKG (electrocardiogram) test before your doctor sends you home with a Holter or event monitor.

An EKG is a simple test that records your heart's electrical activity for a few seconds. The test shows how fast your heart is beating and its rhythm (steady or irregular). An EKG also records the strength and timing of electrical signals as they pass through your heart.

A standard EKG won't detect heart rhythm problems that don't happen during the test. For this reason, your doctor may give you a Holter or event monitor. These monitors are portable. You can wear one while doing your normal daily activities. This increases the chance of recording symptoms that only occur once in a while.

Your doctor will explain how to wear and use the Holter or event monitor. Usually, you'll leave the office wearing it.

Each type of monitor is slightly different, but most have sensors (called electrodes) that attach to the skin on your chest using sticky patches. The sensors need good contact with your skin. Poor contact can cause poor results.

Oil, too much sweat, and hair can keep the patches from sticking to your skin. You may need to shave the area on your chest where your doctor will attach the patches. If you have to replace the patches, you'll need to clean the area with a special prep pad that the doctor will provide.

You may need to use a small amount of special paste or gel to help the patches stick to your skin. Some patches come with paste or gel on them.

What to Expect While Using a Holter or Event Monitor

Your experience while using a Holter or event monitor depends on the type of monitor you have. However, most monitors have some factors in common.

Recording the Heart's Electrical Activity

All monitors record the heart's electrical activity. Thus, maintaining a clear signal between the sensors (electrodes) and the recording device is important.

In most cases, the sensors are attached to your chest using sticky patches. Wires connect the sensors to the monitor. You usually can clip the monitor to your belt or carry it in your pocket. (Postevent recorders and implantable loop recorders don't have chest sensors.)

A good stick between the patches and your skin helps provide a clear signal. Poor contact leads to a poor recording that's hard for your doctor to read.

Oil, too much sweat, and hair can keep the patches from sticking to your skin. You may need to shave the area where your doctor will attach the patches. If you have to replace the patches, you'll need to clean the area with a special prep pad that your doctor will provide.

You may need to use a small amount of special paste or gel to help the patches stick to your skin. Some patches come with paste or gel on them.

Too much movement can pull the patches away from your skin or create "noise" on the EKG (electrocardiogram) strip. An EKG strip is a graph showing the pattern of the heartbeat. Noise looks like a lot of jagged lines; it makes it hard for your doctor to see the real rhythm of your heart.

When you have a symptom, stop what you're doing. This will ensure that the recording shows your heart's activity rather than your movement.

Your doctor will tell you whether you need to adjust your activity level during the testing period. If you exercise, choose a cool location to avoid sweating too much. This will help the patches stay sticky.

Other everyday items also can disrupt the signal between the sensors and the monitor. These items include magnets; metal detectors; microwave ovens; and electric blankets, toothbrushes, and razors. Avoid using these items. Also avoid areas with high voltage.

Cell phones and MP3 players (such as iPods) may interfere with the signal between the sensors and the monitor if they're too close to the monitor. When using any electronic device, try to keep it at least six inches away from the monitor.

Keeping a Diary

While using a Holter or event monitor, your doctor will advise you to keep a diary of your symptoms and activities. Write down what type of symptoms you're having, when they occur, and what you were doing at the time.

The most common symptoms of heart rhythm problems include the following:

• Fainting or feeling dizzy.

• Palpitations. These are feelings that your heart is skipping a beat, fluttering, or beating too hard or fast. You may have these feelings in your chest, throat, or neck.

Make sure to note the time that symptoms occur, because your doctor will match the data with the information in your diary. This allows your doctor to see whether certain activities trigger changes in your heart rate and rhythm.

Also, include details in your diary about when you take any medicine or if you feel stress at certain times during the testing period.

What to Expect with Specific Monitors

Holter Monitors

Holter monitors are about the size of a large deck of cards. You'll wear one for twenty-four to forty-eight hours. You can't get your monitor wet, so you won't be able to bathe or shower. You can take a sponge bath if needed.

When the testing period is done, you'll return the device to your doctor's office. The results will be stored on the device.

The recording period for a standard Holter monitor might be too short to capture a heart rhythm problem. If this is the case, your doctor may recommend a wireless Holter monitor.

Wireless Holter Monitors

Wireless Holter monitors can record for a longer time than standard Holter monitors. You can use a wireless Holter monitor for days or even weeks, until signs or symptoms of a heart rhythm problem occur.

Wireless monitors record for a preset amount of time. Then they automatically send data to your doctor's office or a company that checks the data.

These monitors use wireless cellular technology to send data. However, they still have wires that connect the device to the sensors stuck to your chest.

The batteries in the wireless monitor must be changed every one to two days. You'll need to detach the sensors to shower or bathe and then reattach them.

Event Monitors

Event monitors are slightly smaller than Holter monitors. They can be worn for weeks or until symptoms occur. Most event monitors are worn like Holter monitors—clipped to a belt or carried in a pocket.

When you have symptoms, you simply push a button on your monitor to start recording. Some event monitors start automatically if they detect abnormal heart rhythms.

Postevent Recorders

Postevent recorders can be worn like a wristwatch or carried in a pocket. The pocket version is about the size of a thick credit card. These recorders don't have wires that connect the device to chest sensors.

To start the recorder when you feel a symptom, you hold it to your chest. To start the wristwatch version, you touch a button on the side of the watch.

You send the stored data to your doctor's office using a telephone. Your doctor will explain how to use the monitor before you leave his or her office.

Autodetect Recorders

Autodetect recorders are about the size of the palm of your hand. Wires connect the device to sensors on your chest.

You don't need to start an autodetect recorder. This type of monitor automatically starts recording if it detects abnormal heart rhythms. It then sends the data to your doctor's office.

Implantable Loop Recorders

Implantable loop recorders are about the size of a pack of gum. This type of event monitor is inserted under the skin on your chest. Your doctor will discuss the procedure with you. No chest sensors are used with implantable loop recorders.

Your doctor can program the device to record when you start it during symptoms or automatically if it detects an abnormal heart rhythm.

Devices may differ, so your doctor will tell you how to use your recorder. Sometimes a special card is held close to the device to start it.

What to Expect After Using a Holter or Event Monitor

After you're finished using a Holter or event monitor, you'll return it to your doctor's office or the place where you picked it up.

If you were using an implantable loop recorder, your doctor will need to remove it from your chest. He or she will discuss the procedure with you.

Your doctor will tell you when to expect the results. Once your doctor has reviewed the recordings, he or she will discuss the results with you.

What Does a Holter or Event Monitor Show?

A Holter or event monitor may show what's causing symptoms of an arrhythmia. An arrhythmia is a problem with the rate or rhythm of the heartbeat.

A Holter or event monitor also can show whether a heart rhythm problem is harmless or requires treatment. The monitor might alert your doctor to medical conditions that can result in heart failure, stroke, or sudden cardiac arrest.

If the symptoms of a heart rhythm problem occur often, a Holter or event monitor has a good chance of recording them. You may not have symptoms while using a monitor. Even so, your doctor can learn more about your heart rhythm from the test results.

Sometimes Holter and event monitors can't help doctors diagnose heart rhythm problems. If this happens, talk with your doctor about other steps you can take.

One option might be to try a different type of monitor. Wireless Holter monitors and implantable loop recorders have longer recording periods. This may allow your doctor to get the data he or she needs to make a diagnosis.

What Are the Risks of Using a Holter or Event Monitor?

The sticky patches used to attach the sensors (electrodes) to your chest have a small risk of skin irritation. You also may have an allergic reaction to the paste or gel that's sometimes used to attach the patches. The irritation will go away once the patches are removed.

If you're using an implantable loop recorder, you may get an infection or have pain where the device is placed under the skin. Your doctor can prescribe medicine to treat these problems.

411

Chapter 40

Stress Testing

What Is Stress Testing?

Stress testing provides information about how your heart works during physical stress. Some heart problems are easier to diagnose when your heart is working hard and beating fast.

During stress testing, you exercise (walk or run on a treadmill or pedal a stationary bike) to make your heart work hard and beat fast. Tests are done on your heart while you exercise.

You might have arthritis or another medical problem that prevents you from exercising during a stress test. If so, your doctor may give you medicine to make your heart work hard, as it would during exercise. This is called a pharmacological stress test.

Types of Stress Testing

The two main types of stress testing are a standard exercise stress test and an imaging stress test.

Standard Exercise Stress Test

A standard exercise stress test uses an electrocardiogram (EKG) to detect and record the heart's electrical activity.

Excerpted from "What Is Stress Testing?" National Heart, Lung, and Blood Institute, National Institutes of Health, December 14, 2011.

An EKG shows how fast your heart is beating and the heart's rhythm (steady or irregular). It also records the strength and timing of electrical signals as they pass through your heart.

During a standard stress test, your blood pressure will be checked. You also may be asked to breathe into a special tube during the test. This allows your doctor to see how well you're breathing and measure the gases that you breathe out.

A standard stress test shows changes in your heart's electrical activity. It also can show whether your heart is getting enough blood during exercise.

Imaging Stress Test

As part of some stress tests, pictures are taken of your heart while you exercise and while you're at rest. These imaging stress tests can show how well blood is flowing in your heart and how well your heart pumps blood when it beats.

One type of imaging stress test involves echocardiography (echo). This test uses sound waves to create a moving picture of your heart. An exercise stress echo can show how well your heart's chambers and valves are working when your heart is under stress.

A stress echo also can show areas of poor blood flow to your heart, dead heart muscle tissue, and areas of the heart muscle wall that aren't contracting well. These areas may have been damaged during a heart attack, or they may not be getting enough blood.

Other imaging stress tests use radioactive dye to create pictures of blood flow to your heart. The dye is injected into your bloodstream before the pictures are taken. The pictures show how much of the dye has reached various parts of your heart during exercise and while you're at rest.

Tests that use radioactive dye include a thallium or sestamibi stress test and a positron emission tomography (PET) stress test. The amount of radiation in the dye is considered safe for you and those around you. However, if you're pregnant, you shouldn't have this test because of risks it might pose to your unborn child.

Imaging stress tests tend to detect coronary heart disease (CHD) better than standard (nonimaging) stress tests. Imaging stress tests also can predict the risk of a future heart attack or premature death.

An imaging stress test might be done first (as opposed to a standard exercise stress test) if you:

- can't exercise for enough time to get your heart working at its hardest. (Medical problems, such as arthritis or leg arteries clogged by plaque, might prevent you from exercising long enough.)

- have abnormal heartbeats or other problems that prevent a standard exercise stress test from giving correct results.

- had a heart procedure in the past, such as coronary artery by-pass grafting or angioplasty and stent placement.

Other Names for Stress Testing

- Exercise echocardiogram or exercise stress echo

- Exercise test

- Myocardial perfusion imaging

- Nuclear stress test

- Positron emission tomography (PET) stress test

- Pharmacological stress test

- Sestamibi stress test

- Stress echocardiogram (EKG or ECG)

- Thallium stress test

- Treadmill test

Who Needs Stress Testing?

You may need stress testing if you've had chest pains, shortness of breath, or other symptoms of limited blood flow to your heart.

Imaging stress tests, especially, can show whether you have coronary heart disease (CHD) or a heart valve problem. (Heart valves are like doors; they open and shut to let blood flow between the heart's chambers and into the heart's arteries. So, like CHD, faulty heart valves can limit the amount of blood reaching your heart.)

If you've been diagnosed with CHD or recently had a heart attack, a stress test can show whether you can handle an exercise program. If you've had angioplasty (with or without stent placement) or coronary artery bypass grafting, a stress test can show how well the treatment relieves your CHD symptoms.

You also may need a stress test if, during exercise, you feel faint, have a rapid heartbeat or a fluttering feeling in your chest, or have other symptoms of an arrhythmia (an irregular heartbeat).

If you don't have chest pain when you exercise but still get short of breath, your doctor may recommend a stress test. The test can help show whether a heart problem, rather than a lung problem or being out of shape, is causing your breathing problems.

For such testing, you breathe into a special tube. This allows a technician to measure the gases you breathe out. Breathing into the tube during stress testing also is done before a heart transplant to help assess whether you're a candidate for the surgery.

Stress testing shouldn't be used as a routine screening test for CHD. Usually, you have to have symptoms of CHD before a doctor will recommend stress testing.

However, your doctor may want to use a stress test to screen for CHD if you have diabetes. This disease increases your risk of CHD. Currently, though, no evidence shows that having a stress test will improve your outcome if you have diabetes.

What to Expect Before Stress Testing

Stress testing is done in a doctor's office or at a medical center or hospital. You should wear shoes and clothes in which you can exercise comfortably. Sometimes you're given a gown to wear during the test.

Your doctor might ask you to fast (not eat or drink anything but water) for a short time before the test. If you're diabetic, ask your doctor whether you need to adjust your medicines on the day of the test.

For some stress tests, you can't drink coffee or other caffeinated drinks for a day before the test. Certain over-the-counter or prescription medicines also may interfere with some stress tests. Ask your doctor whether you need to avoid certain drinks or food or change how you take your medicine before the test.

If you use an inhaler for asthma or other breathing problems, bring it to the test. Make sure you let the doctor know that you use it.

What to Expect During Stress Testing

During all types of stress testing, a doctor, nurse, or technician will always be with you to closely check your health status.

Before you start the "stress" part of a stress test, the nurse will put sticky patches called electrodes on the skin of your chest, arms, and legs. To help an electrode stick to the skin, the nurse may have to shave a patch of hair where the electrode will be attached.

The electrodes will be connected to an electrocardiogram (EKG) machine. This machine records your heart's electrical activity. It shows how fast your heart is beating and the heart's rhythm (steady or irregular). An EKG also records the strength and timing of electrical signals as they pass through your heart.

The nurse will put a blood pressure cuff on your arm to check your blood pressure during the stress test. (The cuff will feel tight on your arm when it expands every few minutes.) Also, you might have to breathe into a special tube so the gases you breathe out can be measured.

Next, you'll exercise on a treadmill or stationary bike. If such exercise poses a problem for you, you might turn a crank with your arms instead. During the test, the exercise level will get harder. You can stop whenever you feel the exercise is too much for you.

If you can't exercise, medicine might be injected into a vein in your arm or hand. The medicine will increase blood flow through your coronary arteries and make your heart beat fast, as it would during exercise. You can then have the stress test.

The medicine may make you flushed and anxious, but the effects go away as soon as the test is over. The medicine also may give you a headache.

While you're exercising or getting medicine to make your heart work harder, the nurse will ask you how you're feeling. You should tell him or her if you feel chest pain, short of breath, or dizzy.

The exercise or medicine infusion will continue until you reach a target heart rate, or until you:

- feel moderate to severe chest pain;

- get too out of breath to continue;

- develop abnormally high or low blood pressure or an arrhythmia (an irregular heartbeat);

- become dizzy.

The nurse will continue to check your heart functions and blood pressure after the test until they return to normal levels.

The "stress" part of a stress test (when your heart is working hard) usually lasts about fifteen minutes or less.

However, there's prep time before the test and monitoring time afterward. Both extend the total test time to about an hour for a standard stress test, and up to three hours or more for some imaging stress tests.

Exercise Stress Echocardiogram Test

For an exercise stress echocardiogram (echo) test, the nurse will take pictures of your heart using echocardiography before you exercise and as soon as you finish.

A sonographer (a person who specializes in using ultrasound techniques) will apply gel to your chest. Then, he or she will briefly put a transducer (a wand-like device) against your chest and move it around.

The transducer sends and receives high-pitched sounds that you probably won't hear. The echoes from the sound waves are converted into moving pictures of your heart on a screen.

You might be asked to lie on your side on an exam table for this test. Some stress echo tests also use dye to improve imaging. The dye is injected into your bloodstream while the test occurs.

Sestamibi or Other Imaging Stress Tests Involving Radioactive Dye

For a sestamibi stress test or other imaging stress test that uses radioactive dye, the nurse will inject a small amount of dye into your bloodstream. This is done through a needle placed in a vein in your arm or hand.

You'll get the dye about a half hour before you start exercising or take medicine to make your heart work hard. The amount of radiation in the dye is considered safe for you and those around you. However, if you're pregnant, you shouldn't have this test because of risks it might pose to your unborn child.

Pictures will be taken of your heart at least two times: when it's at rest and when it's working its hardest. You'll lie down on a table, and a special camera or scanner that can detect the dye in your bloodstream will take pictures of your heart.

Some pictures may not be taken until you lie quietly for a few hours after the stress test. Some patients may even be asked to return in a day or so for more pictures.

What to Expect After Stress Testing

After stress testing, you'll be able to return to your normal activities. If you had a test that involved radioactive dye, your doctor may ask you to drink plenty of fluids to flush it out of your body. You shouldn't have certain other imaging tests until the dye is no longer in your body. Your doctor can advise you further.

What Does Stress Testing Show?

Stress testing shows how your heart works during physical stress (exercise) and how healthy your heart is.

A standard exercise stress test uses an EKG (electrocardiogram) to monitor changes in your heart's electrical activity. Imaging stress tests take pictures of blood flow throughout your heart. They also show your heart valves and the movement of your heart muscle.

Doctors use both types of stress tests to look for signs that your heart isn't getting enough blood flow during exercise. Abnormal test results may be due to coronary heart disease (CHD) or other factors, such as poor physical fitness.

If you have a standard exercise stress test and the results are normal, you may not need further testing or treatment. But if your test results are abnormal, or if you're physically unable to exercise, your doctor may want you to have an imaging stress test or other tests.

Even if your standard exercise stress test results are normal, your doctor may want you to have an imaging stress test if you continue having symptoms (such as shortness of breath or chest pain).

Imaging stress tests are more accurate than standard exercise stress tests, but they're much more expensive.

Imaging stress tests show how well blood is flowing in the heart muscle and reveal parts of the heart that aren't contracting strongly. They also can show the parts of the heart that aren't getting enough blood, as well as dead tissue in the heart, where no blood flows. (A heart attack can cause heart tissue to die.)

If your imaging stress test suggests significant CHD, your doctor may want you to have more testing and treatment.

What Are the Risks of Stress Testing?

Stress tests pose little risk of serious harm. The chance of these tests causing a heart attack or death is about one in five thousand. More common, but less serious side effects linked to stress testing include the following:

- An arrhythmia (irregular heartbeat). Often, an arrhythmia will go away quickly once you're at rest. But if it persists, you may need monitoring or treatment in a hospital.

- Low blood pressure, which can cause you to feel dizzy or faint. This problem may go away once your heart stops working hard; it usually doesn't require treatment.

- Jitteriness or discomfort while getting medicine to make your heart work hard and beat fast (you may be given medicine if you can't exercise). These side effects usually go away shortly after you stop getting the medicine. Sometimes the symptoms may last a few hours.

419

Also, some of the medicines used for pharmacological stress tests can cause wheezing, shortness of breath, and other asthma-like symptoms. Sometimes these symptoms are severe and require treatment.

Chapter 41

Tilt Table Testing

What is a tilt-table test?

If you often feel faint or light-headed, your doctor may use a tilt-table test to find out why. During the test, you lie on a table that is slowly tilted upward. The test measures how your blood pressure and heart rate respond to the force of gravity. A nurse or technician keeps track of your blood pressure and your heart rate (pulse) to see how they change during the test.

Why do people have tilt-table tests?

Doctors use this test to trigger your symptoms while watching you. They measure your blood pressure and heart rate during the test to find out what's causing your symptoms. The test is normal if your average blood pressure stays stable as the table tilts upward and your heart rate increases by a normal amount.

If your blood pressure drops and stays low during the test, you may faint or feel lightheaded. This can happen either with an abnormally slow heart rate or with a fast heart rate. That's because your brain isn't getting enough blood for the moment. (This is corrected as soon as you are tilted back to the flat position.) Your heart rate may not be adapting as the table tilts upward, or your blood vessels may not be squeezing hard enough to support your blood pressure.

Feeling lightheaded or fainting may be caused by taking certain medicines, severe dehydration, abnormal heart rhythms (arrhythmias), hypoglycemia (low blood sugar), prolonged bed rest, and certain nervous system disorders that cause low blood pressure.

Are there risks with tilt-table tests?

There are few risks. People rarely faint during tilt-table tests. And even if they do, it's safer than fainting on your own in an uncontrolled situation. If a person does faint, usually they feel well again within a minute or so after the table returns to a flat position.

How do I prepare for a tilt-table test?

- Don't eat or drink for at least four hours before the test.

- If you will have a morning test, your doctor may tell you not to eat or drink after midnight the night before.

- If your test is in the afternoon, you can usually eat a light breakfast. Don't eat lunch.

- If you take medicine, ask your doctor if you should keep taking it on your regular schedule before the test.

What happens during a tilt-table test?

A nurse or technician with special training performs the tilt-table test in a hospital or clinic electrophysiology (EP) lab. The test has two parts.

Part one: The first part of the test shows how your body responds when you change positions:

- You lie on your back on a table. Straps at your waist and knees help you stay in position. An intravenous line (IV) is put in your arm. Small discs with wires are attached to your chest and are connected to an electrocardiograph (ECG) machine to track your heartbeat. A cuff on your arm measures your blood pressure.

- The nurse tilts the table so your head is slightly higher (thirty degrees) than the rest of your body. The nurse checks your blood pressure and your heart rate.

- After about five minutes, the nurse tilts the table more. Now you are lying at a sixty-degree angle or higher. The nurse continues to check your blood pressure and your heart rate for up to forty-five minutes. The nurse will ask you to stay still and quiet during this time, but you should tell the nurse if you feel uncomfortable.

- If your blood pressure drops during this time, the nurse will lower the table and stop the test. You won't need to take the second part of the test. If your blood pressure does not drop after the time is up, the nurse will lower the table and start the second part of the test.

Part two: The second part of the test shows how your body responds to a medicine (isoproterenol) that causes your heart to beat faster and stronger. This medicine is like the hormone adrenaline that your body releases when you are under stress. This medicine may make you feel as if you are exercising. It may make you more sensitive to the tilt-table test if your blood pressure didn't change during the first part of the test:

- The nurse gives you medicine through your IV tube.

- Next, the nurse tilts the table upwards to a sixty-degree angle.

- You may feel your heartbeat increase because of the medicine.

- If your blood pressure drops, the nurse will lower the table to the flat position, stop the medicine, and the test will end.

- If your blood pressure does not drop after about fifteen minutes, the nurse will lower the table and the test will be over.

The tilt-table test can last about ninety minutes if you do both parts of it. If you only do the first part, you may be done in thirty to forty minutes.

What happens after a tilt-table test?

You may feel tired and a little sick to your stomach right after the test. You may stay in a recovery area for thirty to sixty minutes so nurses can keep track of your blood pressure and heart rate. After recovery, most people can drive home and return to their normal activities. However, if you lose consciousness during the test, you may need to have more observation and testing. Don't drive home if you have fainted.

How I do I learn about my results?

You may get your results as soon as the test is over. Sometimes your doctor will give you the results a few days later. Results are either "negative" or "positive":

- If your blood pressure does not fall during the test, and you have no other symptoms, the test results are negative (normal).

- If your blood pressure drops during the test and you feel faint or dizzy, the test is positive. Your doctor may suggest changing your medicines or having more tests. If your fainting is due to a slow heart rate (bradycardia), your doctor may recommend a pacemaker.

How can I learn more about tilt-table tests?

Talk with your doctor. Here are some good questions to ask:

- Why are you using this test instead of a different test?

- Will I feel any effects of the test after it is over?

- What will it feel like when I get medicine during the second part of the test?

- What does it mean if I have a negative test?

- What does it mean if I have a positive test?

- What do you think is causing me to feel lightheaded or faint?

- What can I do to prevent fainting spells?

Chapter 42

Coronary Angiography

What Is Coronary Angiography?

Coronary angiography is a test that uses dye and special x-rays to show the insides of your coronary arteries. The coronary arteries supply oxygen-rich blood to your heart.

A waxy substance called plaque can build up inside the coronary arteries. The buildup of plaque in the coronary arteries is called coronary heart disease (CHD).

Over time, plaque can harden or rupture (break open). Hardened plaque narrows the coronary arteries and reduces the flow of oxygen-rich blood to the heart. This can cause chest pain or discomfort called angina.

If the plaque ruptures, a blood clot can form on its surface. A large blood clot can mostly or completely block blood flow through a coronary artery. This is the most common cause of a heart attack. Over time, ruptured plaque also hardens and narrows the coronary arteries.

Who Needs Coronary Angiography?

Your doctor may recommend coronary angiography if you have any of the following:

Excerpted from "What Is Coronary Angiography?" National Heart, Lung, and Blood Institute, National Institutes of Health, March 2, 2012.

- Angina. This is unexplained pain or pressure in your chest. You also may feel it in your shoulders, arms, neck, jaw, or back. The pain my even feel like indigestion.

- Survived a sudden cardiac arrest (SCA). This is a condition in which your heart suddenly and unexpectedly stops beating.

- Abnormal results from tests such as an electrocardiogram (EKG), exercise stress test, or other test.

Coronary angiography also might be done on an emergency basis, such as during a heart attack. If angiography shows blockages in your coronary arteries, your doctor may do a procedure called angioplasty. This procedure can open blocked heart arteries and prevent further heart damage.

Coronary angiography also can help your doctor plan treatment after you've had a heart attack, especially if you have major heart damage or if you're still having chest pain.

What to Expect Before Coronary Angiography

Before having coronary angiography, talk with your doctor about the following things:

- How the test is done and how to prepare for it.

- Any medicines you're taking, and whether you should stop taking them before the test.

- Whether you have diseases or conditions that may require taking extra steps during or after the test to avoid complications. Examples of such conditions include diabetes and kidney disease.

Your doctor will tell you exactly which procedures will be done. For example, your doctor may recommend coronary angioplasty if the angiography shows a blocked artery.

You will have a chance to ask questions about the procedures. Also, you'll be asked to provide written informed consent to have the procedures.

It's not safe to drive after having cardiac catheterization, which is part of coronary angiography. You'll need to have someone drive you home after the procedure.

What to Expect During Coronary Angiography

During coronary angiography, you're kept on your back and awake. This allows you to follow your doctor's instructions during the test.

You'll be given medicine to help you relax. The medicine might make you sleepy.

Your doctor will numb the area on the arm, groin (upper thigh), or neck where the catheter will enter your blood vessel. Then, he or she will use a needle to make a small hole in the blood vessel. The catheter will be inserted in the hole.

Next, your doctor will thread the catheter through the vessel and into the coronary arteries. Special x-ray movies are taken of the catheter as it's moved into the heart. The movies help your doctor see where to place the tip of the catheter.

Once the catheter is properly placed, your doctor will inject a special type of dye into the tube. The dye will flow through your coronary arteries, making them visible on an x-ray. This x-ray is called an angiogram.

If the angiogram reveals blocked arteries, your doctor may use coronary angioplasty to restore blood flow to your heart.

After your doctor completes the procedure(s), he or she will remove the catheter from your body. The opening left in the blood vessel will then be closed up and bandaged.

A small sandbag or other type of weight might be placed on the bandage to apply pressure. This will help prevent major bleeding from the site.

What to Expect After Coronary Angiography

After coronary angiography, you'll be moved to a special care area in the hospital. You'll be carefully watched for several hours or overnight. During this time, you'll need to limit your movement to avoid bleeding from the site where the catheter was inserted.

While you recover in the special care area, nurses will check your heart rate and blood pressure regularly. They'll also watch for any bleeding at the catheter insertion site.

You may develop a small bruise on your arm, groin (upper thigh), or neck at the catheter insertion site. That area may feel sore or tender for about a week. Let your doctor know if you develop problems such as the following:

- A constant or large amount of blood at the catheter insertion site that can't be stopped with a small bandage

- Unusual pain, swelling, redness, or other signs of infection at or near the catheter insertion site

Your doctor will tell you whether you should avoid certain activities, such as heavy lifting, for a short time after the test.

What Are the Risks of Coronary Angiography?

Coronary angiography is a common medical test. It rarely causes serious problems. However, complications can include the following:

- Bleeding, infection, and pain at the catheter insertion site.

- Damage to blood vessels. Rarely, the catheter may scrape or poke a hole in a blood vessel as it's threaded to the heart.

- An allergic reaction to the dye that's used during the test.

Other, less common complications include the following:

- Arrhythmias (irregular heartbeats). These irregular heartbeats often go away on their own. However, your doctor may recommend treatment if they persist.

- Kidney damage caused by the dye that's used during the test.

- Blood clots that can trigger a stroke, heart attack, or other serious problems.

- Low blood pressure.

- A buildup of blood or fluid in the sac that surrounds the heart. This fluid can prevent the heart from beating properly.

As with any procedure involving the heart, complications can sometimes be fatal. However, this is rare with coronary angiography.

The risk of complications is higher in people who are older and in those who have certain diseases or conditions (such as chronic kidney disease and diabetes).

Chapter 43

Cardiac Computed Tomography (CT)

What Is Cardiac CT?

Cardiac computed tomography, or cardiac CT, is a painless test that uses an x-ray machine to take clear, detailed pictures of the heart. Doctors use this test to look for heart problems.

During a cardiac CT scan, an x-ray machine will move around your body in a circle. The machine will take a picture of each part of your heart. A computer will put the pictures together to make a three-dimensional (3D) picture of the whole heart.

Sometimes an iodine-based dye (contrast dye) is injected into one of your veins during the scan. The contrast dye highlights your coronary (heart) arteries on the x-ray pictures. This type of CT scan is called a coronary CT angiography, or CTA.

What to Expect Before Cardiac CT

Your doctor will tell you how to prepare for the cardiac CT scan. He or she may tell you to avoid caffeine and not eat anything for four hours before the scan. You're usually allowed to drink water before the test.

If you take medicine for diabetes, talk with your doctor about whether you'll need to change how you take it on the day of your cardiac CT scan.

Excerpted from "What Is Cardiac CT?" National Heart, Lung, and Blood Institute, National Institutes of Health, February 29, 2012.

Tell your doctor if you are pregnant or might be pregnant. Even though cardiac CT uses a low radiation dose, the x-rays may harm your fetus. Also let your doctor know if you have asthma or kidney problems or are allergic to any medicines, iodine, or shellfish. These problems can increase your chance of having an allergic reaction to the contrast dye that's sometimes used during cardiac CT.

A technician will ask you to remove your clothes above the waist and wear a hospital gown. You also will be asked to remove any jewelry from around your neck or chest.

If you don't have asthma, chronic obstructive pulmonary disease (COPD), or heart failure, your doctor may give you medicine to slow your heart rate. A slower heart rate will help produce better quality pictures. The medicine will be given by mouth or injected into a vein.

What to Expect During Cardiac CT

Cardiac CT is done in a hospital or outpatient office. A doctor who has experience with CT scanning will supervise the test.

The doctor may want to use an iodine-based dye (contrast dye) during the cardiac CT scan. If so, a needle connected to an intravenous (IV) line will be put in a vein in your hand or arm.

The doctor will inject the contrast dye through the IV line during the scan. You may have a warm feeling when this happens. The dye will make your blood vessels visible on the CT scan pictures.

The technician who runs the cardiac CT scanner will clean areas on your chest and apply sticky patches called electrodes. The patches are attached to an electrocardiogram (EKG) machine. The machine records your heart's electrical activity during the scan.

The CT scanner is a large machine that has a hollow, circular tube in the middle. You will lie on your back on a sliding table. The table can move up and down, and it goes inside the tunnel-like machine.

The table will slide slowly into the opening in the machine. Inside the scanner, an x-ray tube moves around your body to take pictures of different parts of your heart. A computer will put the pictures together to make a three-dimensional (3D) picture of the whole heart.

The technician controls the CT scanner from the next room. He or she can see you through a glass window and talk to you through a speaker.

Moving your body can cause the pictures to blur. You'll be asked to lie still and hold your breath for short moments, while each picture is taken.

A cardiac CT scan usually takes about fifteen minutes to complete. However, it can take more than an hour to get ready for the test and for the medicine to slow your heart rate.

What to Expect After Cardiac CT

After the cardiac CT scan is done, you'll be able to return to your normal activities. Your doctor will discuss the findings with you.

What Does Cardiac CT Show?

Doctors use cardiac CT to detect or evaluate the following things:

- **Coronary heart disease (CHD):** In CHD, a waxy substance called plaque narrows the coronary arteries and limits blood flow to the heart. Contrast dye might be used during a cardiac CT scan to show whether the coronary arteries are narrow or blocked.

- **Calcium buildup in the walls of the coronary arteries:** This type of CT scan is called a coronary calcium scan. Calcium in the coronary arteries may be an early sign of CHD.

- **Problems with the aorta:** The aorta is the main artery that carries oxygen-rich blood from the heart to the body. Cardiac CT can detect an aneurysm or dissection in the aorta.

- **A pulmonary embolism (PE):** A PE is a sudden blockage in a lung artery, usually due to a blood clot.

- **Problems in the pulmonary veins:** The pulmonary veins carry blood from the lungs to the heart. Problems with these veins may lead to an irregular heart rhythm called atrial fibrillation (AF). The pictures that cardiac CT creates of the pulmonary veins can help guide procedures used to treat AF.

- **Problems with heart function and heart valves:** In some cases, doctors may recommend cardiac CT instead of echocardiography or cardiac magnetic resonance imaging (MRI) to look for problems with heart function or heart valves.

- **Pericardial disease:** Cardiac CT can create clear, detailed pictures of the pericardium.

- **Results of coronary artery bypass grafting (CABG):** In CABG, arteries from other areas in your body are used to bypass (that is, go around) narrow coronary arteries. A CT scan can help determine whether the grafted arteries remain open after the surgery.

Doctors also might recommend cardiac CT scans before or after other heart procedures, such as cardiac resynchronization therapy. A

CT scan can help your doctor pinpoint the areas of the heart or blood vessels where the procedure should be done. The scan also can help your doctor check your heart after the procedure.

Because the heart is in motion, a fast type of CT scanner, called multidetector computed tomography (MDCT), might be used to take high-quality pictures of the heart. MDCT also might be used to detect calcium in the coronary arteries.

Another type of CT scanner, called electron-beam computed tomography (EBCT), also is used to detect calcium in the coronary arteries.

What Are the Risks of Cardiac CT?

Cardiac CT involves radiation, although the amount used is considered small. Depending on the type of CT scan you have, the amount of radiation is similar to the amount you're naturally exposed to over one to five years.

There is a small chance that cardiac CT will cause cancer because of the radiation. The risk is higher for people younger than forty years old. New cardiac CT methods are available that reduce the amount of radiation used during the test.

Cardiac CT scans are painless. Some people have side effects from the contrast dye that might be used during the scan. An itchy feeling or a rash may appear after the contrast dye is injected.

Although rare, it is possible to have a serious allergic reaction to the contrast dye. This reaction may cause breathing problems. Doctors use medicine to treat serious allergic reactions.

People who have asthma, chronic obstructive pulmonary disease (COPD), or heart failure may have breathing problems during cardiac CT if they're given beta blockers to slow their heart rates.

Chapter 44

Cardiac Magnetic Resonance Imaging

What Is Cardiac MRI?

Magnetic resonance imaging (MRI) is a safe, noninvasive test that creates detailed pictures of your organs and tissues. "Noninvasive" means that no surgery is done and no instruments are inserted into your body.

MRI uses radio waves, magnets, and a computer to create pictures of your organs and tissues. Unlike other imaging tests, MRI doesn't use ionizing radiation or carry any risk of causing cancer.

Cardiac MRI creates both still and moving pictures of your heart and major blood vessels. Doctors use cardiac MRI to get pictures of the beating heart and to look at its structure and function. These pictures can help them decide the best way to treat people who have heart problems.

Cardiac MRI is a common test. It's used to diagnose and assess many diseases and conditions, including the following:

- Coronary heart disease

- Damage caused by a heart attack

- Heart failure

- Heart valve problems

Excerpted from "What Is Cardiac MRI?" National Heart, Lung, and Blood Institute, National Institutes of Health, February 2, 2012.

- Congenital heart defects (heart defects present at birth)
- Pericarditis (a condition in which the membrane, or sac, around your heart is inflamed)
- Cardiac tumors

Cardiac MRI can help explain results from other tests, such as x-rays and computed tomography scans (also called CT scans).

Doctors sometimes use cardiac MRI instead of invasive procedures or tests that involve radiation (such as x-rays) or dyes containing iodine (these dyes may be harmful to people who have kidney problems).

A contrast agent, such as gadolinium, might be injected into a vein during cardiac MRI. The substance travels to the heart and highlights the heart and blood vessels on the MRI pictures. This contrast agent often is used for people who are allergic to the dyes used in CT scanning.

People who have severe kidney or liver problems may not be able to have the contrast agent. As a result, they may have a noncontrast MRI (an MRI that does not involve contrast agent).

What to Expect Before Cardiac MRI

You'll be asked to fill out a screening form before having cardiac MRI. The form may ask whether you've had any previous surgeries. It also may ask whether you have any metal objects or medical devices (like a cardiac pacemaker) in your body.

Some implanted medical devices, such as man-made heart valves and coronary stents, are safe around the MRI machine, but others are not. For example, the MRI machine can do the following things:

- Cause implanted cardiac pacemakers and defibrillators to malfunction.

- Damage cochlear (inner-ear) implants. Cochlear implants are small, electronic devices that help people who are deaf or who can't hear well understand speech and the sounds around them.

- Cause brain aneurysm clips to move as a result of the MRI's strong magnetic field. This can cause severe injury.

Talk to your doctor or the MRI technician if you have concerns about any implanted devices that may interfere with the MRI.

Your doctor will let you know if you shouldn't have a cardiac MRI because of a medical device. If so, consider wearing a medical ID bracelet or necklace or carrying a medical alert card that states that you shouldn't have an MRI.

If you're pregnant, make sure your doctor knows before you have an MRI. No harmful effects of MRI during pregnancy have been reported; however, more research on the safety of MRI during pregnancy is needed.

Your doctor or technician will tell you whether you need to change into a hospital gown for the test. Don't bring hearing aids, credit cards, jewelry and watches, eyeglasses, pens, removable dental work, or anything that's magnetic near the MRI machine.

Tell your doctor if being in a fairly tight or confined space causes you anxiety or fear. If so, your doctor might give you medicine to help you relax. Your doctor may ask you to fast (not eat) for six hours before you take this medicine on the day of the test.

Some newer cardiac MRI machines are open on all sides. If you're fearful in tight or confined spaces, ask your doctor to help you find a facility that has an open MRI machine.

Your doctor will let you know whether you need to arrange for a ride home after the test.

What to Expect During Cardiac MRI

Cardiac MRI takes place in a hospital or medical imaging facility. A radiologist or other doctor who has special training in medical imaging oversees MRI testing.

Cardiac MRI usually takes thirty to ninety minutes, depending on how many pictures are needed. The test may take less time with some newer MRI machines.

The MRI machine will be located in a special room that prevents radio waves from disrupting the machine. It also prevents the MRI machine's strong magnetic fields from disrupting other equipment.

Traditional MRI machines look like long, narrow tunnels. Newer MRI machines (called short-bore systems) are shorter, wider, and don't completely surround you. Some newer machines are open on all sides. Your doctor will help decide which type of machine is best for you.

Cardiac MRI is painless and harmless. You'll lie on your back on a sliding table that goes inside the tunnel-like machine.

The MRI technician will control the machine from the next room. He or she will be able to see you through a glass window and talk to you through a speaker. Tell the technician if you have a hearing problem.

The MRI machine makes loud humming, tapping, and buzzing noises. Some facilities let you wear earplugs or listen to music during the test.

You will need to remain very still during the MRI. Any movement can blur the pictures. If you're unable to lie still, you may be given medicine to help you relax.

The technician might ask you to hold your breath for ten to fifteen seconds at a time while he or she takes pictures of your heart. Researchers are studying ways that will allow someone having a cardiac MRI to breathe freely during the exam, while achieving the same image quality.

A contrast agent, such as gadolinium, might be used to highlight your blood vessels or heart in the pictures. The substance usually is injected into a vein in your arm using a needle.

You may feel a cool sensation during the injection and discomfort when the needle is inserted. Gadolinium doesn't contain iodine, so it won't cause problems for people who are allergic to iodine.

Your cardiac MRI might include a stress test to detect blockages in your coronary arteries. If so, you'll get other medicines to increase the blood flow in your heart or to increase your heart rate.

What to Expect After Cardiac MRI

You'll be able to return to your normal routine once the cardiac MRI is done.

If you took medicine to help you relax during the test, your doctor will tell you when you can return to your normal routine. The medicine will make you sleepy, so you'll need someone to drive you home.

What Does Cardiac MRI Show?

The doctor supervising your scan will provide your doctor with the results of your cardiac MRI. Your doctor will discuss the findings with you.

Cardiac MRI can reveal various heart diseases and conditions, such as the following:

- Coronary heart disease
- Damage caused by a heart attack
- Heart failure
- Heart valve problems
- Congenital heart defects (heart defects present at birth)
- Pericarditis (a condition in which the membrane, or sac, around your heart is inflamed)
- Cardiac tumors

Cardiac MRI is a fast, accurate tool that can help diagnose a heart attack. The test does this by detecting areas of the heart that don't move normally, have poor blood supply, or are scarred.

Cardiac MRI also can show whether any of the coronary arteries are blocked. A blockage prevents your heart muscle from getting enough oxygen-rich blood, which can lead to a heart attack.

Currently, coronary angiography is the most common procedure for looking at blockages in the coronary arteries. Coronary angiography is an invasive procedure that uses x-rays and iodine-based dye.

Researchers have found that cardiac MRI can sometimes replace coronary angiography, avoiding the need to use x-ray radiation and iodine-based dye. This use of MRI is called MR angiography (MRA).

Echocardiography (echo) is the main test for diagnosing heart valve disease. However, your doctor also might recommend cardiac MRI to assess the severity of valve disease.

A cardiac MRI can confirm information about valve defects or provide more detailed information about heart valve disease.

This information can help your doctor plan your treatment. An MRI also might be done before heart valve surgery to help your surgeon plan for the surgery.

Researchers are finding new ways to use cardiac MRI. In the future, cardiac MRI may replace x-rays as the main way to guide invasive procedures such as cardiac catheterization.

Also, improvements in cardiac MRI will likely lead to better methods for detecting heart disease in the future.

What Are the Risks of Cardiac MRI?

The magnetic fields and radio waves used in cardiac MRI have no side effects. This method of taking pictures of organs and tissues doesn't carry a risk of causing cancer or birth defects.

Serious reactions to the contrast agent used during some MRI tests are very rare. However, side effects are possible and include the following:

- Headache
- Nausea (feeling sick to your stomach)
- Dizziness
- Changes in taste
- Allergic reactions

Rarely, the contrast agent can harm people who have severe kidney or liver disease. The substance may cause a disease called nephrogenic systemic fibrosis.

If your cardiac MRI includes a stress test, more medicines will be used during the test. These medicines may have other side effects that aren't expected during a regular MRI scan, such as the following:

- Arrhythmias, or irregular heartbeats

- Chest pain

- Shortness of breath

- Palpitations (feelings that your heart is skipping a beat, fluttering, or beating too hard or fast)

Chapter 45

Coronary Calcium Scan

What Is a Coronary Calcium Scan?

A coronary calcium scan is a test that looks for specks of calcium in the walls of the coronary (heart) arteries. These specks of calcium are called calcifications.

Calcifications in the coronary arteries are an early sign of coronary heart disease (CHD). CHD is a disease in which a waxy substance called plaque (plak) builds up in the coronary arteries.

Over time, plaque can harden or rupture (break open). Hardened plaque narrows the coronary arteries and reduces the flow of oxygen-rich blood to the heart. This can cause chest pain or discomfort called angina.

If the plaque ruptures, a blood clot can form on its surface. A large blood clot can mostly or completely block blood flow through a coronary artery. This is the most common cause of a heart attack. Over time, ruptured plaque also hardens and narrows the coronary arteries.

CHD also can lead to heart failure and arrhythmias. Heart failure is a condition in which your heart can't pump enough blood to meet your body's needs. Arrhythmias are problems with the rate or rhythm of your heartbeat.

Excerpted from "What Is a Coronary Calcium Scan?" National Heart, Lung, and Blood Institute, National Institutes of Health, March 30, 2012.

What to Expect Before a Coronary Calcium Scan

You don't need to take any special steps before having a coronary calcium scan. However, your doctor may ask you to avoid caffeine and smoking for four hours before the test.

For the scan, you'll remove your clothes above the waist and wear a hospital gown. You also will remove any jewelry from around your neck or chest.

What to Expect During a Coronary Calcium Scan

A coronary calcium scan is done in a hospital or outpatient office. The x-ray machine that's used for the scan is called a computed tomography (CT) scanner.

The technician who runs the scanner will clean areas of your chest and apply sticky patches with sensors called electrodes. The patches are connected to an electrocardiogram (EKG) machine.

The EKG will record your heart's electrical activity during the scan. This makes it possible to take pictures of your heart when it's relaxed between beats.

The CT scanner is a large machine that has a hollow, circular tube in the center. You'll lie on your back on a sliding table. The table can move up and down, and it goes inside the tunnel-like machine.

The table will slowly slide into the opening in the machine. Inside the scanner, an x-ray tube will move around your body to take pictures of your heart. The technician will control the CT scanner from the next room. He or she will be able to see you through a glass window and talk to you through a speaker.

The technician will ask you to lie still and hold your breath for short periods while each picture is taken. You may be given medicine to slow your heart rate. This helps the machine take clearer pictures of your heart. The medicine will be given by mouth or injected into a vein.

The coronary calcium scan will take about ten to fifteen minutes, although the actual scanning will take only a few seconds. During the test, the machine will make clicking and whirring sounds as it takes pictures. The scan causes no discomfort, but the exam room might be chilly to keep the machine working properly.

If you get nervous in enclosed or tight spaces, you might receive medicine to help you stay calm. Your head will remain outside the opening in the machine during the test.

What to Expect After a Coronary Calcium Scan

You'll be able to return to your normal activities after the coronary calcium scan is done. Your doctor will discuss the results of the test with you.

What Does a Coronary Calcium Scan Show?

After a coronary calcium scan, you'll get a calcium score called an Agatston score. The score is based on the amount of calcium found in your coronary (heart) arteries. You may get an Agatston score for each major artery and a total score.

The test is negative if no calcifications are found in your arteries. This means your chance of having a heart attack in the next two to five years is low.

The test is positive if calcifications are found in your arteries. Calcifications are a sign of atherosclerosis and coronary heart disease (CHD). (Atherosclerosis is a condition in which plaque builds up in the arteries.) The higher your Agatston score is, the more severe the atherosclerosis.

An Agatston score of 0 is normal. In general, the higher your score, the more likely you are to have CHD. If your score is high, your doctor may recommend more tests.

What Are the Risks of a Coronary Calcium Scan?

Coronary calcium scans have very few risks. The test isn't invasive, which means that no surgery is done and no instruments are inserted into your body.

Unlike some CT scans, coronary calcium scans don't require an injection of contrast dye to make your heart or arteries visible on x-ray images.

Coronary calcium scans involve radiation, although the amount used is considered small. Electron beam computed tomography (EBCT) uses less radiation than multidetector computed tomography (MDCT).

In either case, the amount of radiation is about equal to the amount of radiation you're naturally exposed to in a single year.

Chapter 46

Nuclear Heart Scan

What Is a Nuclear Heart Scan?

A nuclear heart scan is a test that provides important information about the health of your heart.

For this test, a safe, radioactive substance called a tracer is injected into your bloodstream through a vein. The tracer travels to your heart and releases energy. Special cameras outside of your body detect the energy and use it to create pictures of your heart.

Nuclear heart scans are used for three main purposes:

- To check how blood is flowing to the heart muscle. If part of the heart muscle isn't getting blood, it may be a sign of coronary heart disease (CHD). CHD can lead to chest pain called angina, a heart attack, and other heart problems. When a nuclear heart scan is done for this purpose, it's called myocardial perfusion scanning.

- To look for damaged heart muscle. Damage might be the result of a previous heart attack, injury, infection, or medicine. When a nuclear heart scan is done for this purpose, it's called myocardial viability testing.

- To see how well your heart pumps blood to your body. When a nuclear heart scan is done for this purpose, it's called ventricular function scanning.

"What Is Nuclear Heart Scan?" National Heart, Lung, and Blood Institute, National Institutes of Health, March 9, 2012.

Usually, two sets of pictures are taken during a nuclear heart scan. The first set is taken right after a stress test, while your heart is beating fast.

During a stress test, you exercise to make your heart work hard and beat fast. If you can't exercise, you might be given medicine to increase your heart rate. This is called a pharmacological stress test.

The second set of pictures is taken later, while your heart is at rest and beating at a normal rate.

Types of Nuclear Heart Scans

The two main types of nuclear heart scans are single photon emission computed tomography (SPECT) and cardiac positron emission tomography (PET).

Single Photon Emission Computed Tomography

Doctors use SPECT to help diagnose coronary heart disease (CHD). Combining SPECT with a stress test can show problems with blood flow to the heart. Sometimes doctors can detect these problems only when the heart is working hard and beating fast.

Doctors also use SPECT to look for areas of damaged or dead heart muscle tissue. These areas might be the result of a previous heart attack or other cause.

SPECT also can show how well the heart's lower left chamber (left ventricle) pumps blood to the body. Weak pumping ability might be the result of a heart attack, heart failure, and other causes.

Tracers commonly used during SPECT include thallium-201, technetium-99m sestamibi (Cardiolite®), and technetium-99m tetrofosmin (Myoview™).

Positron Emission Tomography

Doctors can use PET for the same purposes as SPECT—to diagnose CHD, check for damaged or dead heart muscle tissue, and check the heart's pumping strength.

Compared with SPECT, PET takes a clearer picture through thick layers of tissue (such as abdominal or breast tissue). PET also is better at showing whether CHD is affecting more than one of your heart's blood vessels.

Right now, however, there's no clear advantage of using one scan over the other in all situations. Research into advances in both SPECT and PET is ongoing.

PET uses different tracers than SPECT.

What to Expect Before a Nuclear Heart Scan

A nuclear heart scan can take a lot of time. Most scans take between two and five hours, especially if your doctor needs two sets of pictures.

Discuss with your doctor how a nuclear heart scan is done. Talk with him or her about your overall health, including health problems such as asthma, chronic obstructive pulmonary disease (COPD), diabetes, and kidney disease.

If you have lung disease or diabetes, your doctor will give you special instructions before the nuclear heart scan.

If you're having a stress test as part of your nuclear heart scan, wear comfortable walking shoes and loose-fitting clothes for the test. You may be asked to wear a hospital gown during the test.

Let your doctor know about any medicines you take, including prescription and over-the-counter medicines, vitamins, minerals, and other supplements. Some medicines and supplements can interfere with the medicines that might be used during the stress test to raise your heart rate.

What to Expect During a Nuclear Heart Scan

Many nuclear medicine centers are located in hospitals. A doctor who has special training in nuclear heart scans—a cardiologist or radiologist—will oversee the test.

Cardiologists are doctors who specialize in diagnosing and treating heart problems. Radiologists are doctors who have special training in medical imaging techniques.

Before the test begins, the doctor or a technician will use a needle to insert an intravenous (IV) line into a vein in your arm. Through this IV line, he or she will put radioactive tracer into your bloodstream at the right time.

You also will have electrocardiogram (EKG) patches attached to your body to check your heart rate during the test. (An EKG is a simple test that detects and records the heart's electrical activity.)

During the Stress Test

If you're having an exercise stress test as part of your nuclear scan, you'll walk on a treadmill or pedal a stationary bike. During this time, you'll be attached to EKG and blood pressure monitors.

Your doctor will ask you to exercise until you're too tired to continue, short of breath, or having chest or leg pain. You can expect that your heart will beat faster, you'll breathe faster, your blood pressure will increase, and you'll sweat.

Tell your doctor if you have any chest, arm, or jaw pain or discomfort. Also, report any dizziness, light-headedness, or other unusual symptoms.

If you're unable to exercise, your doctor may give you medicine to increase your heart rate. This is called a pharmacological stress test. The medicine might make you feel anxious, sick, dizzy, or shaky for a short time. If the side effects are severe, your doctor may give you other medicine to relieve the symptoms.

Before the exercise or pharmacological stress test ends, the tracer is injected through the IV line.

During the Nuclear Heart Scan

The nuclear heart scan will start shortly after the stress test. You'll lie very still on a padded table.

The nuclear heart scan camera, called a gamma camera, is enclosed in metal housing. The camera can be put in several positions around your body as you lie on the padded table.

For some nuclear heart scans, the metal housing is shaped like a doughnut (with a hole in the middle). You lie on a table that slowly moves through the hole. A computer nearby or in another room collects pictures of your heart.

Usually, two sets of pictures are taken. One will be taken right after the stress test and the other will be taken after a period of rest. The pictures might be taken all in one day or over two days. Each set of pictures takes about fifteen to thirty minutes.

Some people find it hard to stay in one position during the test. Others may feel anxious while lying in the doughnut-shaped scanner. The table may feel hard, and the room may feel chilly because of the air conditioning needed to maintain the machines.

Let your doctor or technician know how you're feeling during the test so he or she can respond as needed.

What to Expect After a Nuclear Heart Scan

Your doctor may ask you to return to the nuclear medicine center on a second day for more pictures. Outpatients will be allowed to go home after the scan or leave the nuclear medicine center between the two scans.

Most people can go back to their daily routines after a nuclear heart scan. The radioactivity will naturally leave your body in your urine or stool. It's helpful to drink plenty of fluids after the test, as your doctor advises.

The cardiologist or radiologist will read and interpret the results of your test. He or she will report the results to your doctor, who will contact you to discuss them. Or, the cardiologist or radiologist may contact you directly to discuss the results.

What Does a Nuclear Heart Scan Show?

The results from a nuclear heart scan can help doctors do the following things:

- Diagnose heart conditions, such as coronary heart disease (CHD), and decide the best course of treatment.

- Manage certain heart diseases, such as CHD and heart failure, and predict short-term or long-term survival.

- Determine your risk for a heart attack.

- Decide whether other heart tests or procedures will help you. Examples of these tests and procedures include coronary angiography and cardiac catheterization.

- Decide whether procedures that increase blood flow to the coronary arteries will help you. Examples of these procedures include angioplasty and coronary artery bypass grafting (CABG).

- Monitor procedures or surgeries that have been done, such as CABG or a heart transplant.

What Are the Risks of a Nuclear Heart Scan?

The radioactive tracer used during nuclear heart scanning exposes the body to a very small amount of radiation. No long-term effects have been reported from these doses.

Radiation dose might be a concern for people who need multiple scans. However, advances in hardware and software may greatly reduce the radiation dose people receive.

Some people are allergic to the radioactive tracer, but this is rare.

If you have coronary heart disease, you may have chest pain during the stress test while you're exercising or taking medicine to raise your heart rate. Medicine can relieve this symptom.

If you're pregnant, tell your doctor or technician before the scan. It might be postponed until after the pregnancy.

447

Chapter 47

Heart Biopsy

Myocardial biopsy is the removal of a small piece of heart muscle for examination.

How the Test Is Performed

Myocardial biopsy is done during cardiac catheterization or similar procedure.

The procedure will take place in a hospital radiology department, special procedures room, or cardiac diagnostics laboratory. You may be given a sedative prior to the procedure to help you relax, but you will remain awake and able to follow instructions during the test. You will lie flat on a stretcher or table while the test is being done.

The skin is scrubbed and a local numbing medicine (anesthetic) is given.

A surgical cut will be made in your arm, neck, or groin. The health care provider inserts a thin tube (catheter) through a vein or artery, depending on whether tissue will be taken from the right or left side of the heart.

If the biopsy is done without another procedure, the catheter is usually placed through a vein in the neck and then carefully threaded into the heart. The doctor uses moving x-ray images (fluoroscopy) to guide the catheter to the correct area. Once in position, a special device with jaws on the tip is used to remove small pieces of tissue from the heart muscle.

The procedure may last one or more hours.

"Myocardial Biopsy," © 2013 A.D.A.M., Inc. Reprinted with permission.

How to Prepare for the Test

You will be told not to eat or drink anything for six to eight hours before the test. The procedure takes place in the hospital. You will usually be admitted the morning of the procedure, but in some cases, you may need to be admitted the night before.

A health care provider will explain the procedure and its risks. You must sign a consent form.

How the Test Will Feel

You may feel some pressure at the biopsy site. You may have some discomfort due to lying still for a long period of time.

Why the Test Is Performed

This procedure is routinely done after heart transplantation to watch for signs of rejection. Your doctor may also order this procedure if you have signs of:

- alcoholic cardiomyopathy;
- cardiac amyloidosis;
- cardiomyopathy;
- hypertrophic cardiomyopathy;
- idiopathic cardiomyopathy;
- ischemic cardiomyopathy;
- myocarditis;
- peripartum cardiomyopathy;
- restrictive cardiomyopathy.

Normal Results

A normal result means there was no abnormal heart muscle tissue.

What Abnormal Results Mean

An abnormal result means abnormal tissue was found. This test may reveal the cause of cardiomyopathy. Abnormal tissue may also be due to:

- amyloidosis;

- myocarditis;
- transplant rejection.

Risks

Risks are moderate and include:

- blood clots;
- bleeding from the biopsy site;
- cardiac arrhythmias;
- infection;
- injury to the recurrent laryngeal nerve;
- injury to the vein or artery;
- pneumothorax;
- rupture of the heart (very rare);
- tricuspid regurgitation.

Alternative Names

Heart biopsy; Biopsy—heart

Chapter 48

Intracardiac Electrophysiology Study

Intracardiac electrophysiology study (EPS) is a test to look at the heart's electrical function. It allows doctors to check for abnormal heartbeats or heart rhythms.

How the Test Is Performed

The study involves placing wire electrodes in the heart. These electrodes measure electrical activity in the heart and its muscle cells.

The procedure is done in a hospital laboratory by trained staff that includes a cardiologist, technicians, and nurses.

A health care provider will clean your groin area and apply a numbing medicine (anesthetic). The cardiologist will then place several intravenous (IV) lines (called sheaths) into the groin or neck area. Once these IVs are in place, wires or electrodes can be passed through the sheaths into your body.

The doctor uses moving x-ray images to carefully guide the catheter up into the heart and place the electrodes into the proper areas.

The electrodes detect the heart's electrical activity and are used to check the heart's electrical system:

- Electrical signals may be used to make the heart skip beats or produce an abnormal heart rhythm. This can help the doctor

---

understand more about what is causing the abnormal heart rhythm or where in the heart it is starting.

- Certain medicines may also be used for the same purpose.

Other procedures that may also be done during the test:

- Placement of a heart pacemaker
- Procedure to destroy small areas in your heart that may be causing your heart rhythm problems (called catheter ablation)

How to Prepare for the Test

You will have to avoid eating or drinking for six to eight hours before the test.

The procedure will take place in a hospital, and you will wear hospital clothing. You must sign a consent form for the procedure.

Your health care provider will instruct you about any changes you must make to your normal medications. Do not stop taking or change any medications without first talking to your health care provider.

You will usually get a mild sedative thirty minutes before the procedure. The procedure may last from one hour to several hours. You may not be able to drive home yourself, even if you are released the same day.

How the Test Will Feel

You will be awake during the test. You may feel some discomfort when the IV is placed into your arm. You may also feel some pressure at the site when the catheter is inserted. You may feel your heart skipping beats or racing at times.

Why the Test Is Performed

Your doctor may order this test if you have signs of an abnormal heart rhythm (arrhythmia). Information from this study helps your doctor learn how severe the arrhythmia is, and the best treatment for it. Before this test is done, your cardiologist may have recommended that you have other tests.

An EPS may be done to:

- test the function of your heart's electrical system;
- pinpoint a known abnormal heart rhythm (arrhythmia) that is starting in the heart, and help decide the best therapy for it;

- determine whether you are at risk for future heart events, especially sudden cardiac death;

- see if medicine is controlling an abnormal heart rhythm;

- see whether you need a pacemaker or implantable cardioverter-defibrillator (ICD).

What Abnormal Results Mean

Abnormal results may be due to slow or fast abnormal heart rhythms, such as:

- atrial fibrillation or flutter;

- heart block;

- sick sinus syndrome;

- supraventricular tachycardia (a collection of abnormal heart rhythms that start in the upper chambers of the heart);

- ventricular fibrillation and ventricular tachycardia;

- Wolff-Parkinson-White syndrome.

This list does not include all causes of abnormal heart rhythms.

The health care provider must find the exact location and type of arrhythmia so that you can get the right treatment. The arrhythmia may start from any area of the heart's electrical system.

Risks

The procedure is generally very safe. Possible risks include:

- arrhythmias;

- bleeding;

- blood clots that lead to embolism;

- cardiac tamponade;

- heart attack;

- infection;

- injury to the vein;

- low blood pressure;

- stroke.

Alternative Names

Electrophysiology study—intracardiac; EPS—intracardiac

References

Miller JM, Zipes DP. Diagnosis of cardiac arrhythmias. In: Bonow RO, Mann DL, Zipes DP, Libby P, eds. *Braunwald's Heart Disease: A Textbook of Cardiovascular Medicine. 9th ed.* Philadelphia, Pa: Saunders Elsevier; 2011:chap 36.

Olgin JE. Approach to the patient with suspected arrhythmia. In: Goldman L, Schafer AI, eds. *Cecil Medicine. 24th ed.* Philadelphia, Pa: Saunders Elsevier; 2011:chap 62.

Part Six

Treating Cardiovascular Disorders

Chapter 49

Medications for Treating Cardiovascular Disorders

Chapter Contents

Section 49.1

Antiarrhythmic Medications

Antiarrhythmic medications are used to treat arrhythmias. An arrhythmia is an abnormal heartbeat that causes your heart to beat too quickly or too slowly. Types of fast arrhythmias include atrial fibrillation, atrial flutter, supraventricular tachycardia, ventricular tachycardia, and premature heartbeats. Slow arrhythmias are called bradycardia and are treated with a pacemaker. Antiarrhythmic medications are used only to treat rapid heart rhythms.

What Are Antiarrhythmic Medications?

Antiarrhythmic medications include several types of medications that are designed to help restore and maintain the normal rhythm of the heart. There are four main types of these medications.

Sodium channel blockers: These medications block the sodium channel of the heart muscle cells, which decreases the speed of electrical conduction. These medications include procainamide (Procan SR, Procanbid, Pronestyl), quinidine (Quinaglute, Quinidex), disopyramide (Norpace), flecainide (Tambocor), and propafenone (Rythmol and Rythmol SR). Each of these medications has a unique set of features and side effects.

Beta blockers: The primary goal of beta blockers is to slow down your heart rate. This will reduce your heart rate during an episode of your abnormally fast heart rhythm. This type of medication is primarily used to control the heart rate during an arrhythmic episode and may also reduce the number of episodes that you experience.

Potassium channel blockers: These medications block the potassium channel in the heart muscle cell and help prevent arrhythmias by lengthening the time of the electrical impulse between heartbeats.

These medications include sotalol (Betapace), dofetilide (Tikosyn) and ibutilide (Corvert, which can be administered only intravenously), amiodarone (Pacerone, Cordarone), and dronedarone (Multaq). Each of these medications has unique side effects.

Calcium channel blockers: These medications are designed to slow the heart rate when experiencing an abnormal heart rhythm. They are also often used to treat high blood pressure. Examples of calcium channel blockers include diltiazem (Cardizem, Cartia) and verapamil (Tiazac, Calan).

Treatment Goals

The goal of therapy with an antiarrhythmic medication is to prevent recurrences of an abnormal, fast arrhythmia. Some patients who take an antiarrhythmic medication will unfortunately still experience some episodes of the heart rhythm problem. Therefore, the goal with these patients is to significantly reduce the frequency and/or duration of an abnormal heart rhythm problem while avoiding side effects of the medication.

Selection of an Antiarrhythmic Medication

To determine the antiarrhythmic medication that will be best for your condition, your physician will consider the health of your heart (as indicated by your ejection fraction or pumping function of the heart muscle, measured through an echocardiogram), your type of heart rhythm problem and any other medical problems you may be experiencing, such as kidney, liver, or lung disease.

Why Might You Need Antiarrhythmic Medications?

If you have been diagnosed with an arrhythmia, the first goal is to restore a normal heart rhythm. One way to do this is through the use of antiarrhythmic medications. These medications are specifically designed to help restore and maintain normal heart rhythm. In addition to use of an antiarrhythmic medication, some patients (for example, patients with a heart rhythm problem called atrial fibrillation or atrial flutter) may also require an electrical cardioversion to restore normal rhythm or a catheter ablation procedure.

What to Expect During Antiarrhythmic Medications

For some patients, it will be suggested that they be admitted to the hospital before starting the antiarrhythmic medication. The main reason for being hospitalized is so your heart rhythm can be continuously monitored and assessed for any changes as a result of the new medication. Most patients experience no symptoms but changes in your heart rhythm may indicate that the dosage or type of medication should be changed.

Antiarrhythmic medications are very useful in helping to control heart rhythm problems but they must be tailored to each individual's specific needs and do have side effects. In order to minimize any side effects, several different tests are performed to monitor the safe use of this medicine even after you are discharged from the hospital.

Section 49.2

Antiplatelet and Anticoagulant Medications

"Anti-Clotting Agents Explained," reprinted with permission from www.heart.org. © 2013 American Heart Association, Inc. All rights reserved.

Antiplatelet and anticoagulant therapies are at the heart of preventing recurrent strokes. Although neither antiplatelet nor anticoagulant drugs can break up a clot (that's a job for tissue plasminogen activator [tPA] and other clot busters being tested), both types of drugs are effective in keeping a clot from forming or stopping the growth of one. A lot of antiplatelets and anticoagulants are available to stroke survivors, and it helps to understand them.

Antiplatelets

Blood platelets are actually fragments of cells—meaning they don't contain all the necessary cellular equipment. When a person gets a cut or scratch, platelets release thromboxane, a chemical that signals other platelets to "help out." Without the release of thromboxane, the platelets won't come (stick) together, no clot will form, and the cut will continue to bleed. If you have a wound, thromboxane is an indispensable self-sealing material; but if you're a stroke survivor, thromboxane's ability to round up "help" to form a blood clot becomes potentially life threatening.

Antiplatelet agents, including aspirin, clopidogrel, dipyridamole, and ticlopidine, work by inhibiting the production of thromboxane. Aspirin is highly recommended for preventing a first stroke, but it and other antiplatelets also have an important role in preventing recurrent strokes.

According to a statement by the American Heart Association, taking aspirin within two days of an ischemic stroke reduces the severity of the stroke. In some cases, it prevents death. For long-term (meaning for the rest of your life unless otherwise specified by your physician) prevention, antiplatelet therapy is recommended primarily for people who have had a transient ischemic attack (TIA or "mini" stroke) or acute ischemic stroke.

Despite the potential benefits, antiplatelet therapy is not for everyone. People with a history of liver or kidney disease, gastrointestinal disease or peptic ulcers, high blood pressure, bleeding disorders, or asthma may not be able to take aspirin or may require special dosage adjustments.

Anticoagulants

While antiplatelets keep clots from forming by inhibiting the production of thromboxane, anticoagulants target clotting factors, which are other agents that are crucial to the blood-clotting process. Clotting factors are proteins made in the liver. These proteins can't be created in the liver without vitamin K—a common vitamin found in cabbage, cauliflower, spinach, and other leafy green vegetables. Anticoagulants, such as warfarin (Coumadin) and heparin, slow clot formation by competing with vitamin K. This inhibits the circulation of certain clotting factors with the exotic names of factors II, VII, IX, and X. Recently two new anticoagulants were U.S. Food and Drug Association (FDA)–approved: dabigatran and rivaroxaban. Both are simpler to use and less risky than warfarin, but their cost restricts their widespread use.

The most important and most effective thing a survivor can do is take their health into their own hands.

Anticoagulants are considered more aggressive drugs than antiplatelets. They are recommended primarily for people with a high risk of stroke and people with atrial fibrillation. More than two million Americans have atrial fibrillation (AF), a rhythmic disorder of the heart where the atria (the heart's pumping chambers) quiver instead of beat. As a result, not all of the blood is pumped out of the heart, allowing pools to collect in the heart chamber, where clots may form.

An embolic stroke is a type of ischemic stroke that occurs when a piece of an atrial blood clot (embolus) is pumped out of the heart, circulates to the brain, and becomes lodged in an artery. The American Heart Association recommends that most AF patients over age sixty-five receive some sort of anticoagulant therapy.

Although anticoagulants tend to be more effective for AF patients, they are generally recommended only for patients with strokes caused by clots originating in the heart. Anticoagulants tend to be more expensive and carry a higher risk of serious side effects, including bruising and skin rash and bleeding in the brain, stomach, and intestines.

When used as directed, however, anticoagulants have proven very effective for AF patients. Although the potential risks seem severe, the life-saving effects give these drugs a bright upside.

Other people who may benefit from anticoagulant therapy for stroke prevention are those with blood that clots easily, and in some cases, patients with intracranial artery blockages that surgery can't remedy.

In comparison to antiplatelets, anticoagulants tend to be affected more by other drugs, vitamins, and even certain foods, making anticoagulant therapy somewhat troublesome for stroke survivors. Because warfarin competes with vitamin K, patients taking it should consult their doctors about possible dietary restrictions, as even some vegetables might cause an imbalance if eaten in excess. Many prescription drugs make warfarin either stronger or weaker.

Anticoagulant therapy with warfarin also requires regular blood tests to ensure the correct drug dose. A weak dosage increases the risk of stroke and heart attack, but too much may cause bleeding. Generic brands may not be the same strength as the one prescribed by your doctor.

Combinations

Given the many benefits of antiplatelet and anticoagulant therapies, it seems logical that a combination of the two might magnify the positive effects. However, researchers have found that a combination of low-dose warfarin and low-dose aspirin is no more effective than aspirin by itself. Furthermore, in the study group, major bleeding episodes (primarily gastrointestinal) occurred nearly twice as often in the combination-therapy patients compared with the aspirin-only patients.

Because of its low cost, availability, and effectiveness, aspirin is the most prescribed and used drug in antiplatelet therapy. Currently, aspirin plus extended-release dipyridamole (an antiplatelet) is the only FDA-approved combination therapy for preventing recurrent stroke.

The End of the Prescription

Anticoagulants and antiplatelets shouldn't be thought of in terms of one therapy being superior to the other. Because all strokes and stroke survivors are unique, secondary prevention must be tailored to fit each survivor's needs. Dr. Philip B. Gorelick, director of the Center for Stroke Research at RUSH Medical College in Chicago, says, "When physicians are deciding which antithrombotic agent to administer in a specific patient, cost, overall efficacy, side-effect profile, and history of underlying disease (e.g., cardiac disease, gastrointestinal bleeding, drug allergy) should be taken into account."

With so many elements factoring into treatments, confusion is inevitable, but this doesn't have to produce helplessness. While antiplatelet and anticoagulant therapies are an important aspect of secondary prevention, they aren't enough. The most important and most effective thing a survivor can do is take their health into their own hands. This means eating a healthy diet, exercising daily, abstaining from smoking, taking prescribed medicines according to doctor's orders and, of course, staying educated.

Section 49.3

Vasodilators

Reprinted from "Vasodilators and Nitrates in Heart Failure." The information in this section is from the U.S. Department of Health and Human Services, Office on Women's Health, 2013. For additional information, visit www.womenshealth.gov or www.hearthealthywomen.org.

What Are Vasodilators and Nitrates?

Vasodilators are a class of medications that cause blood vessels to widen (dilate). Nitrates are the most common type of vasodilator medication. They are sometimes given to people with heart failure to relieve symptoms that persist after treatment with the standard medications.

Nitrates are also combined with the high blood pressure drug hydralazine in a single pill to treat heart failure in African Americans who are already receiving a beta blocker and either an angiotensin-converting enzyme (ACE) inhibitor or angiotensin receptor blocker (ARB). African Americans may not respond as well as whites to ACE inhibitors, the first-choice blood pressure drugs for heart failure, which is why additional medication may be needed in these patients. This combination of nitrates and hydralazine may also be used in other patients who have symptoms despite standard treatment.

Hydralazine is used together with nitrates because nitrates widen the veins and hydralazine widens the arteries, making the combination more effective than either drug alone. Hydralazine may also have other effects that prevent the progression of heart failure.

In people with coronary artery disease, nitrates are used to prevent and relieve chest pain (angina).

Table 49.1. Nitrates

Generic:	Nitroglycerin, Isosorbide mononitrate, Isosorbide dinitrate
Brands:	Nitro-Dur, Nitrostat, Nitrolingual, Imdur, Monoket, Dilatrate, Isordil, Sorbitrate
How it is given:	Pill or tablet, skin patch, spray, injection (in the hospital)
What it is used for:	Prevention of chest pain (angina) due to coronary artery disease Acute relief of an attack of angina due to coronary artery disease Treating heart failure symptoms that have not responded to other treatments
Possible side effects:	Headache, rapid pulse, flushing, sweating, dizziness, lightheadedness, nausea, vomiting
Pregnancy/ Nursing:	The safety of nitrates during pregnancy and nursing is not known. If breastfeeding is desired, do so with caution at higher doses and with prolonged exposure. Observe the infant for signs that they are not receiving enough oxygen (shortness of breath, skin turning blue).

Table 49.2. Hydralazine & Isosorbide Dinitrate

Brands:	BiDil
How it is given:	Pill
What it is used for:	To treat heart failure in African Americans or patients who cannot take ACE inhibitors or ARBs
	Added to standard treatment in women who still have symptoms
	Prevention of chest pain (angina) due to coronary artery disease
You should not be treated with it if:	You have not tried taking ACE inhibitors or ARBs
	You should be monitored carefully if you have coronary artery disease or have suffered a heart attack
Possible side effects:	Headache, dizziness, loss of appetite, nausea, vomiting, diarrhea, pounding/fast heartbeat
Pregnancy/ Nursing:	The safety of this medication during pregnancy is unknown, so it should be used with caution; it is not known if either drug is transferred to breast milk and should be used only if the potential benefits outweigh the risks.

Chapter 50

Procedures to Treat Narrowed or Blocked Arteries

Chapter Contents

Section 50.1

Cardiac Catheterization

Excerpted from "What Is Cardiac Catheter-
ization?" National Heart, Lung, and Blood
Institute, National Institutes of Health,
January 30, 2012.

What Is Cardiac Catheterization?

Cardiac catheterization is a medical procedure used to diagnose and treat some heart conditions.

A long, thin, flexible tube called a catheter is put into a blood vessel in your arm, groin (upper thigh), or neck and threaded to your heart. Through the catheter, your doctor can do diagnostic tests and treatments on your heart.

For example, your doctor may put a special type of dye in the catheter. The dye will flow through your bloodstream to your heart. Then, your doctor will take x-ray pictures of your heart. The dye will make your coronary (heart) arteries visible on the pictures. This test is called coronary angiography.

The dye can show whether a waxy substance called plaque has built up inside your coronary arteries. Plaque can narrow or block the arteries and restrict blood flow to your heart.

The buildup of plaque in the coronary arteries is called coronary heart disease (CHD) or coronary artery disease.

Doctors also can use ultrasound during cardiac catheterization to see blockages in the coronary arteries. Ultrasound uses sound waves to create detailed pictures of the heart's blood vessels.

Doctors may take samples of blood and heart muscle during cardiac catheterization or do minor heart surgery.

Cardiologists (heart specialists) usually do cardiac catheterization in a hospital. You're awake during the procedure, and it causes little or no pain. However, you may feel some soreness in the blood vessel where the catheter was inserted.

Cardiac catheterization rarely causes serious complications.

Who Needs Cardiac Catheterization?

Doctors may recommend cardiac catheterization for various reasons. The most common reason is to evaluate chest pain.

Chest pain might be a symptom of coronary heart disease (CHD). Cardiac catheterization can show whether plaque is narrowing or blocking your coronary arteries.

Doctors also can treat CHD during cardiac catheterization using a procedure called angioplasty.

During angioplasty, a catheter with a balloon at its tip is threaded to the blocked coronary artery. Once in place, the balloon is inflated, pushing the plaque against the artery wall. This creates a wider path for blood to flow to the heart.

Sometimes a stent is placed in the artery during angioplasty. A stent is a small mesh tube that supports the inner artery wall.

Most people who have heart attacks have narrow or blocked coronary arteries. Thus, cardiac catheterization might be used as an emergency procedure to treat a heart attack. When used with angioplasty, the procedure allows your doctor to open up blocked arteries and prevent further heart damage.

Cardiac catheterization also can help your doctor figure out the best treatment plan for you if any of the following are true:

- You recently recovered from a heart attack, but are having chest pain

- You had a heart attack that caused major heart damage

- You had an electrocardiogram (EKG), stress test, or other test with results that suggested heart disease

Cardiac catheterization also might be used if your doctor thinks you have a heart defect or if you're about to have heart surgery. The procedure shows the overall shape of your heart and the four large spaces (heart chambers) inside it. This inside view of the heart will show certain heart defects and help your doctor plan your heart surgery.

Sometimes doctors use cardiac catheterization to see how well the heart valves work. Valves control blood flow in your heart. They open and shut to allow blood to flow between your heart chambers and into your arteries.

Your doctor can use cardiac catheterization to measure blood flow and oxygen levels in different parts of your heart. He or she also can check how well a man-made heart valve is working and how well your heart is pumping blood.

469

If your doctor thinks you have a heart infection or tumor, he or she may take samples of your heart muscle through the catheter. With the help of cardiac catheterization, doctors can even do minor heart surgery, such as repair certain heart defects.

What to Expect Before Cardiac Catheterization

Before having cardiac catheterization, discuss with your doctor the following things:

- How to prepare for the procedure

- Any medicines you're taking, and whether you should stop taking them before the procedure

- Whether you have any conditions (such as diabetes or kidney disease) that may require taking extra steps during or after the procedure to avoid problems

Your doctor will let you know whether you need to arrange for a ride home after the procedure.

What to Expect During Cardiac Catheterization

Cardiac catheterization is done in a hospital. During the procedure, you'll be kept on your back and awake. This allows you to follow your doctor's instructions during the procedure. You'll be given medicine to help you relax, which might make you sleepy.

Your doctor will numb the area on the arm, groin (upper thigh), or neck where the catheter will enter your blood vessel. Then, a needle will be used to make a small hole in the blood vessel. Your doctor will put a tapered tube called a sheath through the hole.

Next, your doctor will put a thin, flexible guide wire through the sheath and into your blood vessel. He or she will thread the wire through your blood vessel to your heart.

Your doctor will use the guide wire to correctly place the catheter. He or she will put the catheter through the sheath and slide it over the guide wire and into the coronary arteries.

Special x-ray movies will be taken of the guide wire and the catheter as they're moved into the heart. The movies will help your doctor see where to put the tip of the catheter.

When the catheter reaches the right spot, your doctor will use it to do tests or treatments on your heart. For example, your doctor may do angioplasty and stenting.

During the procedure, your doctor may put a special type of dye in the catheter. The dye will flow through your bloodstream to your heart. Then, your doctor will take x-ray pictures of your heart. The dye will make your coronary (heart) arteries visible on the pictures. This test is called coronary angiography.

Coronary angiography can show how well the heart's lower chambers, called the ventricles, are pumping blood.

When the catheter is inside your heart, your doctor may use it to take blood and tissue samples or do minor heart surgery.

To get a more detailed view of a blocked coronary artery, your doctor may do intracoronary ultrasound. For this test, your doctor will thread a tiny ultrasound device through the catheter and into the artery. This device gives off sound waves that bounce off the artery wall (and its blockage). The sound waves create a picture of the inside of the artery.

If the angiogram or intracoronary ultrasound shows blockages in the coronary arteries, your doctor may use angioplasty to treat the blocked arteries.

After your doctor does all of the needed tests or treatments, he or she will pull back the catheter and take it out along with the sheath. The opening left in the blood vessel will be closed up and bandaged.

A small weight might be put on top of the bandage for a few hours to apply more pressure. This will help prevent major bleeding from the site.

What to Expect After Cardiac Catheterization

After cardiac catheterization, you will be moved to a special care area. You will rest there for several hours or overnight. During that time, you'll have to limit your movement to avoid bleeding from the site where the catheter was inserted.

While you recover in this area, nurses will check your heart rate and blood pressure regularly. They also will check for bleeding from the catheter insertion site.

A small bruise might form at the catheter insertion site, and the area may feel sore or tender for about a week. Let your doctor know if you have problems such as the following:

- A constant or large amount of bleeding at the insertion site that can't be stopped with a small bandage

- Unusual pain, swelling, redness, or other signs of infection at or near the insertion site

471

Talk to your doctor about whether you should avoid certain activities, such as heavy lifting, for a short time after the procedure.

What Are the Risks of Cardiac Catheterization?

Cardiac catheterization is a common medical procedure. It rarely causes serious problems. However, complications can include the following:

- Bleeding, infection, and pain at the catheter insertion site.

- Damage to blood vessels. Rarely, the catheter may scrape or poke a hole in a blood vessel as it's threaded to the heart.

- An allergic reaction to the dye that's used during coronary angiography.

Other, less common complications include the following:

- Arrhythmias (irregular heartbeats). These irregular heartbeats often go away on their own. However, your doctor may recommend treatment if they persist.

- Kidney damage caused by the dye used during coronary angiography.

- Blood clots that can trigger a stroke, heart attack, or other serious problems.

- Low blood pressure.

- A buildup of blood or fluid in the sac that surrounds the heart. This fluid can prevent the heart from beating properly.

As with any procedure involving the heart, complications sometimes can be fatal. However, this is rare with cardiac catheterization.

The risks of cardiac catheterization are higher in people who are older and in those who have certain diseases or conditions (such as chronic kidney disease and diabetes).

Section 50.2

Carotid Endarterectomy

Excerpted from "What Is Carotid Endarterectomy?"
National Heart, Lung, and Blood Institute, National Institutes
of Health, December 1, 2010.

What Is Carotid Endarterectomy?

Carotid endarterectomy, or CEA, is a type of surgery that is used to prevent strokes in people who have carotid artery disease.

Carotid artery disease occurs if plaque builds up in the two large arteries on each side of your neck (the carotid arteries). The carotid arteries supply your brain with oxygen-rich blood.

Plaque is made up of fat, cholesterol, calcium, and other substances found in the blood. Over time, plaque hardens and narrows the carotid arteries. This limits or blocks the flow of oxygen-rich blood to your brain, which can lead to a stroke.

A stroke also can occur if the plaque in a carotid artery cracks or ruptures (bursts). Blood cell fragments called platelets stick to the site of the injury and may clump together to form blood clots. Blood clots can partly or fully block a carotid artery.

A piece of plaque or a blood clot also can break away from the wall of the carotid artery. The plaque or clot can travel through the bloodstream and get stuck in one of the brain's smaller arteries. This can block blood flow in the artery and cause a stroke.

Who Needs Carotid Endarterectomy?

Your doctor may recommend carotid endarterectomy (CEA) if you have carotid artery disease. CEA can help prevent strokes in people who have this disease.

CEA is most helpful for people who have carotid artery disease and one or more of the following:

- A prior stroke.

- A prior transient ischemic attack (TIA), also called a "mini-stroke." During a TIA, you may have some or all of the symptoms of a stroke. However, the symptoms usually last less than one to two hours (although they may last up to twenty-four hours).

- Severely blocked carotid arteries (even if you don't have stroke symptoms).

Other Treatments for Carotid Artery Disease

Anticlotting medicines, such as aspirin and clopidogrel, also are used to treat people who have carotid artery disease. These medicines help reduce blood clotting and lower the risk of stroke.

A procedure called carotid angioplasty may be used instead of CEA to treat blocked carotid arteries. For this procedure, a thin tube with a balloon on the end is threaded to the narrowed or blocked carotid artery.

Once in place, the balloon is inflated to push the plaque outward against the wall of the artery. Usually, the doctor then places a small metal stent (tube) in the artery. The stent reduces the risk that the artery will become blocked again.

What to Expect Before Carotid Endarterectomy

Your doctor will tell you how to prepare for carotid endarterectomy (CEA). Before CEA, you may have one or more tests to examine your carotid arteries. These tests can show whether your arteries are narrowed and how much they're narrowed.

What to Expect During Carotid Endarterectomy

Carotid endarterectomy (CEA) is done in a hospital. The surgery usually takes about two hours.

You will have anesthesia during the surgery so you don't feel pain. The term "anesthesia" refers to a loss of feeling and awareness. General anesthesia temporarily puts you to sleep. Local anesthesia numbs only certain areas of your body.

Your surgeon may choose to give you local anesthesia so he or she can talk to you during the surgery. This allows the surgeon to check your brain's reaction to the decrease in blood flow that occurs during the surgery.

During CEA, your surgeon will make an incision (cut) in your neck to expose the blocked section of the carotid artery. He or she will put a clamp on your artery to stop blood from flowing through it.

During the procedure, your brain gets blood from the carotid artery on the other side of your neck. However, your surgeon also may use a tube called a shunt to move blood around the narrowed or blocked carotid artery.

Next, your surgeon will make a cut in the blocked part of the artery. To remove the plaque, he or she will remove the inner lining of the artery around the blockage.

Finally, your surgeon will close the artery with stitches and stop any bleeding. He or she will then close the incision in your neck.

If you have small arteries or have already had a CEA, your surgeon might place a patch over the cut in the artery before closing the incision in your neck. The patch may reduce the risk of stroke for some patients.

Some surgeons use another technique called eversion carotid endarterectomy. For this surgery, one of the branches of the carotid artery is cut and turned inside out. The plaque is then cleaned out and the artery is reattached.

What to Expect After Carotid Endarterectomy

After carotid endarterectomy (CEA), you may stay in the hospital for one to two days. This allows you to safely recover from the procedure.

If your surgery takes place early in the day and you're doing well, you may be able to go home the same day.

Recovery

For a few days after the surgery, your neck may hurt. You also may find it hard to swallow. Your doctor may advise you to eat soft foods that are easy to swallow until your neck isn't as sore. Your doctor may prescribe medicine to help control any pain or discomfort.

Talk with your doctor about when it's safe for you to go back to your normal activities after having CEA.

Ongoing Care

After CEA, ongoing care and treatment are important. Discuss your treatment needs with your doctor. Ask him or her when you should schedule follow-up visits.

Talk with your doctor about when to seek emergency care. Problems that require urgent care may include severe headaches and swelling in the neck. Signs or symptoms that suggest a stroke or transient ischemic attack (TIA, or "mini-stroke") also require urgent care. These signs and symptoms may include the following:

• Numbness or weakness of the face, arms, or legs, especially on one side of the body

- Confusion and trouble speaking or understanding speech

- Trouble seeing in one or both eyes

- Dizziness, trouble walking, loss of balance or coordination, and unexplained falls

- Severe headache with no clear cause

Let your doctor know if you have questions about any of your medicines or how to take them. After CEA, your doctor may prescribe anti-clotting medicines, such as low-dose aspirin and clopidogrel. These medicines help prevent blood clots from forming or getting larger.

What Are the Risks of Carotid Endarterectomy?

Carotid endarterectomy (CEA) is fairly safe when done by surgeons who have experience with it. However, serious complications, such as stroke and death, can occur.

CEA also can cause less serious complications. For example, you may have a bad reaction to the anesthesia, bleeding, or infection. Short-term nerve injury may cause numbness in your face or tongue.

Certain factors may raise your risk of having CEA complications. For example, women are at higher risk of complications than men. Other risk factors include having diabetes or other serious medical conditions. People who are older than seventy-five and have other risk factors also are at higher risk.

Talk with your doctor about the risks of CEA. He or she can help you decide whether the surgery may benefit you.

Section 50.3

Coronary Angioplasty

Excerpted from "What Is Coronary Angioplasty?" National Heart, Lung,
and Blood Institute, National Institutes of Health, February 1, 2012.

What Is Coronary Angioplasty?

Coronary angioplasty is a procedure used to open narrow or blocked
coronary (heart) arteries. The procedure restores blood flow to the
heart muscle.

Who Needs Coronary Angioplasty?

Your doctor may recommend coronary angioplasty if you have narrow or blocked coronary arteries as a result of coronary heart disease
(CHD).

Angioplasty is one treatment for CHD. Other treatments include
medicines and coronary artery bypass grafting (CABG). CABG is a
type of surgery in which a healthy artery or vein from the body is connected, or grafted, to a blocked coronary artery.

The grafted artery or vein bypasses (that is, goes around) the blocked
portion of the coronary artery. This improves blood flow to the heart.

Compared with CABG, some advantages of angioplasty are that it:

- doesn't require open-heart surgery;

- doesn't require general anesthesia (that is, you won't be given
  medicine to make you sleep during the procedure);

- has a shorter recovery time.

However, angioplasty isn't for everyone. For some people, CABG
might be a better option. For example, CABG might be used to treat
people who have severe CHD, narrowing of the left main coronary
artery, or poor function in the lower left heart chamber.

Your doctor will consider many factors when deciding which
treatment(s) to recommend.

Angioplasty also is used as an emergency treatment for heart attack. As plaque builds up in the coronary arteries, it can rupture. This can cause a blood clot to form on the surface of the plaque and block blood flow to the heart muscle.

Quickly opening the blockage restores blood flow and reduces heart muscle damage during a heart attack.

How Is Coronary Angioplasty Done?

Before you have coronary angioplasty, your doctor will need to know the location and extent of the blockages in your coronary (heart) arteries. To find this information, your doctor will use coronary angiography. This test uses dye and special x-rays to show the insides of your arteries.

During angiography, a small tube (or tubes) called a catheter is inserted into an artery, usually in the groin (upper thigh). The catheter is threaded to the coronary arteries.

Special dye, which is visible on x-ray pictures, is injected through the catheter. The x-ray pictures are taken as the dye flows through your coronary arteries. The dye shows whether blockages are present and their location and severity.

For the angioplasty procedure, another catheter with a balloon at its tip (a balloon catheter) is inserted in the coronary artery and placed in the blockage. Then, the balloon is expanded. This pushes the plaque against the artery wall, relieving the blockage and improving blood flow.

A small mesh tube called a stent usually is placed in the artery during angioplasty. The stent is wrapped around the deflated balloon catheter before the catheter is inserted into the artery.

When the balloon is inflated to compress the plaque, the stent expands and attaches to the artery wall. The stent supports the inner artery wall and reduces the chance of the artery becoming narrow or blocked again.

Some stents are coated with medicine that is slowly and continuously released into the artery. They are called drug-eluting stents. The medicine helps prevent scar tissue from blocking the artery following angioplasty.

What to Expect Before Coronary Angioplasty

Coronary angioplasty is done in a hospital. A cardiologist will perform the procedure. A cardiologist is a doctor who specializes in diagnosing and treating heart diseases and conditions.

If angioplasty isn't done as an emergency treatment, you'll meet with your cardiologist beforehand. He or she will go over your medical history (including the medicines you take), do a physical exam, and talk to you about the procedure.

Your doctor also may recommend tests, such as blood tests, an electrocardiogram (EKG), and a chest x-ray.

Once the angioplasty is scheduled, your doctor will advise you about the following things:

- When to begin fasting (not eating or drinking) before the procedure. Often, you have to stop eating and drinking six to eight hours before the procedure.

- What medicines you should and shouldn't take on the day of the procedure.

- When to arrive at the hospital and where to go.

Even though angioplasty takes only one to two hours, you'll likely need to stay in the hospital overnight. Your doctor may advise you to not drive for a certain amount of time after the procedure. Thus, you'll probably need to arrange a ride home.

What to Expect During Coronary Angioplasty

Coronary angioplasty is done in a special part of the hospital called the cardiac catheterization laboratory. The "cath lab" has special video screens and x-ray machines.

Your doctor will use this equipment to see enlarged pictures of the blockages in your coronary arteries.

Preparation

In the cath lab, you'll lie down. An intravenous (IV) line will be placed in your arm to give you fluids and medicines. The medicines will relax you and help prevent blood clots from forming.

The area where your doctor will insert the catheter will be shaved. The catheter usually is inserted in your groin (upper thigh). The shaved area will be cleaned and then numbed. The numbing medicine may sting as it's going in.

The Procedure

During angioplasty, you'll be awake but sleepy.

479

Your doctor will use a needle to make a small hole in an artery in your arm or groin. A thin, flexible guide wire will be inserted into the artery through the small hole. Then, your doctor will remove the needle and place a tapered tube called a sheath over the guide wire and into the artery.

Next, your doctor will put a long, thin, flexible tube called a guiding catheter through the sheath and slide it over the guide wire. The catheter is moved to the opening of a coronary artery, and the guide wire is removed.

Your doctor will inject special dye through the catheter. The dye will help show the inside of the coronary artery and any blockages on an x-ray picture called an angiogram.

Another guide wire is then put through the catheter into the coronary artery and threaded past the blockage. A thin catheter with a balloon at its tip (a balloon catheter) is threaded over the wire and through the guiding catheter.

The balloon catheter is positioned in the blockage. Then, the balloon is inflated. This pushes the plaque against the artery wall, relieving the blockage and improving blood flow through the artery. Sometimes the balloon is inflated and deflated more than once to widen the artery.

Your doctor may put a stent (small mesh tube) in your artery to help keep it open. If so, the stent will be wrapped around the balloon catheter.

When your doctor inflates the balloon, the stent will expand against the wall of the artery. When the balloon is deflated and pulled out of the artery with the catheter, the stent remains in place in the artery.

After angioplasty is done, the sheath, guide wires, and catheters are removed from your artery. Pressure is applied to stop bleeding at the catheter insertion site. Sometimes a special device is used to seal the hole in the artery.

During angioplasty, you'll receive strong antiplatelet medicines through your IV line. These medicines help prevent blood clots from forming in the artery or on the stent. Your doctor may start you on antiplatelet medicines before the angioplasty.

What to Expect After Coronary Angioplasty

After coronary angioplasty, you'll be moved to a special care unit. You'll stay there for a few hours or overnight. You must lie still for a few hours to allow the blood vessel in your arm or groin (upper thigh) to seal completely.

While you recover, someone on your health care team will check your blood pressure, heart rate, oxygen level, and temperature. The site where the catheters were inserted also will be checked for bleeding. That area may feel sore or tender for a while.

Going Home

Most people go home the day after the procedure. When your doctor thinks you're ready to leave the hospital, you'll get instructions to follow at home, such as the following:

- How much activity or exercise you can do. (Most people are able to walk the day after the angioplasty.)

- When you should follow up with your doctor.

- What medicines you should take.

- What you should look for daily when checking for signs of infection around the catheter insertion site. Signs of infection include redness, swelling, and drainage.

- When you should call your doctor. For example, you may need to call if you have shortness of breath; a fever; or signs of infection, pain, or bleeding.

- When you should call 9-1-1 (for example, if you have any chest pain).

Your doctor will prescribe medicine to help prevent blood clots from forming. Take all of your medicine as your doctor prescribes.

If you got a stent during angioplasty, the medicine reduces the risk that blood clots will form in the stent. Blood clots in the stent can block blood flow and cause a heart attack.

Recovery and Recuperation

Most people recover from angioplasty and return to work within a week of leaving the hospital.

Your doctor will want to check your progress after you leave the hospital. During the follow-up visit, your doctor will examine you, make changes to your medicines (if needed), do any necessary tests, and check your overall recovery.

Use this time to ask questions you may have about activities, medicines, or lifestyle changes, or to talk about any other issues that concern you.

Lifestyle Changes

Although angioplasty can reduce the symptoms of coronary heart disease (CHD), it isn't a cure for CHD or the risk factors that led to it. Making healthy lifestyle changes can help treat CHD and maintain the good results from angioplasty.

Talk with your doctor about your risk factors for CHD and the lifestyle changes you should make. Lifestyle changes might include changing your diet, quitting smoking, being physically active, losing weight or maintaining a healthy weight, and reducing stress.

Cardiac Rehabilitation

Your doctor may recommend cardiac rehabilitation (rehab). Cardiac rehab is a medically supervised program that helps improve the health and well-being of people who have heart problems.

Cardiac rehab includes exercise training, education on heart healthy living, and counseling to reduce stress and help you return to an active life. Your doctor can tell you where to find a cardiac rehab program near your home.

What Are the Risks of Coronary Angioplasty?

Coronary angioplasty is a common medical procedure. Serious complications don't occur often. However, they can happen no matter how careful your doctor is or how well he or she does the procedure.

Angioplasty complications can include the following:

- Discomfort and bleeding at the catheter insertion site.

- Blood vessel damage from the catheters.

- An allergic reaction to the dye used during the angioplasty.

- An arrhythmia (irregular heartbeat).

- The need for emergency coronary artery bypass grafting during the procedure (less than 3 percent of people). This may occur if an artery closes down instead of opening up.

- Kidney damage caused by the dye used during the angioplasty.

- Heart attack (3 to 5 percent of people).

- Stroke (less than 1 percent of people).

Sometimes chest pain can occur during angioplasty because the balloon briefly blocks blood supply to the heart.

As with any procedure involving the heart, complications can sometimes be fatal. However, this is rare with coronary angioplasty. Less than 2 percent of people die during the procedure.

The risk of complications is higher in the following groups:

• People aged sixty-five and older

• People who have chronic kidney disease

• People who are in shock

• People who have extensive heart disease and blockages in their coronary (heart) arteries

Research on angioplasty is ongoing to make it safer and more effective and to prevent treated arteries from narrowing again.

Section 50.4

Coronary Artery Bypass Grafting

Excerpted from "What Is Coronary Artery Bypass Grafting?"
National Heart, Lung, and Blood Institute, National Institutes of
Health, February 23, 2012.

What Is Coronary Artery Bypass Grafting?

Coronary artery bypass grafting (CABG) is a type of surgery that improves blood flow to the heart. Surgeons use CABG to treat people who have severe coronary heart disease (CHD).

CHD is a disease in which a waxy substance called plaque builds up inside the coronary arteries. These arteries supply oxygen-rich blood to your heart.

Over time, plaque can harden or rupture (break open). Hardened plaque narrows the coronary arteries and reduces the flow of oxygen-rich blood to the heart. This can cause chest pain or discomfort called angina.

If the plaque ruptures, a blood clot can form on its surface. A large blood clot can mostly or completely block blood flow through a coronary artery. This is the most common cause of a heart attack. Over time, ruptured plaque also hardens and narrows the coronary arteries.

CABG is one treatment for CHD. During CABG, a healthy artery or vein from the body is connected, or grafted, to the blocked coronary artery. The grafted artery or vein bypasses (that is, goes around) the blocked portion of the coronary artery. This creates a new path for oxygen-rich blood to flow to the heart muscle.

Surgeons can bypass multiple coronary arteries during one surgery.

Types of Coronary Artery Bypass Grafting

There are several types of coronary artery bypass grafting (CABG). Your doctor will recommend the best option for you based on your needs.

Traditional Coronary Artery Bypass Grafting

Traditional CABG is used when at least one major artery needs to be bypassed. During the surgery, the chest bone is opened to access the heart.

Medicines are given to stop the heart; a heart-lung bypass machine keeps blood and oxygen moving throughout the body during surgery. This allows the surgeon to operate on a still heart.

After surgery, blood flow to the heart is restored. Usually, the heart starts beating again on its own. Sometimes mild electric shocks are used to restart the heart.

Off-Pump Coronary Artery Bypass Grafting

This type of CABG is similar to traditional CABG because the chest bone is opened to access the heart. However, the heart isn't stopped, and a heart-lung bypass machine isn't used. Off-pump CABG sometimes is called beating heart bypass grafting.

Minimally Invasive Direct Coronary Artery Bypass Grafting

This type of surgery differs from traditional CABG because the chest bone isn't opened to reach the heart. Instead, several small cuts are made on the left side of the chest between the ribs. This type of surgery mainly is used to bypass blood vessels at the front of the heart.

Minimally invasive bypass grafting is a fairly new procedure. It isn't right for everyone, especially if more than one or two coronary arteries need to be bypassed.

Who Needs Coronary Artery Bypass Grafting?

Coronary artery bypass grafting (CABG) is used to treat people who have severe coronary heart disease (CHD) that could lead to a heart attack. CABG also might be used during or after a heart attack to treat blocked arteries.

Your doctor may recommend CABG if other treatments, such as lifestyle changes or medicines, haven't worked. He or she also may recommend CABG if you have severe blockages in your large coronary (heart) arteries, especially if your heart's pumping action has already grown weak.

CABG also might be a treatment option if you have blockages in your coronary arteries that can't be treated with angioplasty.

Your doctor will decide whether you're a candidate for CABG based on factors such as the following:

- The presence and severity of CHD symptoms

- The severity and location of blockages in your coronary arteries

- Your response to other treatments

- Your quality of life

- Any other medical problems you have

What to Expect Before Coronary Artery Bypass Grafting

You may have tests to prepare you for coronary artery bypass grafting (CABG). For example, you may have blood tests, an electrocardiogram (EKG), echocardiography, a chest x-ray, cardiac catheterization, and coronary angiography.

Your doctor will tell you how to prepare for CABG surgery. He or she will advise you about what you can eat or drink, which medicines to take, and which activities to stop (such as smoking). You'll likely be admitted to the hospital on the same day as the surgery.

If tests for coronary heart disease show that you have severe blockages in your coronary (heart) arteries, your doctor may admit you to the hospital right away. You may have CABG that day or the day after.

What to Expect During Coronary Artery Bypass Grafting

Coronary artery bypass grafting (CABG) requires a team of experts. A cardiothoracic surgeon will do the surgery with support from an

485

anesthesiologist, perfusionist (heart-lung bypass machine specialist), other surgeons, and nurses.

There are several types of CABG. They range from traditional surgery to newer, less-invasive methods.

Traditional Coronary Artery Bypass Grafting

This type of surgery usually lasts three to six hours, depending on the number of arteries being bypassed. Many steps take place during traditional CABG.

You'll be under general anesthesia for the surgery. The term "anesthesia" refers to a loss of feeling and awareness. General anesthesia temporarily puts you to sleep.

During the surgery, the anesthesiologist will check your heartbeat, blood pressure, oxygen levels, and breathing. A breathing tube will be placed in your lungs through your throat. The tube will connect to a ventilator (a machine that supports breathing).

The surgeon will make an incision (cut) down the center of your chest. He or she will cut your chest bone and open your rib cage to reach your heart.

You'll receive medicines to stop your heart. This allows the surgeon to operate on your heart while it's not beating. You'll also receive medicines to protect your heart function during the time that it's not beating.

A heart-lung bypass machine will keep oxygen-rich blood moving throughout your body during the surgery.

The surgeon will take an artery or vein from your body—for example, from your chest or leg—to use as the bypass graft. For surgeries with several bypasses, both artery and vein grafts are commonly used:

- **Artery grafts:** These grafts are much less likely than vein grafts to become blocked over time. The left internal mammary artery most often is used for an artery graft. This artery is located inside the chest, close to the heart. Arteries from the arm or other places in the body also are used.

- **Vein grafts:** Although veins are commonly used as grafts, they're more likely than artery grafts to become blocked over time. The saphenous vein—a long vein running along the inner side of the leg—typically is used.

When the surgeon finishes the grafting, he or she will restore blood flow to your heart. Usually, the heart starts beating again on its own. Sometimes mild electric shocks are used to restart the heart.

You'll be disconnected from the heart-lung bypass machine. Then, tubes will be inserted into your chest to drain fluid.

The surgeon will use wire to close your chest bone (much like how a broken bone is repaired). The wire will stay in your body permanently. After your chest bone heals, it will be as strong as it was before the surgery.

Stitches or staples will be used to close the skin incision. The breathing tube will be removed when you're able to breathe without it.

Nontraditional Coronary Artery Bypass Grafting

Nontraditional CABG includes off-pump CABG and minimally invasive CABG.

Off-pump coronary artery bypass grafting: Surgeons can use off-pump CABG to bypass any of the coronary (heart) arteries. Off-pump CABG is similar to traditional CABG because the chest bone is opened to access the heart.

However, the heart isn't stopped and a heart-lung-bypass machine isn't used. Instead, the surgeon steadies the heart with a mechanical device.

Off-pump CABG sometimes is called beating heart bypass grafting.

Minimally invasive direct coronary artery bypass grafting: There are several types of minimally invasive direct coronary artery bypass (MIDCAB) grafting. These types of surgery differ from traditional bypass surgery because the chest bone isn't opened to reach the heart. Also, a heart-lung bypass machine isn't always used for these procedures.

These procedures are as follows:

- *MIDCAB procedure:* This type of surgery mainly is used to bypass blood vessels at the front of the heart. Small incisions are made between your ribs on the left side of your chest, directly over the artery that needs to be bypassed. The incisions usually are about three inches long. (The incision made in traditional CABG is at least six to eight inches long.) The left internal mammary artery most often is used for the graft in this procedure. A heart-lung bypass machine isn't used during MIDCAB grafting.

- *Port-access coronary artery bypass procedure:* The surgeon does this procedure through small incisions (ports) made in your chest. Artery or vein grafts are used. A heart-lung bypass machine is used during this procedure.

- *Robot-assisted technique:* This type of procedure allows for even smaller, keyhole-sized incisions. A small video camera is inserted in one incision to show the heart, while the surgeon uses remote-controlled surgical instruments to do the surgery. A heart-lung bypass machine sometimes is used during this procedure.

What to Expect After Coronary Artery Bypass Grafting

Recovery in the Hospital

After surgery, you'll typically spend one or two days in an intensive care unit (ICU). Your health care team will check your heart rate, blood pressure, and oxygen levels regularly during this time.

An intravenous (IV) line will likely be inserted into a vein in your arm. Through the IV line, you may get medicines to control blood flow and blood pressure. You also will likely have a tube in your bladder to drain urine and a tube in your chest to drain fluid.

You may receive oxygen therapy (oxygen given through nasal prongs or a mask) and a temporary pacemaker while in the ICU. A pacemaker is a small device that's placed in the chest or abdomen to help control abnormal heart rhythms.

Your doctor also might recommend that you wear compression stockings on your legs. These stockings are tight at the ankle and become looser as they go up the legs. This creates gentle pressure that keeps blood from pooling and clotting.

While in the ICU, you'll also have bandages on your chest incision (cut) and on the areas where arteries or veins were removed for grafting.

After you leave the ICU, you'll be moved to a less intensive care area of the hospital for three to five days before going home.

Recovery at Home

Your doctor will give you instructions for recovering at home, such as the following:

- How to care for your healing incisions
- How to recognize signs of infection or other complications
- When to call the doctor right away
- When to make follow-up appointments

You'll also learn how to deal with common side effects from surgery. Side effects often go away within four to six weeks after surgery, but may include the following:

- Discomfort or itching from healing incisions
- Swelling of the area where arteries or veins were removed for grafting
- Muscle pain or tightness in the shoulders and upper back
- Fatigue (tiredness), mood swings, or depression
- Problems sleeping or loss of appetite
- Constipation
- Chest pain at the site of the chest bone incision (more frequent with traditional CABG)

Full recovery from traditional CABG may take six to twelve weeks or more. Nontraditional CABG doesn't require as much recovery time.

Your doctor will tell you when you can become active again. It varies from person to person, but there are some typical timeframes.

Often, people can resume sexual activity and return to work after about six weeks. Some people may need to find less physically demanding types of work or work a reduced schedule at first.

Talk with your doctor about when you can resume activity, including sexual activity, working, and driving.

Ongoing Care

Care after surgery may include periodic checkups with doctors. During these visits, you may have tests to see how your heart is working. Tests may include an EKG (electrocardiogram), stress testing, echocardiography, and a cardiac computed tomography (CT) scan.

CABG is not a cure for coronary heart disease (CHD). After the surgery, your doctor may recommend a treatment plan that includes lifestyle changes. Following the plan can help you stay healthy and lower the risk of CHD getting worse.

Lifestyle changes might include changing your diet, quitting smoking, being physically active, losing weight or maintaining a healthy weight, and reducing stress.

Your doctor also may refer you to cardiac rehabilitation (rehab). Cardiac rehab is a medically supervised program that helps improve the health and well-being of people who have heart problems.

Cardiac rehab includes exercise training, education on heart healthy living, and counseling to reduce stress and help you return to an active life. Your doctor can tell you where to find a cardiac rehab program near your home.

Taking medicines as prescribed also is important after CABG. Your doctor may prescribe medicines to manage pain during recovery, lower your cholesterol and blood pressure, reduce the risk of blood clots forming, manage diabetes, or treat depression.

What Are the Risks of Coronary Artery Bypass Grafting?

As with any type of surgery, coronary artery bypass grafting (CABG) has risks. The risks of CABG include the following:

- Wound infection and bleeding

- Reactions to anesthesia

- Fever

- Pain

- Stroke, heart attack, or even death

Some patients have a fever associated with chest pain, irritability, and decreased appetite. This is due to inflammation involving the lung and heart sac.

This complication sometimes occurs after surgeries that involve cutting through the pericardium (the outer covering of the heart). The problem usually is mild, but some patients may develop fluid buildup around the heart that requires treatment.

Memory loss and other issues, such as problems concentrating or thinking clearly, might occur in some people.

These problems are more likely to affect older patients and women. These issues often improve within six to twelve months of surgery.

In general, the risk of complications is higher if CABG is done in an emergency situation (for example, during a heart attack). The risk also is higher if you have other diseases or conditions, such as diabetes, kidney disease, lung disease, or peripheral arterial disease (P.A.D.).

Section 50.5

Stents to Keep Coronary Arteries Open

A stent is a tiny wire mesh tube. It props open an artery and is left there permanently. When a coronary artery (an artery feeding the heart muscle) is narrowed by a buildup of fatty deposits called plaque, it can reduce blood flow. If blood flow is reduced to the heart muscle, chest pain can result. If a clot forms and completely blocks the blood flow to part of the heart muscle, a heart attack results.

Stents help keep coronary arteries open and reduce the chance of a heart attack.

How are arteries opened?

To open a narrowed artery, a doctor may do a procedure called a percutaneous coronary intervention (PCI) or angioplasty. In it, a balloon-tipped tube (catheter) is inserted into an artery and moved to the point of blockage. Then the balloon is inflated. This compresses the plaque and opens the narrowed spot. When the opening in the vessel has been widened, the balloon is deflated and the catheter is withdrawn.

How are stents used?

When a stent is used, it's collapsed and put over the balloon catheter. It's then moved into the area of the blockage. When the balloon is inflated, the stent expands, locks in place, and forms a scaffold. This holds the artery open. The stent stays in the artery permanently and holds it open. This improves blood flow to the heart muscle and relieves symptoms (usually chest pain).

Stents are used depending on certain features of the artery blockage. Factors that affect whether a stent can be used include the size of the artery and where the blockage is.

Stenting has become fairly common. Most angioplasty procedures are done using stents.

What are the advantages of using a stent?

In certain patients, stents reduce the renarrowing that sometimes occurs after balloon angioplasty or other procedures that use catheters.

Patients who have angioplasty and stents recover from these procedures much faster than patients who have coronary artery bypass surgery (CABG). They have much less discomfort, too.

Can stented arteries reclose?

In about a third of patients who've had angioplasty without a stent, the artery that was opened begins to become narrowed again within months of the procedure. This renarrowing is called restenosis.

Stents help prevent this. In recent years, doctors have used new types of stents called drug-eluting stents. These stents are covered with drugs that help keep the blood vessel from reclosing. Stents not coated with drugs are called bare metal stents. It's important that patients with either type of stent take their anti-clotting medicines as directed.

If stents don't work and the arteries reclose, you may need coronary artery bypass surgery (CABG).

What precautions should be taken after a stent procedure?

Patients who've had a stent procedure must take one or more blood-thinning agents. Examples are aspirin and clopidogrel. These medications help reduce the risk of a blood clot developing in the stent and blocking the artery:

- Aspirin is used indefinitely.

- Clopidogrel is used for one to twelve months (or perhaps even longer) after the procedure (depending on the type of stent).

- Clopidogrel can cause side effects, so blood tests will be done periodically. It's important that you don't stop taking this medication for any reason without consulting your cardiologist who has been treating your coronary artery disease.

- For the next four weeks a magnetic resonance imaging (MRI) scan should not be done without a cardiologist's approval. But metal detectors don't affect the stent.

Chapter 51

Procedures to Treat Heart Rhythm Disorders

Chapter Contents

Section 51.1

Cardiac Resynchronization Therapy

Millions of people worldwide suffer from congestive heart failure (CHF), a serious and common problem that is often due to weak pumping of the heart muscle. Poor heart pumping function can cause fatigue, leg swelling, trouble exercising, and difficulty breathing. Lifestyle changes, medications, and heart surgery can sometimes help with symptoms, but because many people with CHF also have an arrhythmia, or heart rhythm problem, they need even more help to keep their hearts functioning properly.

What is cardiac resynchronization therapy?

Cardiac resynchronization therapy (CRT) can relieve CHF symptoms by improving the timing of the heart's contractions, or beats, which protects patients from abnormally slow and fast heart rhythms.

CRT uses a biventricular pacemaker (or defibrillator) with two wires in the lower chambers of the heart to overcome this slow or abnormal conduction. By delivering simultaneous or near simultaneous electrical impulses to both lower heart chambers (the right and left ventricles), it causes the heart to beat in a more synchronized, efficient manner. Biventricular pacing improves the symptoms of about two-thirds of the patients undergoing this procedure and also improves survival.

As people with heart muscle damage also may have dangerously fast heart rhythms, biventricular pacing is often combined with a defibrillator.

How does a CRT device work?

The procedure to put in a resynchronization device is a little more complicated than putting in a regular pacemaker or defibrillator. The extra or third wire required is usually positioned in a very small vein that goes to the left side of the heart. Although most people have a vein that can be used for this purpose, this is not true of everyone. Therefore, occasionally this extra wire is placed on the outside of the heart during a surgical procedure or at the time of another heart operation such as valve surgery or a coronary bypass operation.

Like all pacemakers and defibrillators, biventricular devices require monitoring to be certain that they are functioning in the best possible way. Their batteries also gradually wear down, and they need to be changed—generally a small operation—every five to seven years.

Section 51.2

Cardioversion

Excerpted from "What is Cardioversion?" National Heart, Lung, and Blood Institute, National Institutes of Health, May 25, 2012.

What Is Cardioversion?

Cardioversion is a procedure that can restore a fast or irregular heartbeat to a normal rhythm. A fast or irregular heartbeat is called an arrhythmia.

Arrhythmias can prevent your heart from pumping enough blood to your body. They also can raise your risk for stroke, heart attack, and sudden cardiac arrest.

Who Needs Cardioversion?

Your doctor may recommend cardioversion if you have an arrhythmia that's causing troublesome symptoms. These symptoms may include dizziness, shortness of breath, extreme fatigue (tiredness), and chest discomfort.

Atrial fibrillation, or AF, is a common type of arrhythmia treated with cardioversion. In AF, the heart's electrical signals travel through the heart's upper chambers (the atria) in a fast and disorganized way. This causes the atria to quiver instead of contract.

Atrial flutter, which is similar to AF, also might be treated with cardioversion. In atrial flutter, the heart's electrical signals travel through the atria in a fast, but regular rhythm.

Cardioversion sometimes is used to treat rapid heart rhythms in the lower heart chambers (the ventricles).

Cardioversion usually is a scheduled procedure. However, you may need an emergency cardioversion if your symptoms are severe.

For some people who have other heart conditions in addition to arrhythmias, cardioversion might not be the best treatment option. Talk with your doctor about whether cardioversion is an option for you.

What to Expect Before Cardioversion

You usually can't have any food or drinks for about twelve hours before having cardioversion (as your doctor advises).

You're at higher risk for dangerous blood clots during and after a cardioversion. The procedure can dislodge blood clots that have formed as the result of an arrhythmia.

Your doctor may prescribe anticlotting medicine to prevent dangerous clots. He or she may recommend that you take this medicine for several weeks before and after the cardioversion procedure.

To find out whether you need anticlotting medicine, you might have transesophageal echocardiography (TEE) before the cardioversion. TEE is a special type of ultrasound. An ultrasound is a test that uses sound waves to look at the organs and structures in the body.

TEE involves a flexible tube with a device at its tip that sends sound waves. Your doctor will guide the tube down your throat and into your esophagus (the passage leading from your mouth to your stomach). You'll be given medicine to make you sleep during the procedure.

Your doctor will place the tube close to your heart, and the sound waves will create pictures of your heart. Your doctor will look at these pictures to see whether you have any blood clots.

The TEE will be done at the same time as the cardioversion or just before the procedure. If your doctor finds blood clots, he or she may delay your cardioversion for a few weeks. During this time, you'll take anticlotting medicine.

Even if no blood clots are found, your doctor may prescribe anticlotting medicine during and after the cardioversion to prevent dangerous blood clots from forming.

Before the cardioversion procedure, you'll be given medicine to make you sleep. This medicine can affect your awareness when you wake up. So, you'll need to arrange for someone to drive you home after the procedure.

What to Expect During Cardioversion

A nurse or technician will stick soft pads called electrodes on your chest and possibly on your back. He or she may need to shave some areas on your skin to get the pads to stick.

The electrodes will be attached to a cardioversion machine. The machine will record your heart's electrical activity and send low-energy shocks through the pads to restore a normal heart rhythm.

Your nurse will use a needle to insert an intravenous (IV) line into a vein in your arm. Through this line, you'll get medicine that will make you fall asleep.

While you're asleep, a cardiologist (heart specialist) will send one or more low-energy electrical shocks to your heart. You won't feel any pain from the shocks.

Your health care team will closely watch your heart rhythm and blood pressure during the procedure for any signs of complications.

Cardioversion takes just a few minutes. However, you'll likely be in the hospital for a few hours due to the prep time and monitoring after the procedure.

What to Expect After Cardioversion

Your health care team will closely watch you after the procedure for any signs of complications. Your doctor or nurse will let you know when you can go home. You'll likely be able to go home the same day as the procedure.

You may feel drowsy for several hours after the cardioversion because of the medicine used to make you sleep. You shouldn't drive or operate heavy machinery the day of the procedure.

You'll need to arrange for someone to drive you home from the hospital. Until the medicine wears off, it also may affect your awareness and ability to make decisions.

You may have some redness or soreness on your chest where the electrodes were placed. This may last for a few days after the procedure. You also may have slight bruising or soreness at the site where the intravenous (IV) line was inserted.

Your doctor will likely prescribe anticlotting medicine for several weeks after the procedure to prevent blood clots. During this time, you also may take medicine to prevent repeat arrhythmias.

What Are the Risks of Cardioversion?

Although uncommon, cardioversion does have risks. The procedure can sometimes worsen arrhythmias. Rarely, it can cause life-threatening arrhythmias. These irregular heartbeats are treated with electrical shocks or medicines.

Cardioversion can dislodge blood clots in the heart. These clots can travel to organs and tissues in the body and cause a stroke or other problems. Taking anticlotting medicines before and after cardioversion can reduce this risk.

Section 51.3

Catheter Ablation

Excerpted from "What Is Catheter Ablation?" National Heart, Lung, and Blood Institute, National Institutes of Health, March 5, 2012.

What Is Catheter Ablation?

Catheter ablation is a medical procedure used to treat some types of arrhythmia. An arrhythmia is a problem with the rate or rhythm of the heartbeat.

During catheter ablation, a series of catheters (thin, flexible wires) are put into a blood vessel in your arm, groin (upper thigh), or neck. The wires are guided into your heart through the blood vessel.

A special machine sends energy to your heart through one of the catheters. The energy destroys small areas of heart tissue where abnormal heartbeats may cause an arrhythmia to start.

Catheter ablation often involves radiofrequency (RF) energy. This type of energy uses radio waves to produce heat that destroys the heart tissue. Studies have shown that RF energy works well and is safe.

Who Needs Catheter Ablation?

Your doctor may recommend catheter ablation if any of the following are true:

• You have an arrhythmia that medicine can't control.

• You can't tolerate the medicine your doctor has prescribed for your arrhythmia.

- You have certain types of arrhythmia. (Your doctor can tell you whether catheter ablation can help treat your arrhythmia.)

- You have faulty electrical activity in your heart that raises your risk of ventricular fibrillation (v-fib) and sudden cardiac arrest (SCA). V-fib is a life-threatening arrhythmia. SCA is a condition in which your heart suddenly stops beating.

What to Expect Before Catheter Ablation

Before you have catheter ablation, your doctor may review your medical history, do a physical exam, and recommend tests and procedures.

Your doctor will want to know about any medicines you're taking. Some medicines can interfere with catheter ablation. If you take any of these medicines, your doctor may advise you to stop taking them before the procedure.

Your doctor also may ask whether you have diabetes, kidney disease, or other conditions. If so, he or she might need to take extra steps during or after the procedure to help you avoid complications.

Before catheter ablation, you may have tests such as the following:

- **An electrocardiogram (EKG):** This simple, painless test records your heart's electrical activity. The test shows how fast your heart is beating and its rhythm (steady or irregular). An EKG also records the strength and timing of electrical signals as they pass through your heart.

- **Echocardiography:** This is a painless test that uses sound waves to create moving pictures of your heart. The pictures show the size and shape of your heart. They also show how well your heart's chambers and valves are working.

- **Stress testing:** Some heart problems are easier to diagnose when your heart is working hard and beating fast. During stress testing, you exercise to make your heart work hard and beat fast while heart tests are done. If you can't exercise, you may be given medicine to raise your heart rate.

Less often, your doctor may recommend cardiac catheterization, coronary angiography, or a test to rule out an overactive thyroid. (An arrhythmia can be a symptom of an untreated overactive thyroid.)

If you're pregnant, let your doctor know before having catheter ablation. The procedure involves radiation, which can harm the fetus.

Talk with your doctor about whether the benefits of the procedure outweigh the risks.

If you're a woman of childbearing age, your doctor might recommend a pregnancy test before catheter ablation to make sure you're not pregnant.

Once the procedure is scheduled, your doctor will tell you how to prepare for it. You'll likely need to stop eating and drinking by midnight before the procedure. Your doctor will give you specific instructions.

Some people go home the same day as the procedure. Others need to stay in the hospital longer. Driving after the procedure might not be safe. Your doctor will let you know whether you need to arrange for someone to drive you home.

What to Expect During Catheter Ablation

Catheter ablation is done in a hospital. Doctors who do this procedure have special training in cardiac electrophysiology (the heart's electrical system) and ablation (destruction) of diseased heart tissue.

Before the Procedure

Before the procedure, you'll be given medicine through an intravenous (IV) line inserted into a vein in your arm. The medicine will help you relax and might make you sleepy. You'll also be connected to several machines that will check your heart's activity during the procedure.

Once you're drowsy, your doctor will numb an area on your arm, groin (upper thigh), or neck. He or she will use a needle to make a small hole in one of your blood vessels. Your doctor will put a tapered tube called a sheath through this hole.

Next, your doctor will put a series of catheters (thin, flexible wires) through the sheath and into your blood vessel. He or she will thread the wires to the correct place in your heart.

An imaging method called fluoroscopy will help your doctor see the wires as they're moved into your heart. Fluoroscopy uses real-time x-ray images.

During the Procedure

Electrodes at the end of the catheters will stimulate your heart and record its electrical activity. This will help your doctor learn where abnormal heartbeats are starting in your heart.

After your doctor pinpoints the source of the abnormal heartbeats, he or she will aim the tip of a special catheter at the small area of heart tissue. A machine will send energy through the catheter to create a scar line, also called an ablation line.

The scar line will create a barrier between the damaged heart tissue and the surrounding healthy heart tissue. This will stop abnormal electrical signals from traveling to the rest of the heart and causing arrhythmias.

What You Might Feel

You might sleep on and off during the procedure. You generally will not feel anything except for the following:

- A burning sensation when your doctor injects medicine into the area where he or she will insert the catheters

- Discomfort or burning in your chest when your doctor applies the energy

- A faster heartbeat when your doctor stimulates your heart to find out where abnormal heartbeats are starting

The procedure lasts three to six hours. When it's over, your doctor will remove the catheters and the sheath. He or she will close the opening in your blood vessel and bandage it. Pressure will be applied to the site to help prevent major bleeding.

What to Expect After Catheter Ablation

After catheter ablation, you'll be moved to a special care unit where you'll lie still for four to six hours of recovery. Lying still prevents bleeding from the catheter insertion site.

You'll be connected to devices that measure your heart's electrical activity and blood pressure. Nurses will regularly check these monitors. Nurses also will check to make sure that you're not bleeding from the catheter insertion site.

Going Home

Your doctor will decide whether you need to stay overnight in the hospital. Some people go home the same day as the procedure. Others need to stay in the hospital longer.

Before you go home, your doctor will tell you the following things:

- Which medicines you need to take

- How much physical activity you can do

- How to care for the catheter insertion site

- When to schedule follow-up care

Driving after the procedure might not be safe. Your doctor will let you know whether you need to arrange for someone to drive you home.

Recovery and Recuperation

Recovery from catheter ablation usually is quick. You may feel stiff and achy from lying still after the procedure.

Also, a small bruise may form at the catheter insertion site. The area may feel sore or tender for about a week. Most people can return to their normal activities within a few days.

Your doctor will talk with you about signs and symptoms to watch for. Let your doctor know whether you have problems such as the following:

- A constant or large amount of bleeding at the catheter insertion site that you can't stop with a small bandage

- Unusual pain, swelling, redness, or other signs of infection at or near the catheter insertion site

- Strong, rapid, or other irregular heartbeats

- Fainting

What Are the Risks of Catheter Ablation?

Catheter ablation has some risks. The procedure may cause any of the following:

- Bleeding, infection, and pain at the catheter insertion site.

- Damage to blood vessels. Rarely, the catheters may scrape or poke a hole in a blood vessel as they're threaded to the heart.

- Puncture of the heart.

- Damage to the heart's electrical system, which may cause you to need a permanent pacemaker. A pacemaker is a small device that's placed under the skin of your chest or abdomen to help control arrhythmias.

- Blood clots, which could lead to a stroke or other problems.

- Narrowing of the veins that carry blood from the lungs to the heart. This narrowing is called stenosis.

Also, catheter ablation involves radiation. Thus, the procedure may increase the risk of cancer, although the risk is small.

As with any procedure involving the heart, complications sometimes can be fatal. However, this is rare with catheter ablation.

Section 51.4

Implantable Cardioverter Defibrillator

Excerpted from "What Is an Implantable Cardioverter Defibrillator?" National Heart, Lung, and Blood Institute, National Institutes of Health, November 9, 2011.

What Is an Implantable Cardioverter Defibrillator?

An implantable cardioverter defibrillator (ICD) is a small device that's placed in the chest or abdomen. Doctors use the device to help treat irregular heartbeats called arrhythmias.

An ICD uses electrical pulses or shocks to help control life-threatening arrhythmias, especially those that can cause sudden cardiac arrest (SCA).

SCA is a condition in which the heart suddenly stops beating. If the heart stops beating, blood stops flowing to the brain and other vital organs. SCA usually causes death if it's not treated within minutes.

Who Needs an Implantable Cardioverter Defibrillator?

Implantable cardioverter defibrillators (ICDs) are used in children, teens, and adults. Your doctor may recommend an ICD if you're at risk for certain types of arrhythmia.

ICDs are used to treat life-threatening ventricular arrhythmias, such as those that cause the ventricles to beat too fast or quiver. You may be considered at high risk for a ventricular arrhythmia if either of the following is true:

- You have had a ventricular arrhythmia before

- You have had a heart attack that has damaged your heart's electrical system

Doctors often recommend ICDs for people who have survived sudden cardiac arrest (SCA). They also may recommend them for people who have certain heart conditions that put them at high risk for SCA.

For example, some people who have long QT syndrome, Brugada syndrome, or congenital heart disease may benefit from an ICD, even if they've never had ventricular arrhythmias before.

Some people who have heart failure may need a CRT-D device. This device combines a type of pacemaker called a cardiac resynchronization therapy (CRT) device with a defibrillator (D). CRT-D devices help both ventricles work together. This allows them to do a better job of pumping blood out of the heart.

How Does an Implantable Cardioverter Defibrillator Work?

An implantable cardioverter defibrillator (ICD) has wires with electrodes on the ends that connect to one or more of your heart's chambers. These wires carry the electrical signals from your heart to a small computer in the ICD. The computer monitors your heart rhythm.

If the ICD detects an irregular rhythm, it sends low-energy electrical pulses to prompt your heart to beat at a normal rate. If the low-energy pulses restore your heart's normal rhythm, you might avoid the high-energy pulses or shocks of the defibrillator (which can be painful).

Single-chamber ICDs have a wire that goes to either the right atrium or right ventricle. The wire senses electrical activity and corrects faulty electrical signaling within that chamber.

Dual-chamber ICDs have wires that go to both an atrium and a ventricle. These ICDs provide low-energy pulses to either or both chambers. Some dual-chamber ICDs have three wires. They go to an atrium and both ventricles.

The wires on an ICD connect to a small metal box implanted in your chest or abdomen. The box contains a battery, pulse generator, and small computer. When the computer detects irregular heartbeats, it triggers the ICD's pulse generator to send electrical pulses. Wires carry these pulses to the heart.

The ICD also can record the heart's electrical activity and heart rhythms. The recordings can help your doctor fine-tune the programming of your ICD so it works better to correct irregular heartbeats.

The type of ICD you get is based on your heart's pumping abilities, it's structural defects, and the type of irregular heartbeats you've had. Your ICD will be programmed to respond to the type of arrhythmia you're most likely to have.

What to Expect During Implantable Cardioverter Defibrillator Surgery

Placing an implantable cardioverter defibrillator (ICD) requires minor surgery, which usually is done in a hospital. You'll be given medicine right before the surgery that will help you relax and might make you fall asleep.

Your doctor will give you medicine to numb the area where he or she will put the ICD. He or she also may give you antibiotics to prevent infections.

First, your doctor will thread the ICD wires through a vein to the correct place in your heart. An x-ray "movie" of the wires as they pass through your vein and into your heart will help your doctor place them.

Once the wires are in place, your doctor will make a small cut into the skin of your chest or abdomen. He or she will then slip the ICD's small metal box through the cut and just under your skin. The box contains the battery, pulse generator, and computer.

Once the ICD is in place, your doctor will test it. You'll be given medicine to help you sleep during this testing so you don't feel any electrical pulses. Then your doctor will sew up the cut. The entire surgery takes a few hours.

What to Expect After Implantable Cardioverter Defibrillator Surgery

Expect to stay in the hospital one to two days after implantable cardioverter defibrillator (ICD) surgery. This allows your health care team to check your heartbeat and make sure your ICD is working well.

You'll need to arrange for a ride home from the hospital because you won't be able to drive for at least a week while you recover from the surgery.

For a few days to weeks after the surgery, you may have pain, swelling, or tenderness in the area where your ICD was placed. The pain usually is mild, and over-the-counter medicines can help relieve it. Talk to your doctor before taking any pain medicines.

Your doctor may ask you to avoid high-impact activities and heavy lifting for about a month after ICD surgery. Most people return to their normal activities within a few days of having the surgery.

What Are the Risks of Having an Implantable Cardioverter Defibrillator?

Unnecessary Electrical Pulses

Implantable cardioverter defibrillators (ICDs) can sometimes give electrical pulses or shocks that aren't needed.

A damaged wire or a very fast heart rate due to extreme physical activity may trigger unnecessary pulses. These pulses also can occur if you forget to take your medicines.

Children tend to be more physically active than adults. Thus, younger people who have ICDs are more likely to receive unnecessary pulses than older people.

Pulses sent too often or at the wrong time can damage the heart or trigger an irregular, sometimes dangerous heartbeat. They also can be painful and upsetting.

If needed, your doctor can reprogram your ICD or prescribe medicine so unnecessary pulses occur less often.

Risks Related to Surgery

Although rare, some ICD risks are related to the surgery used to place the device. These risks include the following:

- Swelling, bruising, or infection at the area where the ICD was placed

- Bleeding from the site where the ICD was placed

- Blood vessel, heart, or nerve damage

- A collapsed lung

- A bad reaction to the medicine used to make you relax or sleep during the surgery

Other Risks

People who have ICDs may be at higher risk for heart failure. Heart failure is a condition in which your heart can't pump enough blood to meet your body's needs. It's not clear whether an ICD increases the risk of heart failure, or whether heart failure is just more common in people who need ICDs.

Although rare, an ICD may not work properly. This will prevent the device from correcting irregular heartbeats. If this happens, your doctor may be able to reprogram the device. If that doesn't work, you doctor might have to replace the ICD.

The longer you have an ICD, the more likely it is that you'll have some of the related risks.

How Will an Implantable Cardioverter Defibrillator Affect My Lifestyle?

The low-energy electrical pulses your implantable cardioverter defibrillator (ICD) gives aren't painful. You may not notice them, or you may feel a fluttering in your chest.

The high-energy pulses or shocks your ICD gives last only a fraction of a second. They may feel like thumping or a painful kick in the chest, depending on their strength.

Your doctor may give you medicine to decrease the number of irregular heartbeats you have. This will reduce the number of high-energy pulses sent to your heart. Such medicines include amiodarone or sotalol and beta blockers.

Your doctor may want you to call his or her office or come in within twenty-four hours of getting a strong shock from your ICD. See your doctor or go to an emergency room right away if you get many strong shocks within a short time.

Devices That Can Disrupt Implantable Cardioverter Defibrillator Functions

Once you have an ICD, you have to avoid close or prolonged contact with electrical devices or devices that have strong magnetic fields. Devices that can interfere with an ICD include the following:

* Cell phones and MP3 players (for example, iPods)

* Household appliances, such as microwave ovens

* High-tension wires

* Metal detectors

* Industrial welders

* Electrical generators

These devices can disrupt the electrical signaling of your ICD and prevent it from working well. You may not be able to tell whether your ICD has been affected.

How likely a device is to disrupt your ICD depends on how long you're exposed to it and how close it is to your ICD.

To be on the safe side, some experts recommend not putting your cell phone or MP3 player in a shirt pocket over your ICD (if they're turned on). You may want to hold your cell phone up to the ear that's opposite the site where your ICD was implanted. If you strap your MP3 player to your arm while listening to it, put it on the arm that's farther from your ICD.

You can still use household appliances, but avoid close and prolonged contact, as it may interfere with your ICD.

You can walk through security system metal detectors at your normal pace. Someone can check you with a metal detector wand as long as it isn't held for too long over your ICD site. You should avoid sitting or standing close to a security system metal detector. Notify airport screeners if you have an ICD.

Stay at least two feet away from industrial welders or electrical generators. Rarely, ICDs have caused unnecessary shocks during long, high-altitude flights.

Procedures That Can Disrupt Implantable Cardioverter Defibrillator Functions

Some medical procedures can disrupt your ICD. These procedures include the following:

- Magnetic resonance imaging (MRI)

- Shock-wave lithotripsy to treat kidney stones

- Electrocauterization to stop bleeding during surgery

Let all of your doctors, dentists, and medical technicians know that you have an ICD. Your doctor can give you a card that states what kind of ICD you have. Carry this card in your wallet. You might want to wear a medical ID bracelet or necklace that states that you have an ICD.

Maintaining Daily Activities

Physical activity: An ICD usually won't limit you from taking part in sports and exercise, including strenuous activities.

You may need to avoid full-contact sports, such as football. Such contact could damage your ICD or shake loose the wires in your heart. Ask your doctor how much and what kinds of physical activity are safe for you.

Driving: You'll have to avoid driving for at least a week while you recover from ICD surgery. If you've had sudden cardiac arrest, a ventricular arrhythmia, or certain symptoms of a ventricular arrhythmia (such as fainting), your doctor may ask you to not drive until you have gone six months without fainting. Some people may still faint even with an ICD.

Commercial driving isn't permitted with an ICD.

Ongoing Care

Your doctor will want to check your ICD regularly. Over time, your ICD may stop working well for one of the following reasons:

- Its wires get dislodged or broken

- Its battery fails

- Your heart disease progresses

- Other devices have disrupted its electrical signaling

To check your ICD, your doctor may ask you to come in for an office visit several times a year. Some ICD functions can be checked over the phone or through a computer connection to the internet.

Your doctor also may recommend an electrocardiogram (EKG) to check for changes in your heart's electrical activity.

Battery Replacement

ICD batteries last between five and seven years. Your doctor will replace the generator along with the battery before the battery begins to run down.

Replacing the generator/battery is less involved surgery than the original surgery to implant the ICD. The wires of your ICD also may need to be replaced eventually. Your doctor can tell you whether you need to replace your ICD or its wires.

What Are the Benefits of Having an Implantable Cardioverter Defibrillator?

An ICD works well at detecting and stopping certain life-threatening arrhythmias. An ICD can work better than drug therapy at preventing sudden cardiac arrest, depending on the cause of the arrest.

An ICD can't cure heart disease. However, it can lower the risk of dying from SCA.

Section 51.5

Pacemaker

Excerpted from "What Is a Pacemaker?" National Heart, Lung, and
Blood Institute, National Institutes of Health, February 28, 2012.

What Is a Pacemaker?

A pacemaker is a small device that's placed in the chest or abdomen
to help control abnormal heart rhythms. This device uses electrical
pulses to prompt the heart to beat at a normal rate.

Pacemakers are used to treat arrhythmias. Arrhythmias are problems with the rate or rhythm of the heartbeat. During an arrhythmia,
the heart can beat too fast, too slow, or with an irregular rhythm.

A heartbeat that's too fast is called tachycardia. A heartbeat that's
too slow is called bradycardia.

During an arrhythmia, the heart may not be able to pump enough
blood to the body. This can cause symptoms such as fatigue (tiredness),
shortness of breath, or fainting. Severe arrhythmias can damage the
body's vital organs and may even cause loss of consciousness or death.

A pacemaker can relieve some arrhythmia symptoms, such as fatigue and fainting. A pacemaker also can help a person who has abnormal heart rhythms resume a more active lifestyle.

Who Needs a Pacemaker?

Doctors recommend pacemakers for many reasons. The most common reasons are bradycardia and heart block.

Bradycardia is a heartbeat that is slower than normal. Heart block
is a disorder that occurs if an electrical signal is slowed or disrupted
as it moves through the heart.

Heart block can happen as a result of aging, damage to the heart
from a heart attack, or other conditions that disrupt the heart's electrical activity. Some nerve and muscle disorders also can cause heart
block, including muscular dystrophy.

Your doctor also may recommend a pacemaker if any of the following are true:

- Aging or heart disease damages your sinus node's ability to set the correct pace for your heartbeat. Such damage can cause slower than normal heartbeats or long pauses between heartbeats. The damage also can cause your heart to switch between slow and fast rhythms. This condition is called sick sinus syndrome.

- You've had a medical procedure to treat an arrhythmia called atrial fibrillation. A pacemaker can help regulate your heartbeat after the procedure.

- You need to take certain heart medicines, such as beta blockers. These medicines can slow your heartbeat too much.

- You faint or have other symptoms of a slow heartbeat. For example, this may happen if the main artery in your neck that supplies your brain with blood is sensitive to pressure. Just quickly turning your neck can cause your heart to beat slower than normal. As a result, your brain might not get enough blood flow, causing you to feel faint or collapse.

- You have heart muscle problems that cause electrical signals to travel too slowly through your heart muscle. Your pacemaker may provide cardiac resynchronization therapy (CRT) for this problem. CRT devices coordinate electrical signaling between the heart's lower chambers.

- You have long QT syndrome, which puts you at risk for dangerous arrhythmias.

Doctors also may recommend pacemakers for people who have certain types of congenital heart disease or for people who have had heart transplants. Children, teens, and adults can use pacemakers.

Before recommending a pacemaker, your doctor will consider any arrhythmia symptoms you have, such as dizziness, unexplained fainting, or shortness of breath. He or she also will consider whether you have a history of heart disease, what medicines you're currently taking, and the results of heart tests.

How Does a Pacemaker Work?

A pacemaker consists of a battery, a computerized generator, and wires with sensors at their tips. (The sensors are called electrodes.) The battery powers the generator, and both are surrounded by a thin metal box. The wires connect the generator to the heart.

A pacemaker helps monitor and control your heartbeat. The electrodes detect your heart's electrical activity and send data through the wires to the computer in the generator.

If your heart rhythm is abnormal, the computer will direct the generator to send electrical pulses to your heart. The pulses travel through the wires to reach your heart.

Newer pacemakers can monitor your blood temperature, breathing, and other factors. They also can adjust your heart rate to changes in your activity.

The pacemaker's computer also records your heart's electrical activity and heart rhythm. Your doctor will use these recordings to adjust your pacemaker so it works better for you.

Your doctor can program the pacemaker's computer with an external device. He or she doesn't have to use needles or have direct contact with the pacemaker.

Pacemakers have one to three wires that are each placed in different chambers of the heart:

- The wires in a single-chamber pacemaker usually carry pulses from the generator to the right ventricle (the lower right chamber of your heart).

- The wires in a dual-chamber pacemaker carry pulses from the generator to the right atrium (the upper right chamber of your heart) and the right ventricle. The pulses help coordinate the timing of these two chambers' contractions.

- The wires in a biventricular pacemaker carry pulses from the generator to an atrium and both ventricles. The pulses help coordinate electrical signaling between the two ventricles. This type of pacemaker also is called a cardiac resynchronization therapy (CRT) device.

Types of Pacemaker Programming

The two main types of programming for pacemakers are demand pacing and rate-responsive pacing.

A demand pacemaker monitors your heart rhythm. It sends electrical pulses to your heart only if your heart is beating too slow or if it misses a beat.

A rate-responsive pacemaker will speed up or slow down your heart rate depending on how active you are. To do this, the device monitors your sinus node rate, breathing, blood temperature, and other factors to determine your activity level.

Your doctor will work with you to decide which type of pacemaker is best for you.

What to Expect During Pacemaker Surgery

Placing a pacemaker requires minor surgery. The surgery usually is done in a hospital or special heart treatment laboratory.

Before the surgery, an intravenous (IV) line will be inserted into one of your veins. You will receive medicine through the IV line to help you relax. The medicine also might make you sleepy.

Your doctor will numb the area where he or she will put the pacemaker so you don't feel any pain. Your doctor also may give you antibiotics to prevent infection.

First, your doctor will insert a needle into a large vein, usually near the shoulder opposite your dominant hand. Your doctor will then use the needle to thread the pacemaker wires into the vein and to correctly place them in your heart.

An x-ray "movie" of the wires as they pass through your vein and into your heart will help your doctor place them. Once the wires are in place, your doctor will make a small cut into the skin of your chest or abdomen.

He or she will slip the pacemaker's small metal box through the cut, place it just under your skin, and connect it to the wires that lead to your heart. The box contains the pacemaker's battery and generator.

Once the pacemaker is in place, your doctor will test it to make sure it works properly. He or she will then sew up the cut. The entire surgery takes a few hours.

What to Expect After Pacemaker Surgery

Expect to stay in the hospital overnight so your health care team can check your heartbeat and make sure your pacemaker is working well. You'll likely have to arrange for a ride to and from the hospital because your doctor may not want you to drive yourself.

For a few days to weeks after surgery, you may have pain, swelling, or tenderness in the area where your pacemaker was placed. The pain usually is mild; over-the-counter medicines often can relieve it. Talk to your doctor before taking any pain medicines.

Your doctor may ask you to avoid vigorous activities and heavy lifting for about a month after pacemaker surgery. Most people return to their normal activities within a few days of having the surgery.

What Are the Risks of Pacemaker Surgery?

Pacemaker surgery generally is safe. If problems do occur, they may include the following:

- Swelling, bleeding, bruising, or infection in the area where the pacemaker was placed

- Blood vessel or nerve damage

- A collapsed lung

- A bad reaction to the medicine used during the procedure

Talk with your doctor about the benefits and risks of pacemaker surgery.

How Will a Pacemaker Affect My Lifestyle?

Once you have a pacemaker, you have to avoid close or prolonged contact with electrical devices or devices that have strong magnetic fields. Devices that can interfere with a pacemaker include the following:

- Cell phones and MP3 players (for example, iPods)

- Household appliances, such as microwave ovens

- High-tension wires

- Metal detectors

- Industrial welders

- Electrical generators

These devices can disrupt the electrical signaling of your pacemaker and stop it from working properly. You may not be able to tell whether your pacemaker has been affected.

How likely a device is to disrupt your pacemaker depends on how long you're exposed to it and how close it is to your pacemaker.

To be safe, some experts recommend not putting your cell phone or MP3 player in a shirt pocket over your pacemaker (if the devices are turned on).

You may want to hold your cell phone up to the ear that's opposite the site where your pacemaker is implanted. If you strap your MP3 player to your arm while listening to it, put it on the arm that's farther from your pacemaker.

You can still use household appliances, but avoid close and prolonged exposure, as it may interfere with your pacemaker.

You can walk through security system metal detectors at your normal pace. Security staff can check you with a metal detector wand as long as it isn't held for too long over your pacemaker site. You should avoid sitting or standing close to a security system metal detector. Notify security staff if you have a pacemaker.

Also, stay at least two feet away from industrial welders and electrical generators.

Some medical procedures can disrupt your pacemaker. These procedures include the following:

- Magnetic resonance imaging, or MRI

- Shock-wave lithotripsy to get rid of kidney stones

- Electrocauterization to stop bleeding during surgery

Let all of your doctors, dentists, and medical technicians know that you have a pacemaker. Your doctor can give you a card that states what kind of pacemaker you have. Carry this card in your wallet. You may want to wear a medical ID bracelet or necklace that states that you have a pacemaker.

Physical Activity

In most cases, having a pacemaker won't limit you from doing sports and exercise, including strenuous activities.

You may need to avoid full-contact sports, such as football. Such contact could damage your pacemaker or shake loose the wires in your heart. Ask your doctor how much and what kinds of physical activity are safe for you.

Ongoing Care

Your doctor will want to check your pacemaker regularly (about every three months). Over time, a pacemaker can stop working properly for the following reasons:

- Its wires get dislodged or broken

- Its battery gets weak or fails

- Your heart disease progresses

- Other devices have disrupted its electrical signaling

To check your pacemaker, your doctor may ask you to come in for an office visit several times a year. Some pacemaker functions can be checked remotely using a phone or the internet.

Your doctor also may ask you to have an electrocardiogram (EKG) to check for changes in your heart's electrical activity.

Battery Replacement

Pacemaker batteries last between five and fifteen years (average six to seven years), depending on how active the pacemaker is. Your doctor will replace the generator along with the battery before the battery starts to run down.

Replacing the generator and battery is less-involved surgery than the original surgery to implant the pacemaker. Your pacemaker wires also may need to be replaced eventually.

Your doctor can tell you whether your pacemaker or its wires need to be replaced when you see him or her for follow-up visits.

Chapter 52

Procedures to Treat Heart Valve Problems

Chapter Contents

Section 52.1

Balloon Valvuloplasty

Balloon valvuloplasty, also called percutaneous balloon valvuloplasty, is a surgical procedure that opens a narrowed heart valve, without need for open heart surgery. It's also sometimes referred to as balloon enlargement of a narrowed heart valve.

What Is Balloon Valvuloplasty?

A balloon valvuloplasty is a procedure in which the narrowed heart valve is stretched open without need for open heart surgery.

During this procedure, a cardiologist uses echocardiography and x-ray images to guide a balloon into the narrowed opening of the mitral valve. The deflated balloon is positioned in the valve opening and inflated repeatedly. The inflated balloon widens the valve's opening by splitting the valve leaflets apart, thereby reducing the obstruction to blood flow.

Once the valve is widened, the balloon-tipped catheter is removed.

Why Have a Balloon Valvuloplasty?

Balloon valvuloplasty is performed on patients who have a narrowed heart valve, a condition called stenosis. It is used primarily to treat pulmonary valve stenosis or mitral valve stenosis when other medical treatment has not corrected or relieved the related problems.

The goal of the procedure is to improve valve function and blood flow by enlarging the valve opening. It is sometimes used to avoid or delay open heart surgery and valve replacement.

What to Expect During Balloon Valvuloplasty

Preparing for Your Procedure

Prior to balloon valvuloplasty, you'll meet with your physician to discuss your medical history, medications you take, and any questions you have. Avoid eating or drinking for at least six hours before the procedure.

During Your Procedure

An intravenous line is inserted so medications can be given. These medications may include anticoagulants to prevent clot formation and radioactive dye for x-rays. Your groin area is shaved and cleaned with an antiseptic. You are given an oral sedative medication about an hour before surgery to help you relax.

After Your Procedure

After your procedure, you spend several hours in the recovery room. Your vital signs, such as heart rate, breathing, and heart sounds are monitored. Electrical leads attached to electrocardiogram (EKG/ECG) equipment are placed on your chest and limbs so your health care team can monitor your status.

The site where the catheter was inserted is observed for bleeding until the catheter is removed. The leg in which the catheter was inserted is temporarily prevented from moving.

Intravenous fluids are given to help eliminate the x-ray dye. In addition, pain medication is available if needed. Your physician will determine how long you need to keep taking anticoagulant medications based on your particular symptoms and treatment.

After discharge from the hospital, you can usually resume normal activities. A balloon valvuloplasty requires lifelong follow-up with your physician because valves can degenerate and narrowing can recur (restenosis). An echocardiogram may be performed to assess the results of the procedure.

Section 52.2

Heart Valve Surgery

Heart valve surgery is done to replace or repair heart valves that aren't working correctly. Most valve replacements involve the aortic and mitral valves. The aortic valve separates the left ventricle (your heart's main pumping chamber) and the aorta (the major artery that carries blood to your body). The mitral valve separates the left atrium from the left ventricle.

What do heart valves do?

The four valves in your heart are made of thin (but strong) flaps of tissue that open and close as your heart pumps. They make sure that blood flows through your heart in the right direction. Your valves work hard as they stretch back and forth with every heartbeat.

What are the types of valve problems?

Heart valve problems make the heart work too hard. This can lead to heart failure. In some cases, valves:

- don't open enough (stenosis).

- don't let enough blood flow through (also called stenosis).

- don't close properly, and let blood leak where it shouldn't. This is called incompetence, insufficiency or regurgitation.

- prolapse—mitral valve flaps don't close properly (more common in women). As pressure builds inside the left ventricle, it pushes the mitral valve flap back into the left atrium, which may cause a small leak.

What causes valve problems?

- A small birth defect that's not repaired may get worse later in life and cause problems.

- Aging can make valves weaken or harden.

- Certain diseases can scar or destroy a valve.

What can be done?

- Yearly check-ups with your doctor, living a healthy lifestyle, or medication may be all that's needed.

- In some cases, an operation may be needed to repair a damaged valve.

- Sometimes the valve must be taken out and replaced with a new, artificial one. Ask your doctor about the different kinds used.

What is valve surgery like?

With some heart valve problems, the best treatment is surgery. Your doctor will tell you more, but here are some things you can expect:

- You'll be asleep during the operation. It can take three to five hours.

- After surgery, you'll go to an intensive care unit (ICU).

- Your family can visit you briefly in the ICU.

What about afterwards?

- After you leave the ICU, you'll move to a hospital room.

- You'll be sore and stiff from the incision.

- To clear the fluids in your lungs, you must breathe deeply and cough hard.

- You'll be given medicine.

- In a day or two, you'll be able to sit up and start walking around.

- You can eat normally, though salt may be restricted.

- You'll feel a little better and stronger each day

Chapter 53

Aneurysm Repair

An aneurysm is a weakened area of an artery that bulges or expands. The greatest concern with an aneurysm is that it may rupture. Aneurysms that rupture can cause severe internal bleeding, which can be fatal.

Most aneurysms occur in the aorta, the main artery that runs through the chest to the abdomen. There are two primary types of aortic aneurysms:

- An abdominal aortic aneurysm occurs in the part of the aorta that passes through the middle to lower abdomen.

- A thoracic aortic aneurysm occurs on the section of the aorta that passes through the chest cavity.

Aneurysms that occur in arteries other than the aorta are called peripheral aneurysms. These types of aneurysms most commonly develop in the legs.

Treatment of an aneurysm depends on its size and on the symptoms an individual may be experiencing. The goal of treatment is to prevent the aneurysm from rupturing or, in the case of a peripheral aneurysm, to prevent blood clots from developing. Aneurysms can be repaired or removed with traditional open surgery or with a minimally invasive procedure.

What Is Aneurysm Repair Surgery?

An aneurysm can be repaired with an endovascular stent graft or with open surgical repair. The best method to repair each aneurysm depends on factors such as the location and size of the aneurysm, as well as the overall health of the individual.

Endovascular repair makes use of a catheter that guides a stent graft through small incisions in the groin. The graft is inserted into the aneurysm and seals the aneurysm from within. This procedure can eliminate the need for open surgical repair.

Open surgical repair may be recommended if the aneurysm anatomy does not allow for endovascular repair. In this procedure, the damaged area is removed and replaced with a stent graft, which is made of synthetic material.

Aneurysms can be monitored or corrected surgically while the bulge is intact but require emergency surgery when they rupture. If your aneurysm is small, your physician may recommend watching and waiting, which means that you will be monitored every six to twelve months for signs of changes in the aneurysm size.

Why Have an Aneurysm Repair Surgery?

An aneurysm may or may not cause symptoms or problems. Aneurysms often do not cause symptoms and may be found incidentally during an examination for another condition. Physicians and patients must discuss and decide if the risk of surgery is less than the risk of possible bleeding if an aneurysm is not repaired.

A physician may recommend emergency surgery if an aneurysm causes symptoms, such as abdominal or back pain, because the aneurysm may be on the verge of bursting. A ruptured aneurysm is a very dangerous condition. Although it is possible to repair a ruptured aneurysm surgically, it is important to identify and treat aneurysms before a rupture occurs. An aneurysm that causes internal bleeding requires open surgery aneurysm repair.

What to Expect During Aneurysm Repair Surgery

Preparing for Your Procedure

Before surgery you'll meet with your physician to discuss your medical history, the medicines you take, and any questions you have. Your physician may also schedule routine tests including:

- **CT scan (computed tomography scan, also called CAT scan):** An imaging procedure that uses x-rays and computer technology to produce cross-sectional, detailed images of the body, including bones, muscles, fat and organs.

- **MRI (magnetic resonance imaging):** A noninvasive, sophisticated imaging procedure that uses large magnets and a computer to produce detailed images of organs and structures inside the body.

- **Ultrasound:** A test that uses high-frequency sound waves to evaluate blood flow in a vessel.

A vascular surgeon will give you instructions to follow before the surgery, such as fasting and when to stop taking medications you normally take.

During Your Procedure

There are two types of aneurysm repair surgeries. You and your surgeon will determine which procedure is right for your condition:

- **Endovascular repair:** During this procedure, repairs are made using small incisions in the groin to avoid a large abdominal or chest incision. Through the femoral artery in the leg, the surgeon inserts a catheter to position an artificial graft inside the artery. The stent graft provides a permanent alternative path for blood flow, bypassing the aneurysm.

- **Open surgery repair:** During this procedure, the surgeon makes an incision in the skin in the area above the aneurysm. Once the aneurysm is located, the surgeon places clamps on it, below and above the bulge. The surgeon cuts open the aneurysm and attaches an artificial graft to the sides of the artery. This tube connects the artery above and below the aneurysm. After the surgeon wraps the wall of the aneurysm around the graft, the clamps are removed to allow blood to flow.

After Your Procedure

You may be connected to the following equipment after surgery:

- A heart monitor
- Oxygen given through a tube in the nose and an oxygen monitor on your finger

- A Foley catheter, a tube that goes into the bladder to drain urine

- An intravenous line (IV) to provide fluids

Your physician may schedule you for an imaging study to make sure that your aneurysm is not redeveloping and that the graft is functioning properly.

You may stay in the hospital for seven to ten days after your surgery, depending on the site of your incision and your general health. Your physician or vascular surgeon will give you any special instructions you need to follow after the surgery.

Chapter 54

Heart Defect Repair

Congenital heart defect corrective surgery fixes or treats a heart defect that a child is born with. A baby born with one or more heart defects has congenital heart disease. Surgery is needed if the defect is dangerous to the child's health or well-being.

There are different types of pediatric heart surgery.

Patent Ductus Arteriosus (PDA) Ligation

- Before birth, the baby has a blood vessel that runs between the aorta (the main artery to the body) and the pulmonary artery (the main artery to the lungs), called the ductus arteriosus. This opening usually closes shortly after birth. A PDA occurs when this opening does not close after birth.

- In most cases, the doctor will use medicine to close off the opening. If this does not work, then other techniques are used to close the opening.

- Sometimes the PDA can be closed with a procedure that does not involve surgery. The procedure is usually done in a laboratory that uses x-rays. In this procedure, the surgeon inserts a wire into an artery in the leg and passes it up to the heart. There are no cuts, except for a tiny hole in the groin. Then, a small metal coil or another device is passed through the wire into the infant's arteriosus artery. The coil or other device blocks the blood flow, and this corrects the problem.

- Another method is to make a small surgical cut on the left side of the chest. The surgeon finds the PDA and then ties off or clips the ductus arteriosus, or divides and cuts it. Tying off the ductus arteriosus is called ligation. This procedure may be done in the neonatal intensive care unit (NICU).

Coarctation of the Aorta Repair

- Coarctation of the aorta occurs when a part of the aorta has a very narrow section, like in an hourglass timer.

- To repair this defect, a cut is usually made on the left side of the chest, between the ribs. There are many ways to repair coarctation of the aorta.

- The most common way to repair it is to cut the narrow section and make it bigger with a patch made of Gore-Tex, a man-made (synthetic) material.

- Another way to repair this problem is to remove the narrow section of the aorta and stitch the remaining ends together. This can usually be done in older children.

- A third way to repair this problem is called a subclavian flap. First, a cut is made in the narrow part of the aorta. Then, a patch is taken from the left subclavian artery (the artery to the arm) to enlarge the narrow section of the aorta.

- A fourth way to repair the problem is to connect a tube to the normal sections of the aorta, on either side of the narrow section. Blood flows through the tube and bypasses the narrow section.

- A newer method does not require surgery. A small wire is placed through an artery in the groin and up to the aorta. A small balloon is then opened up in the narrow area. A stent or small tube is left there to help keep the artery open. The procedure is done in a laboratory with x-rays. This procedure is often used when the coarctation occurs after it has already been fixed.

Atrial Septal Defect (ASD) Repair

- The atrial septum is the wall between the left and right atria (upper chambers) of the heart. There is a natural opening before birth that usually closes on its own when a baby is born. When the flap does not close, the child has an ASD.

- Sometimes an ASD can be closed without open-heart surgery. First, the surgeon makes a tiny cut in the groin. Then the surgeon inserts a wire into a blood vessel that goes to the heart. Next, two small umbrella-shaped "clamshell" devices are placed on the right and left sides of the septum. These two devices are attached to each other. This closes the hole in the heart. Not all medical centers do this procedure.

- Open-heart surgery may also be done to repair ASD. Using open-heart surgery, the septum can be closed using stitches. Another way to cover the hole is with a patch.

Ventricular Septal Defect (VSD) Repair

- The ventricular septum is the wall between the left and right ventricles (lower chambers) of the heart. A hole in the ventricular septum is called a VSD.

- By age one, most small VSDs close on their own. However, those VSDs that do stay open after this age must be closed.

- Larger VSDs, small ones in certain parts of the ventricular septum, or ones that cause heart failure or endocarditis (inflammation) need open-heart surgery. The hole in the septum is usually closed with a patch.

- Some septal defects can be closed without surgery. The procedure involves passing a small wire into the heart and placing a patch over the defect. The surgeon is guided by x-rays.

Tetralogy of Fallot Repair

- Tetralogy of Fallot is a heart defect that exists from birth (congenital). It usually includes four defects in the heart and causes the baby to turn a bluish color (cyanosis).

- Open-heart surgery is needed, and it is often done when the child is between six months and two years old.

- The surgery involves:
    - closing the ventricular septal defect with a patch;
    - opening the pulmonary valve and removing the thickened muscle (stenosis);

529

- placing a patch on the right ventricle and main pulmonary artery to improve blood flow to the lungs.

- The child may have a shunt procedure done first. A shunt moves blood from one area to another. This is done if the open-heart surgery needs to be delayed because the child is too sick to go through surgery:

  - During a shunt procedure, the surgeon makes a surgical cut in the left side of the chest.

  - Once the child is older, the shunt is closed and the main repair in the heart is performed.

Transposition of the Great Vessels Repair

- In a normal heart, the aorta comes from the left side of the heart, and the pulmonary artery comes from the right side. In transposition of the great vessels, these arteries come from the opposite sides of the heart. The child may also have other birth defects.

- Correcting transposition of the great vessels requires open-heart surgery. If possible, this surgery is done shortly after birth.

- The most common repair is called an arterial switch. The aorta and pulmonary artery are divided. The pulmonary artery is connected to the right ventricle, where it belongs. Then, the aorta and coronary arteries are connected to the left ventricle, where they belong.

Truncus Arteriosus Repair

- Truncus arteriosus is a rare condition that occurs when the aorta, coronary arteries, and pulmonary artery all come out of one common trunk. The disorder may be very simple, or very complex. In all cases, it requires open-heart surgery to repair the defect.

- Repair is usually done in the first few days or weeks of the infant's life. The pulmonary arteries are separated from the aortic trunk, and any defects are patched. Usually, children also have a ventricular septal defect, and that is also closed. A connection is then placed between the right ventricle and the pulmonary arteries.

- Most children need one or two more surgeries as they grow.

Tricuspid Atresia Repair

- The tricuspid valve is found between the upper and lower chambers on the right side of the heart. Tricuspid atresia occurs when this valve is deformed, narrow, or missing.

- Babies born with tricuspid atresia are blue because they cannot get blood to the lungs to pick up oxygen.

- To get to the lungs, blood must cross an atrial septal defect (ASD), ventricular septal defect (VSD), or a patent ductus artery (PDA). (These conditions are described above.) This condition severely restricts blood flow to the lungs.

- Soon after birth, the baby may be given a medicine called prostaglandin E. This medicine will help keep the patent ductus arteriosus open so that blood can continue to flow to the lungs. However, this will only work for a while. The child will eventually need surgery.

- The child may need a series of shunts and surgeries to correct this defect. The goal of this surgery is to allow blood from the body to flow into the lungs. The surgeon may have to repair the tricuspid valve, replace the valve, or put in a shunt so that blood can get to the lungs.

Total Anomalous Pulmonary Venous Return (TAPVR) Correction

- TAPVR occurs when the pulmonary veins bring oxygen-rich blood from the lungs back to the right side of the heart, instead of the left side of the heart, where it usually goes in healthy people.

- This condition must be corrected with surgery. When the surgery is done depends on how sick the baby is. The surgery may be done in the newborn period if the infant has severe symptoms. If it is not done right after birth, it is done in the first six months of the baby's life.

- TAPVR repair requires open-heart surgery. The pulmonary veins are routed back to the left side of the heart, where they belong, and any abnormal connections are closed.

- If a PDA is present, it is tied off and divided.

Hypoplastic Left Heart Repair

- This is a very severe heart defect that is caused by a very poorly developed left heart. If it is not treated, it causes death in most babies who are born with it. Unlike babies with other heart defects, those with hypoplastic left heart do not have any other defects. Operations to treat this defect are done at specialized medical centers. Usually surgery corrects this defect.

- A series of three heart operations is usually needed. The first operation is done in the first week of the baby's life. This is a complicated surgery where one blood vessel is created from the pulmonary artery and the aorta. This new vessel carries blood to the lungs and the rest of the body.

- The second operation is usually done when the baby is four to six months old (Fontan operation).

- The third operation is done a year after the second operation.

- A heart transplant is another option for this condition. But finding a donor heart for an infant is very difficult. Infant heart transplants can be done at only a few medical centers.

Chapter 55

Total Artificial Heart

What Is a Total Artificial Heart?

A total artificial heart (TAH) is a device that replaces the two lower chambers of the heart. These chambers are called ventricles. You might benefit from a TAH if both of your ventricles don't work due to end-stage heart failure.

Heart failure is a condition in which the heart can't pump enough blood to meet the body's needs. "End stage" means the condition has become so severe that all treatments, except heart transplant, have failed. (A heart transplant is surgery to remove a person's diseased heart and replace it with a healthy heart from a deceased donor.)

Overview

You might need a TAH for one of two reasons:

- To keep you alive while you wait for a heart transplant
- If you're not eligible for a heart transplant, but you have end-stage heart failure in both ventricles

The TAH is attached to your heart's upper chambers—the atria. Between the TAH and the atria are mechanical valves that work like the heart's own valves. Valves control the flow of blood in the heart.

Excerpted from "What Is a Total Artificial Heart?" National Heart, Lung, and Blood Institute, National Institutes of Health, July 6, 2012.

Currently, the two types of TAHs are the CardioWest and the Abio-Cor. The main difference between these TAHs is that the CardioWest is connected to an outside power source and the AbioCor isn't.

The CardioWest has tubes that, through holes in the abdomen, run from inside the chest to an outside power source.

The AbioCor TAH is completely contained inside the chest. A battery powers this TAH. The battery is charged through the skin with a special magnetic charger.

Energy from the external charger reaches the internal battery through an energy transfer device called transcutaneous energy transmission, or TET.

An implanted TET device is connected to the implanted battery. An external TET coil is connected to the external charger. Also, an implanted controller monitors and controls the pumping speed of the heart.

Outlook

A TAH usually extends life for months beyond what is expected with end-stage heart failure. If you're waiting for a heart transplant, a TAH can keep you alive while you wait for a donor heart. A TAH also can improve your quality of life. However, a TAH is a very complex device. It's challenging for surgeons to implant, and it can cause complications.

Currently, TAHs are used only in a small number of people. Researchers are working to make even better TAHs that will allow people to live longer and have fewer complications.

Who Needs a Total Artificial Heart?

You might benefit from a total artificial heart (TAH) if both of your ventricles don't work due to end-stage heart failure.

If you're waiting for a heart transplant, a TAH can help you survive longer. It also can improve your quality of life. If your life expectancy is less than thirty days and you're not eligible for a heart transplant, a TAH may extend your life beyond the expected thirty days.

A TAH is a "last resort" device. This means only people who have tried every other type of treatment, except heart transplant, can get it. TAHs aren't used for people who may benefit from medicines or other procedures.

TAHs also have a size limit. These devices are fairly large and can fit into only large chest areas. Currently, no TAHs are available that can fit into children's chests. However, researchers are trying to make smaller models.

The U.S. Food and Drug Administration (FDA) has approved the TAH for certain types of patients. Your doctor will discuss with you whether you meet the conditions for getting a TAH.

If you and your doctor decide that a TAH is a good option for you, you also will discuss which of the two types of TAH will work best for you.

What to Expect Before Total Artificial Heart Surgery

Before you get a total artificial heart (TAH), you'll likely spend at least a week in the hospital to prepare for the surgery. You might already be in the hospital getting treatment for heart failure.

During this time, you'll learn about the TAH and how to live with it. You and your loved ones will spend time with your surgeons, cardiologist (heart specialist), and nurses to make sure you have all the information you need before surgery. You can ask to see what the device looks like and how it will be attached inside your body.

Your doctors will make sure that your body is strong enough for the surgery. If they think your body is too weak, you may need to get extra nutrition through a feeding tube before the surgery.

You also will have tests to make sure you're ready for the surgery.

What to Expect During Total Artificial Heart Surgery

Total artificial heart (TAH) surgery is complex and can take between five and nine hours. It requires many experts and assistants. As many as fifteen people might be in the operating room during surgery.

Before the surgery, you're given medicine to make you sleep. During the surgery, the anesthesiologist checks your heartbeat, blood pressure, oxygen levels, and breathing.

A breathing tube is placed in your windpipe through your throat. This tube is connected to a ventilator (a machine that supports breathing).

A cut is made down the center of your chest. The chest bone is then cut and your ribcage is opened so the surgeon can reach your heart.

Medicines are used to stop your heart. This allows the surgeons to operate on your heart while it's still. A heart-lung bypass machine keeps oxygen-rich blood moving through your body during surgery.

What to Expect After Total Artificial Heart Surgery

Recovery in the Hospital

Recovery time after total artificial heart (TAH) surgery depends a lot on your condition before the surgery.

If you had severe heart failure for a while before getting the TAH, your body may be weak and your lungs may not work very well. Thus, you may still need a ventilator (a machine that supports breathing) after surgery. You also may need to continue getting nutrition through a feeding tube.

Your hospital stay could last a month or longer after TAH surgery.

Right after surgery, you'll be in the hospital's intensive care unit. An intravenous (IV) line will be inserted into a vein in your arm to give you fluids and nutrition. You'll also have a tube in your bladder to drain urine.

After a few days or more, depending on how quickly your body recovers, you'll move to a regular hospital room. Nurses who have experience with TAHs and similar devices will take care of you.

The nurses will help you get out of bed, sit, and walk around. As you get stronger, the feeding and urine tubes will be removed. You'll be able to go to the bathroom on your own and have a regular diet. You'll also be able to take a shower. You'll learn how to do this while taking care of your TAH device.

Nurses and physical therapists will help you gain your strength through a slow increase in activity. You'll also learn how to care for your TAH device at home.

Having family or friends visit you at the hospital can be very helpful. They can help you with various activities. They also can learn about caring for the TAH device so they can help you when you go home.

Going Home

Activity level: When you go home after TAH surgery, you'll likely be able to do more activities than you could before. You'll probably be able to get out of bed, get dressed, and move around the house. You may even be able to drive. Your health care team will advise you on the level of activity that's safe for you.

Bathing: If you have an AbioCor TAH, you can shower or swim, as long as the device is charged.

If you have a CardioWest TAH, you'll have tubes connected to a power source outside of your body. The tubes go through an opening in your skin. This opening can let in bacteria and increase your risk of infections.

You'll need to take special steps before you bathe to make sure the tubes going through your abdomen don't get wet. Your health care team will explain how to do this.

Caring for the TAH: If you have an AbioCor TAH, you'll need to keep it charged with its magnetic charger. When it's charged, you can do activities that feel comfortable to you (as your doctor advises).

If you have a CardioWest TAH, it will be attached to an external power source, also called a driver. The driver is portable, so you'll be able to walk around and do activities.

Nutrition and exercise: While you recover from TAH surgery, it's very important to get good nutrition. Talk with your health care team about following a proper eating plan for recovery.

Your health care team may recommend a supervised exercise program. Exercise can give your body the strength it needs to recover.

During the months or years when your heart wasn't working well (before surgery), the muscles in your body weakened. Building up the muscles again will allow you to do more activities and feel less tired.

Ongoing Care

You'll have regular checkups with your health care team. The team will want to check your progress and make sure your TAH is working well.

If you have an AbioCor TAH, your health care team can check it remotely. This means that if you think something is wrong, you can hook up the device to a computer with internet access.

The computer will transfer data to your health care team so they can see how your TAH is working. Certain problems may require you to see your doctor in person.

The CardioWest TAH can't be checked remotely.

Your health care team will explain warning signs to watch for. If these signs occur, or if you start feeling sick, you'll need to see your doctor right away.

Cardiac rehab: Your health care team may recommend cardiac rehabilitation (rehab). This is a medically supervised program that helps improve the health and well-being of people who have heart problems.

Rehab programs include exercise training, education on heart healthy living, and counseling to reduce stress and help you return to a more active life.

Medicines: You'll need to take medicine to prevent dangerous blood clots for as long as you have a TAH. Regular blood tests will show whether the medicine is working.

You also will need to take medicine to try to prevent infections. Your doctor may ask you to take your temperature every day to make sure you don't have a fever. A fever can be a warning sign of infection.

Make sure to take all your medicines as prescribed and report any side effects to your doctor.

Heart transplant: If you're on the waiting list for a heart transplant, you'll likely be in close contact with the transplant center. Most donor hearts must be transplanted within four hours after removal from the donor.

The transplant center staff may give you a pager so they can contact you at any time. You need to be prepared to arrive at the hospital within two hours of being notified about a donor heart.

Emotional issues: Getting a TAH may cause fear, anxiety, and stress. If you're waiting for a heart transplant, you may worry that the TAH won't keep you alive long enough to get a new heart. You may feel overwhelmed or depressed.

All of these feelings are normal for someone going through major heart surgery. Talk about how you feel with your health care team. Talking to a professional counselor also can help. If you're very depressed, your doctor may recommend medicines or other treatments that can improve your quality of life.

Support from family and friends also can help relieve stress and anxiety. Let your loved ones know how you feel and what they can do to help you.

What Are the Risks of a Total Artificial Heart?

Getting a total artificial heart (TAH) involves some serious risks. These risks include blood clots, bleeding, infection, and device malfunctions. Because of these risks, only a small number of people currently have TAHs.

There's a small risk of dying during TAH surgery. There's also a small risk that your body may respond poorly to the medicine used to put you to sleep during the surgery. However, most patients survive and recover from TAH surgery.

If you're eligible for a TAH, you'll work with your doctor to decide whether the benefits of the device outweigh the risks.

Researchers are working to improve TAHs and lessen the risks of using these devices.

Blood Clots

When your blood comes into contact with something that isn't a natural part of your body, such as a TAH, it tends to clot more than normal. Blood clots can disrupt blood flow and may block blood vessels leading to important organs in the body.

Blood clots can lead to severe complications or even death. For this reason, you need to take anticlotting medicine for as long as you have a TAH.

Bleeding

The surgery to implant a TAH is very complex. Bleeding can occur in your chest during and after the surgery.

Anticlotting medicine also raises your risk of bleeding because it thins your blood. Balancing the anticlotting medicine with the risk of bleeding can be hard. Make sure to take your medicine exactly as your doctor prescribes.

Infection

One of the two available TAHs, the CardioWest, attaches to a power source outside your body through holes in your abdomen. These holes increase the risk of bacteria getting in and causing an infection.

With permanent tubes running through your skin, the risk of infection is serious. You'll need to take medicine to try to prevent infections.

Your health care team will watch you very closely if you have any signs of infection, such as a fever. You may need to check your temperature several times a day as part of your ongoing care.

With both types of TAH, you're at risk for infection after surgery. Your doctor will prescribe medicine to reduce the risk.

Device Malfunctions

Because TAHs are so complex, they can malfunction (not work properly) in different ways. A TAH's:

- pumping action may not be exactly right;
- power may fail;
- parts may stop working well.

This doesn't mean a TAH is bound to fail. In fact, TAHs that have been implanted in people in recent years have generally worked very well. However, problems with the device can occur.

Chapter 56

Heart Transplant

What Is a Heart Transplant?

A heart transplant is surgery to remove a person's diseased heart and replace it with a healthy heart from a deceased donor. Most heart transplants are done on patients who have end-stage heart failure.

Overview

Heart transplants are done as a life-saving measure for end-stage heart failure.

Because donor hearts are in short supply, patients who need heart transplants go through a careful selection process. They must be sick enough to need a new heart, yet healthy enough to receive it.

Survival rates for people receiving heart transplants have improved, especially in the first year after the transplant.

About 88 percent of patients survive the first year after transplant surgery, and 75 percent survive for five years. The ten-year survival rate is about 56 percent.

After the surgery, most heart transplant patients can return to their normal levels of activity. However, less than 30 percent return to work for many different reasons.

Excerpted from "What Is a Heart Transplant?" National Heart, Lung, and Blood Institute, National Institutes of Health, January 3, 2012.

What to Expect Before a Heart Transplant

The Heart Transplant Waiting List

Patients who are eligible for a heart transplant are added to a waiting list for a donor heart. This waiting list is part of a national allocation system for donor organs. The Organ Procurement and Transplantation Network (OPTN) runs this system.

OPTN has policies in place to make sure donor hearts are given out fairly. These policies are based on urgency of need, available organs, and the location of the patient who is receiving the heart (the recipient).

Organs are matched for blood type and size of donor and recipient.

The Donor Heart

Guidelines for how a donor heart is selected require that the donor meet the legal requirement for brain death and that the correct consent forms are signed.

Guidelines suggest that the donor should be younger than sixty-five years old, have little or no history of heart disease or trauma to the chest, and not be exposed to hepatitis or human immunodeficiency virus (HIV).

The guidelines recommend that the donor heart should not be without blood circulation for more than four hours.

Waiting Times

About three thousand people in the United States are on the waiting list for a heart transplant on any given day. About two thousand donor hearts are available each year. Wait times vary from days to several months and will depend on a recipient's blood type and condition.

A person might be taken off the list for some time if he or she has a serious medical event, such as a stroke, infection, or kidney failure.

Time spent on the waiting list plays a part in who receives a donor heart. For example, if two patients have equal need, the one who has been waiting longer will likely get the first available donor heart.

Ongoing Medical Treatment

Patients on the waiting list for a donor heart get ongoing treatment for heart failure and other medical conditions.

For example, doctors may treat them for arrhythmias (irregular heartbeats). Arrhythmias can cause sudden cardiac arrest in people who have heart failure.

The doctors at the transplant centers may place implantable cardioverter defibrillators (ICDs) in patients before surgery. ICDs are small devices that are placed in the chest or abdomen. They help control life-threatening arrhythmias.

Another possible treatment for waiting list patients is a ventricular assist device (VAD). A VAD is a mechanical pump that helps support heart function and blood flow.

Routine outpatient care for waiting list patients may include frequent exercise testing, testing the strength of the heartbeat, and right cardiac catheterization (a test to measure blood pressure in the right side of the heart).

You also might start a cardiac rehabilitation (rehab) program. Cardiac rehab is a medically supervised program that helps improve the health and well-being of people who have heart problems.

The program can help improve your physical condition before the transplant. Also, you will learn the types of exercises used in the program, which will help you take part in cardiac rehab after the transplant.

Contact with the Transplant Center During the Wait

Patients on the waiting list often are in close contact with their transplant centers. Most donor hearts must be transplanted within four hours after removal from the donor.

At some heart transplant centers, patients get a pager so the center can contact them at any time. They're asked to tell the transplant center staff if they're going out of town. Patients often need to be prepared to arrive at the hospital within two hours of being notified about a donor heart.

Not all patients who are called to the hospital will get a heart transplant. Sometimes, at the last minute, doctors find that a donor heart isn't suitable for a patient. Other times, patients from the waiting list are called to come in as possible backups, in case something happens with the selected recipient.

What to Expect During a Heart Transplant

Just before heart transplant surgery, the patient will get general anesthesia. The term "anesthesia" refers to a loss of feeling and awareness. General anesthesia temporarily puts you to sleep.

Surgeons use open-heart surgery to do heart transplants. The surgeon will make a large incision (cut) in the patient's chest to open the rib cage and operate on the heart.

A heart-lung bypass machine is hooked up to the heart's arteries and veins. The machine pumps blood through the patient's lungs and body during the surgery.

The surgeon removes the patient's diseased heart and sews the healthy donor heart into place. The patient's aorta and pulmonary arteries are not replaced as part of the surgery.

What to Expect After a Heart Transplant

Staying in the Hospital

The amount of time a heart transplant recipient spends in the hospital varies. Recovery often involves one to two weeks in the hospital and three months of monitoring by the transplant team at the heart transplant center.

Monitoring may include frequent blood tests, lung function tests, electrocardiograms (EKGs), echocardiograms, and biopsies of the heart tissue.

A heart biopsy is a standard test that can show whether your body is rejecting the new heart. This test is often done in the weeks after a transplant.

During a heart biopsy, a tiny grabbing device is inserted into a vein in the neck or groin (upper thigh). The device is threaded through the vein to the right atrium of the new heart to take a small tissue sample. The tissue sample is checked for signs of rejection.

While in the hospital, your health care team may suggest that you start a cardiac rehabilitation (rehab) program. Cardiac rehab is a medically supervised program that helps improve the health and well-being of people who have heart problems.

Cardiac rehab includes counseling, education, and exercise training to help you recover. Rehab may start with a member of the rehab team helping you sit up in a chair or take a few steps. Over time, you'll increase your activity level.

Watching for Signs of Rejection

Your body will regard your new heart as a foreign object. You'll need medicine to prevent your immune system from attacking the heart.

You and the transplant team will work together to protect the new heart. You'll watch for signs and symptoms that your body is rejecting the organ. These signs and symptoms include the following:

- Shortness of breath
- Fever

- Fatigue (tiredness)

- Weight gain (retaining fluid in the body)

- Reduced amounts of urine (problems in the kidneys can cause this sign)

You and the team also will work together to manage the transplant medicines and their side effects, prevent infections, and continue treatment of ongoing medical conditions.

Your doctors may ask you to check your temperature, blood pressure, and pulse when you go home.

Preventing Rejection

You'll need to take medicine to suppress your immune system so that it doesn't reject the new heart. These medicines are called immunosuppressants.

Immunosuppressants are a combination of medicines that are tailored to your situation. Often, they include cyclosporine, tacrolimus, mycophenolate mofetil (MMF), and steroids (such as prednisone).

Your doctors may need to change or adjust your transplant medicines if they aren't working well or if you have too many side effects.

Managing Transplant Medicines and Their Side Effects

You'll have to manage multiple medicines after having a heart transplant. It's helpful to set up a routine for taking medicines at the same time each day and for refilling prescriptions. It's crucial to never run out of medicine. Always using the same pharmacy may help.

Keep a list of all your medicines with you at all times in case of an accident. When traveling, keep extra doses of medicine with you (not packed in your luggage). Bring your medicines with you to all doctor visits.

Side effects from medicines can be serious. Side effects include risk of infection, diabetes, osteoporosis (thinning of the bones), high blood pressure, kidney disease, and cancer—especially lymphoma and skin cancer.

Discuss any side effects of the medicines with your transplant team. Your doctors may change or adjust your medicines if you're having problems. Make sure your doctors know all of the medicines you're taking.

Preventing Infection

Some transplant medicines can increase your risk of infection. You may be asked to watch for signs of infection, including fever, sore throat, cold sores, and flu-like symptoms.

Signs of possible chest or lung infections include shortness of breath, cough, and a change in the color of sputum (spit).

Watching closely for these signs is important because transplant medicines can sometimes mask them. Also, pay close attention to signs of infection at the site of your incision (cut). These signs can include redness, swelling, or drainage.

Ask your doctor what steps you should take to reduce your risk of infection. For example, your doctor may suggest that you avoid contact with animals or crowds of people in the first few months after your transplant.

Regular dental care also is important. Your doctor or dentist may prescribe antibiotics before any dental work to prevent infections.

What Are the Risks of a Heart Transplant?

Although heart transplant surgery is a life-saving measure, it has many risks. Careful monitoring, treatment, and regular medical care can prevent or help manage some of these risks.

The risks of having a heart transplant include the following:

- Failure of the donor heart
- Complications from medicines
- Infection
- Cancer

Failure of the Donor Heart

Over time, the new heart may fail due to the same reasons that caused the original heart to fail. Failure of the donor heart also can occur if your body rejects the donor heart or if cardiac allograft vasculopathy (CAV) develops. CAV is a blood vessel disease.

Patients who have a heart transplant that fails can be considered for another transplant (called a retransplant).

Primary graft dysfunction: The most frequent cause of death in the first thirty days after transplant is primary graft dysfunction. This occurs if the new donor heart fails and isn't able to function.

Factors such as shock or trauma to the donor heart or narrow blood vessels in the recipient's lungs can cause primary graft dysfunction. Doctors may prescribe medicines (for example, inhaled nitric oxide and intravenous nitrates) to treat this condition.

Rejection of the donor heart: Rejection is one of the leading causes of death in the first year after transplant. The recipient's immune system sees the new heart as a foreign object and attacks it.

During the first year, heart transplant patients have an average of one to three episodes of rejection. Rejection is most likely to occur within six months of the transplant surgery.

Cardiac allograft vasculopathy (CAV): CAV is a chronic (ongoing) disease in which the walls of the coronary arteries in the new heart become thick, hard, and less stretchy. CAV can destroy blood circulation in the new heart and cause serious damage.

CAV is a leading cause of donor heart failure and death in the years following transplant surgery. CAV can cause heart attack, heart failure, dangerous arrhythmias, and sudden cardiac arrest.

To detect CAV, your doctor may recommend coronary angiography yearly and other tests, such as stress echocardiography or intravascular ultrasound.

Complications from Medicines

Taking daily medicines that stop the immune system from attacking the new heart is crucial, even though the medicines have serious side effects.

Cyclosporine and other medicines can cause kidney damage. Kidney damage affects more than 25 percent of patients in the first year after transplant.

Infection

When the immune system—the body's defense system—is suppressed, the risk of infection increases. Infection is a major cause of hospital admission for heart transplant patients. It also is a leading cause of death in the first year after transplant.

Cancer

Suppressing the immune system leaves patients at risk for cancers and malignancies. Malignancies are a major cause of late death in heart transplant patients.

The most common malignancies are tumors of the skin and lips (patients at highest risk are older, male, and fair-skinned) and malignancies in the lymph system, such as non-Hodgkin lymphoma.

Other Complications

High blood pressure develops in more than 70 percent of heart transplant patients in the first year after transplant and in nearly 95 percent of patients within five years.

High levels of cholesterol and triglycerides in the blood develop in more than 50 percent of heart transplant patients in the first year after transplant and in 84 percent of patients within five years.

Osteoporosis can develop or worsen in heart transplant patients. This condition thins and weakens the bones.

Chapter 57

Rehabilitation after Heart Attack or Stroke

Chapter Contents

Section 57.1

Cardiac Rehabilitation

Excerpted from "What Is Cardiac Rehabilitation?" National Heart, Lung, and Blood Institute, National Institutes of Health, February 22, 2012.

What Is Cardiac Rehabilitation?

Cardiac rehabilitation (rehab) is a medically supervised program that helps improve the health and well-being of people who have heart problems.

Rehab programs include exercise training, education on heart healthy living, and counseling to reduce stress and help you return to an active life.

Cardiac rehab can help you do the following things:

- Recover after a heart attack or heart surgery.

- Prevent future hospital stays, heart problems, and death related to heart problems.

- Address risk factors that can lead to coronary heart disease and other heart problems. These risk factors include high blood pressure, high blood cholesterol, overweight or obesity, diabetes, smoking, lack of physical activity, and depression and other emotional health concerns.

- Adopt healthy lifestyle changes. These changes may include following a heart healthy diet, being physically active, and learning how to manage stress.

- Improve your health and quality of life.

Your cardiac rehab program will be designed to meet your needs.

What to Expect When Starting Cardiac Rehabilitation

Your doctor may refer you to cardiac rehabilitation (rehab) during an office visit or while you're in the hospital recovering from a heart attack or heart surgery. If your doctor doesn't mention it, ask him or her whether cardiac rehab might benefit you.

Rehab activities will vary depending on your condition. If you're recovering from major heart surgery, rehab will likely start with a member of the rehab team helping you sit up in a chair or take a few steps.

You'll work on range-of-motion exercises, such as moving your fingers, hands, arms, legs, and feet. Over time, you'll increase your activity level.

Once you leave the hospital, rehab will continue in a rehab center. The rehab center might be part of the hospital or located elsewhere.

Try to find a center close to home that offers services at a convenient time. If no centers are near your home, or if it's too hard to get to them, ask your doctor about home-based rehab.

For the first two to three months, you'll go to rehab regularly to learn how to reduce risk factors and start an exercise program. After that, your rehab team may recommend less frequent visits.

Overall, you may work with the rehab team for three months or longer. The length of time you continue cardiac rehab depends on your situation.

Health Assessment

Before you start cardiac rehab, your rehab team will assess your health. This includes taking your medical history and doing a physical exam and tests.

What to Expect During Cardiac Rehabilitation

During cardiac rehabilitation (rehab), you'll learn how to do the following things:

- Increase your physical activity level and exercise safely
- Follow a heart healthy diet
- Reduce risk factors for future heart problems
- Improve your emotional health

Your rehab team will work with you to create a plan that meets your needs. Each part of cardiac rehab will help lower your risk for future heart problems.

What Are the Benefits and Risks of Cardiac Rehabilitation?

Benefits

Cardiac rehabilitation (rehab) has many benefits. It can do the following things:

- Reduce your overall risk of dying, the risk of future heart problems, and the risk of dying from a heart attack

- Decrease pain and the need for medicines to treat heart or chest pain

- Lessen the chance that you'll have to go back to the hospital or emergency room for a heart problem

- Improve your overall health by reducing your risk factors for heart problems

- Improve your quality of life and make it easier for you to work, take part in social activities, and exercise

Going to cardiac rehab regularly also can reduce stress, improve your ability to move around, and help you stay independent.

Risks

The lifestyle changes that you make during cardiac rehab have few risks.

At first, physical activity is safer in the rehab setting than at home. Members of the rehab team are trained and have experience teaching people who have heart problems how to exercise.

Your rehab team will watch you to make sure you're safe. They'll check your blood pressure several times during your exercise training. They also may use an electrocardiogram (EKG) to see how your heart reacts and adapts to exercise. After some training, most people learn to exercise safely at home.

Very rarely, physical activity during rehab causes serious problems. These problems can include injuries to your muscles and bones or heart rhythm problems that can lead to a heart attack or death.

Your rehab team will tell you about signs and symptoms of possible problems to watch for while exercising at home. If you notice these signs and symptoms, you should stop the activity and contact your doctor.

Section 57.2

Stroke Rehabilitation

Excerpted from "Post-Stroke Rehabilitation," National Institute of
Neurological Disorders and Stroke, National Institutes of Health,
July 26, 2011.

In the United States more than seven hundred thousand people
suffer a stroke[1] each year, and approximately two-thirds of these individuals survive and require rehabilitation. The goals of rehabilitation
are to help survivors become as independent as possible and to attain
the best possible quality of life. Even though rehabilitation does not
"cure" the effects of stroke in that it does not reverse brain damage,
rehabilitation can substantially help people achieve the best possible
long-term outcome.

What is post-stroke rehabilitation?

Rehabilitation helps stroke survivors relearn skills that are lost
when part of the brain is damaged. For example, these skills can
include coordinating leg movements in order to walk or carrying out
the steps involved in any complex activity. Rehabilitation also teaches
survivors new ways of performing tasks to circumvent or compensate
for any residual disabilities. Individuals may need to learn how to
bathe and dress using only one hand, or how to communicate effectively when their ability to use language has been compromised.
There is a strong consensus among rehabilitation experts that the
most important element in any rehabilitation program is carefully
directed, well-focused, repetitive practice—the same kind of practice
used by all people when they learn a new skill, such as playing the
piano or pitching a baseball.

Rehabilitative therapy begins in the acute-care hospital after the
person's overall condition has been stabilized, often within twenty-four
to forty-eight hours after the stroke. The first steps involve promoting
independent movement because many individuals are paralyzed or
seriously weakened. Patients are prompted to change positions frequently while lying in bed and to engage in passive or active range of

motion exercises to strengthen their stroke-impaired limbs. ("Passive" range-of-motion exercises are those in which the therapist actively helps the patient move a limb repeatedly, whereas "active" exercises are performed by the patient with no physical assistance from the therapist.) Depending on many factors—including the extent of the initial injury—patients may progress from sitting up and being moved between the bed and a chair to standing, bearing their own weight, and walking, with or without assistance. Rehabilitation nurses and therapists help patients who are able to perform progressively more complex and demanding tasks, such as bathing, dressing, and using a toilet, and they encourage patients to begin using their stroke-impaired limbs while engaging in those tasks. Beginning to reacquire the ability to carry out these basic activities of daily living represents the first stage in a stroke survivor's return to independence.

For some stroke survivors, rehabilitation will be an ongoing process to maintain and refine skills and could involve working with specialists for months or years after the stroke.

What disabilities can result from a stroke?

The types and degrees of disability that follow a stroke depend upon which area of the brain is damaged and how much is damaged. It is difficult to compare one individual's disability to another, since every stroke can damage slightly different parts and amounts of the brain. Generally, stroke can cause five types of disabilities: paralysis or problems controlling movement; sensory disturbances including pain; problems using or understanding language; problems with thinking and memory; and emotional disturbances.

Paralysis or problems controlling movement (motor control): Paralysis is one of the most common disabilities resulting from stroke. The paralysis is usually on the side of the body opposite the side of the brain damaged by stroke, and may affect the face, an arm, a leg, or the entire side of the body. This one-sided paralysis is called hemiplegia if it involves complete inability to move or hemiparesis if it is less than total weakness. Stroke patients with hemiparesis or hemiplegia may have difficulty with everyday activities such as walking or grasping objects. Some stroke patients have problems with swallowing, called dysphagia, due to damage to the part of the brain that controls the muscles for swallowing. Damage to a lower part of the brain, the cerebellum, can affect the body's ability to coordinate movement, a disability called ataxia, leading to problems with body posture, walking, and balance.

Sensory disturbances including pain: Stroke patients may lose the ability to feel touch, pain, temperature, or position. Sensory deficits also may hinder the ability to recognize objects that patients are holding and can even be severe enough to cause loss of recognition of one's own limb. Some stroke patients experience pain, numbness, or odd sensations of tingling or prickling in paralyzed or weakened limbs, a symptom known as paresthesias.

The loss of urinary continence is fairly common immediately after a stroke and often results from a combination of sensory and motor deficits. Stroke survivors may lose the ability to sense the need to urinate or the ability to control bladder muscles. Some may lack enough mobility to reach a toilet in time. Loss of bowel control or constipation also may occur. Permanent incontinence after a stroke is uncommon, but even a temporary loss of bowel or bladder control can be emotionally difficult for stroke survivors.

Stroke survivors frequently have a variety of chronic pain syndromes resulting from stroke-induced damage to the nervous system (neuropathic pain). In some stroke patients, pathways for sensation in the brain are damaged, causing the transmission of false signals that result in the sensation of pain in a limb or side of the body that has the sensory deficit. The most common of these pain syndromes is called "thalamic pain syndrome" (caused by a stroke to the thalamus, which processes sensory information from the body to the brain), which can be difficult to treat even with medications. Finally, some pain that occurs after stroke is not due to nervous system damage, but rather to mechanical problems caused by the weakness from the stroke. Patients who have a seriously weakened or paralyzed arm commonly experience moderate to severe pain that radiates outward from the shoulder. Most often, the pain results from lack of movement in a joint that has been immobilized for a prolonged period of time (such as having your arm or shoulder in a cast for weeks) and the tendons and ligaments around the joint become fixed in one position. This is commonly called a "frozen" joint; "passive" movement (the joint is gently moved or flexed by a therapist or caregiver rather than by the individual) at the joint in a paralyzed limb is essential to prevent painful "freezing" and to allow easy movement if and when voluntary motor strength returns.

Problems using or understanding language (aphasia): At least one-fourth of all stroke survivors experience language impairments, involving the ability to speak, write, and understand spoken and written language. A stroke-induced injury to any of the brain's language-control centers can severely impair verbal communication. The dominant centers for language are in the left side of the brain for right-handed individuals and many left-handers as well. Damage to a language center located on the dominant side of the brain, known as Broca area, causes expressive aphasia. People with this type of aphasia have difficulty conveying their thoughts through words or writing. They lose the ability to speak the words they are thinking and to put words together in coherent, grammatically correct sentences. In contrast, damage to a language center located in a rear portion of the brain, called Wernicke area, results in receptive aphasia. People with this condition have difficulty understanding spoken or written language and often have incoherent speech. Although they can form grammatically correct sentences, their utterances are often devoid of meaning. The most severe form of aphasia, global aphasia, is caused by extensive damage to several areas of the brain involved in language function. People with global aphasia lose nearly all their linguistic abilities; they cannot understand language or use it to convey thought.

Problems with thinking and memory: Stroke can cause damage to parts of the brain responsible for memory, learning, and awareness. Stroke survivors may have dramatically shortened attention spans or may experience deficits in short-term memory. Individuals also may lose their ability to make plans, comprehend meaning, learn new tasks, or engage in other complex mental activities. Two fairly common deficits resulting from stroke are anosognosia, an inability to acknowledge the reality of the physical impairments resulting from stroke, and neglect, the loss of the ability to respond to objects or sensory stimuli located on the stroke-impaired side. Stroke survivors who develop apraxia (loss of ability to carry out a learned purposeful movement) cannot plan the steps involved in a complex task and act on them in the proper sequence. Stroke survivors with apraxia also may have problems following a set of instructions. Apraxia appears to be caused by a disruption of the subtle connections that exist between thought and action.

Emotional disturbances: Many people who survive a stroke feel fear, anxiety, frustration, anger, sadness, and a sense of grief for their physical and mental losses. These feelings are a natural response to the psychological trauma of stroke. Some emotional disturbances and personality changes are caused by the physical effects of brain damage. Clinical depression, which is a sense of hopelessness that disrupts an individual's ability to function, appears to be the emotional disorder most commonly experienced by stroke survivors. Signs of clinical depression include sleep disturbances, a radical change in eating patterns that may lead to sudden weight loss or gain, lethargy, social withdrawal, irritability, fatigue, self-loathing, and suicidal thoughts. Post-stroke depression can be treated with antidepressant medications and psychological counseling.

What medical professionals specialize in post-stroke rehabilitation?

Post-stroke rehabilitation involves physicians; rehabilitation nurses; physical, occupational, recreational, speech-language, and vocational therapists; and mental health professionals.

Physicians: Physicians have the primary responsibility for managing and coordinating the long-term care of stroke survivors, including recommending which rehabilitation programs will best address individual needs. Physicians also are responsible for caring for the stroke survivor's general health and providing guidance aimed at preventing a second stroke, such as controlling high blood pressure or diabetes and eliminating risk factors such as cigarette smoking, excessive weight, a high-cholesterol diet, and high alcohol consumption.

Rehabilitation nurses: Nurses specializing in rehabilitation help survivors relearn how to carry out the basic activities of daily living. They also educate survivors about routine health care, such as how to follow a medication schedule, how to care for the skin, how to move out of a bed and into a wheelchair, and special needs for people with diabetes. Rehabilitation nurses also work with survivors to reduce risk factors that may lead to a second stroke, and provide training for caregivers.

Physical therapists: Physical therapists help survivors regain the use of stroke-impaired limbs, teach compensatory strategies to reduce the effect of remaining deficits, and establish ongoing exercise programs to help people retain their newly learned skills. Disabled people tend to avoid using impaired limbs, a behavior called learned non-use. However, the repetitive use of impaired limbs encourages brain plasticity[2] and helps reduce disabilities.

Occupational and recreational therapists: Like physical therapists, occupational therapists are concerned with improving motor and sensory abilities and ensuring patient safety in the post-stroke period. They help survivors relearn skills needed for performing self-directed activities (also called occupations) such as personal grooming, preparing meals, and housecleaning. Therapists can teach some survivors how to adapt to driving and provide on-road training. They often teach people to divide a complex activity into its component parts, practice each part, and then perform the whole sequence of actions. This strategy can improve coordination and may help people with apraxia relearn how to carry out planned actions.

Occupational therapists also teach people how to develop compensatory strategies and change elements of their environment that limit activities of daily living. For example, people with the use of only one hand can substitute hook and loop fasteners (such as Velcro) for buttons on clothing. Occupational therapists also help people make changes in their homes to increase safety, remove barriers, and facilitate physical functioning, such as installing grab bars in bathrooms.

Speech-language pathologists: Speech-language pathologists help stroke survivors with aphasia relearn how to use language or develop alternative means of communication. They also help people improve their ability to swallow, and they work with patients to develop problem-solving and social skills needed to cope with the after-effects of a stroke.

When can a stroke patient get rehabilitation?

Rehabilitation should begin as soon as a stroke patient is stable, sometimes within twenty-four to forty-eight hours after a stroke. This first stage of rehabilitation can occur within an acute-care hospital; however, it is very dependent on the unique circumstances of the individual patient.

Recently, in the largest stroke rehabilitation study in the United States, researchers compared two common techniques to help stroke patients improve their walking. Both methods—training on a body-weight-supported treadmill or working on strength and balance exercises at home with a physical therapist—resulted in equal improvements in the individual's ability to walk by the end of one year. Researchers found that functional improvements could be seen as late as one year after the stroke, which goes against the conventional wisdom that most recovery is complete by six months. The trial showed that 52 percent of the participants made significant improvements in walking, everyday function, and quality of life, regardless of how severe their impairment was, or whether they started the training at two or six months after the stroke.

Where can a stroke patient get rehabilitation?

At the time of discharge from the hospital, the stroke patient and family coordinate with hospital social workers to locate a suitable living arrangement. Many stroke survivors return home, but some move into some type of medical facility.

Inpatient rehabilitation units: Inpatient facilities may be freestanding or part of larger hospital complexes. Patients stay in the facility, usually for two to three weeks, and engage in a coordinated, intensive program of rehabilitation. Such programs often involve at least three hours of active therapy a day, five or six days a week. Inpatient facilities offer a comprehensive range of medical services, including full-time physician supervision and access to the full range of therapists specializing in post-stroke rehabilitation.

Outpatient units: Outpatient facilities are often part of a larger hospital complex and provide access to physicians and the full range of therapists specializing in stroke rehabilitation. Patients typically spend several hours, often three days each week, at the facility taking part in coordinated therapy sessions and return home at night. Comprehensive outpatient facilities frequently offer treatment programs as intense as those of inpatient facilities, but they also can offer less demanding regimens, depending on the patient's physical capacity.

Nursing facilities: Rehabilitative services available at nursing facilities are more variable than are those at inpatient and outpatient units. Skilled nursing facilities usually place a greater emphasis on rehabilitation, whereas traditional nursing homes emphasize residential care. In addition, fewer hours of therapy are offered compared to outpatient and inpatient rehabilitation units.

Home-based rehabilitation programs: Home rehabilitation allows for great flexibility so that patients can tailor their program of rehabilitation and follow individual schedules. Stroke survivors may participate in an intensive level of therapy several hours per week or follow a less demanding regimen. These arrangements are often best suited for people who require treatment by only one type of rehabilitation therapist. Patients dependent on Medicare coverage for their rehabilitation must meet Medicare's "homebound" requirements to qualify for such services; at this time lack of transportation is not a valid reason for home therapy. The major disadvantage of home-based rehabilitation programs is the lack of specialized equipment. However, undergoing treatment at home gives people the advantage of practicing skills and developing compensatory strategies in the context of their own living environment. In the recent stroke rehabilitation trial, intensive balance and strength rehabilitation in the home was equivalent to treadmill training at a rehabilitation facility in improving walking.

Notes

1. An ischemic stroke or "brain attack" occurs when brain cells die because of inadequate blood flow. When blood flow is interrupted, brain cells are robbed of vital supplies of oxygen and nutrients. About 80 percent of strokes are caused by the blockage of an artery in the neck or brain. A hemorrhagic stroke is caused by a burst blood vessel in the brain that causes bleeding into or around the brain.

2. Functions compromised when a specific region of the brain is damaged by stroke can sometimes be taken over by other parts of the brain. This ability to adapt and change is known as neuroplasticity.

Part Seven

Preventing Cardiovascular Disorders

Chapter 58

Preventing Heart Disease at Any Age

You're never too young—or too old—to take care of your heart.

Preventing heart disease (and all cardiovascular diseases) means making smart choices now that will pay off the rest of your life.

Lack of exercise, a poor diet, and other bad habits can take their toll over the years. Anyone at any age can benefit from simple steps to keep their heart healthy during each decade of life. Here's how.

What You Can Do to Prevent Heart Disease

All Age Groups

No matter what your age, everyone can benefit from a healthy diet and adequate physical activity.

Choose a healthy eating plan. The food you eat can decrease your risk of heart disease and stroke. Choose foods low in saturated fat, trans fat, cholesterol, sodium, and added sugars and sweeteners. As part of a healthy diet, eat plenty of fruits and vegetables, fiber-rich whole grains, fish (preferably oily fish—at least twice per week), nuts, legumes, and seeds. Also try eating some meals without meat. Select fat-free and low-fat dairy products and lean meats and poultry (skinless). Limit sugar-sweetened beverages.

Be physically active. You can slowly work up to at least two and a half hours (150 minutes) of moderate-intensity aerobic physical activity (like brisk walking) every week or an hour and fifteen minutes (75 minutes) of vigorous intensity aerobic physical activity (such as jogging or running) or a combination of both every week. Additionally, on two or more days a week you need muscle-strengthening activities that work all major muscle groups (legs, hips, back, abdomen, chest, shoulders, and arms).

In Your Twenties

Getting smart about your heart early on puts you far ahead of the curve. The things you do—and don't—are a tell-tale sign of how long and how well you're going to live, said Richard Stein, M.D. "There's no one I know who said: 'I felt better being sedentary. I felt better eating a terrible diet,'" said Stein, a cardiologist and professor of medicine at New York University School of Medicine. "All these things actually make you feel better while they help you."

Find a doctor and have regular wellness exams. Healthy people need doctors, too. Establishing a relationship with a physician means you can start heart-health screenings now. Talk to your doctor about your diet, lifestyle, and checking your blood pressure, cholesterol, heart rate, body mass index, and waist circumference. You may also need your blood sugar checked if you are pregnant, overweight, or have diabetes. Knowing where your numbers stand early makes it easier to spot a possible change in the future.

Be physically active. It's a lot easier to be active and stay active if you start at a young age. "If you're accustomed to physical activity, you'll sustain it," Dr. Stein said. Keep your workout routine interesting by mixing it up and finding new motivators.

Don't smoke and avoid secondhand smoke. If you picked up smoking as a teen, it's time to quit smoking. Even exposure to secondhand smoke poses a serious health hazard. Nonsmokers are up to 30 percent more likely to develop heart disease or lung cancer from secondhand smoke exposure at home or work, according to a U.S. Surgeon General report.

In Your Thirties

Juggling family and career leaves many adults with little time to worry about their hearts. Here are some ways to balance all three.

Make heart-healthy living a family affair. Create and sustain heart-healthy habits in your kids and you'll reap the benefits, too.

Spend less time on the couch and more time on the move. Explore a nearby park on foot or bike. Shoot some hoops or walk the dog. Plant a vegetable and fruit garden together in the yard, and invite your kids into the kitchen to help cook.

Know your family history. Shake your family tree to learn about heart health. Having a relative with heart disease increases your risk, especially if the relative is a parent or sibling. That means you need to focus on risk factors you can control by maintaining a healthy weight, exercising regularly, not smoking, and eating right. Also, keep your doctor informed about any heart problems you learn about in your family.

Tame your stress. Long-term stress causes an increase in heart rate and blood pressure that may damage the artery walls. Learning stress management techniques benefits your body and your quality of life. Try deep-breathing exercises and find time each day to do something you enjoy. Giving back through volunteering also does wonders for knocking out stress.

In Your Forties

If heart health hasn't been a priority, don't worry. Healthy choices you make now can strengthen your heart for the long haul. Understand why you need to make lifestyle changes and have the confidence to make them. Then, tackle them one at a time. "Each success makes you more confident to take on the next one," said Dr. Stein, who is also an American Heart Association volunteer.

Watch your weight. In your forties, your metabolism starts slowing down. But you can avoid weight gain by following a heart-healthy diet and getting plenty of exercise. The trick is to find a workout routine you enjoy. If you need motivation to get moving, find a workout buddy or join American Heart Association Walking Paths and Walking Clubs.

Have your blood sugar level checked. In addition to blood pressure checks and other heart-health screenings, you should have a fasting blood glucose test by the time you're forty-five. This first test serves as a baseline for future tests, which you should have every three years. Testing may be done earlier or more often if you are overweight, diabetic, or at risk for becoming diabetic.

Don't brush off snoring. Listen to your sleeping partner's complaints about your snoring. One in five adults has at least mild sleep apnea, a condition that causes pauses in breathing during sleep. If not properly treated, sleep apnea can contribute to high blood pressure, heart disease, and stroke.

In Your Fifties

Unlike the emergence of wrinkles and gray hair, what you can't see as you get older is the impact aging has on your heart. So starting in the fifties, you need to take extra steps.

Eat a healthy diet. It's easy to slip into some unhealthy eating habits, so refresh your eating habits eating plenty of fruits and vegetables, fiber-rich whole grains, fish (preferably oily fish—at least twice per week), nuts, legumes, and seeds and try eating some meals without meat.

Learn the warning signs of a heart attack and stroke. Now is the time to get savvy about symptoms. Not everyone experiences sudden numbness with a stroke or severe chest pain with a heart attack. And heart attack symptoms in women can be different than men.

Follow your treatment plan. By now, you may have been diagnosed with high blood pressure, high cholesterol, diabetes, or other conditions that increase your risk for heart disease or stroke. Lower your risk by following your prescribed treatment plan, including medications and lifestyle and diet changes.

In Your Sixties-Plus

With age comes an increased risk for heart disease. Your blood pressure, cholesterol, and other heart-related numbers tend to rise. Watching your numbers closely and managing any health problems that arise—along with the requisite healthy eating and exercise—can help you live longer and better.

Have an ankle-brachial index test. Starting in your sixties, an ankle-brachial index test should be done every one to two years as part of a physical exam. The test assesses the pulses in the feet to help diagnose peripheral artery disease (PAD), a lesser-known cardiovascular disease in which plaque builds up in the leg arteries.

Watch your weight. Your body burns fewer calories as you get older. Excess weight causes your heart to work harder and increases the risk for heart disease, high blood pressure, diabetes, and high cholesterol. Exercising regularly and eating smaller portions of nutrient-rich foods may help you maintain a healthy weight.

Learn the warning signs of a heart attack and stroke. Heart attack symptoms in women can be different than in men. Knowing when you're having a heart attack or stroke means you're more likely to get immediate help. Quick treatment can save your life and prevent serious disability.

Chapter 59

Controlling High Blood Pressure

What Is High Blood Pressure?

High blood pressure (HBP) is a serious condition that can lead to coronary heart disease, heart failure, stroke, kidney failure, and other health problems.

"Blood pressure" is the force of blood pushing against the walls of the arteries as the heart pumps blood. If this pressure rises and stays high over time, it can damage the body in many ways.

Overview

About one in three adults in the United States has HBP. The condition itself usually has no signs or symptoms. You can have it for years without knowing it. During this time, though, HBP can damage your heart, blood vessels, kidneys, and other parts of your body.

Knowing your blood pressure numbers is important, even when you're feeling fine. If your blood pressure is normal, you can work with your health care team to keep it that way. If your blood pressure is too high, treatment may help prevent damage to your body's organs.

Reprinted from "What Is High Blood Pressure?" and "How Is High Blood Pressure Treated?" National Heart, Lung, and Blood Institute, National Institutes of Health, August 2, 2012.

Blood Pressure Numbers

Blood pressure is measured as systolic and diastolic pressures. "Systolic" refers to blood pressure when the heart beats while pumping blood. "Diastolic" refers to blood pressure when the heart is at rest between beats.

You most often will see blood pressure numbers written with the systolic number above or before the diastolic number, such as 120/80 mmHg. (The mmHg is millimeters of mercury—the units used to measure blood pressure.)

Table 59.1 shows normal blood pressure numbers for adults. It also shows which numbers put you at greater risk for health problems.

Table 59.1. Categories for Blood Pressure Levels in Adults (measured in millimeters of mercury, or mmHg)

Category	*Systolic (top number)*		*Diastolic (bottom number)*
Normal	Less than 120	And	Less than 80
Prehypertension	120–139	Or	80–89
High blood pressure			
Stage 1	140–159	Or	90–99
Stage 2	160 or higher	Or	100 or higher

The ranges in the table apply to most adults (aged eighteen and older) who don't have short-term serious illnesses.

Blood pressure doesn't stay the same all the time. It lowers as you sleep and rises when you wake up. Blood pressure also rises when you're excited, nervous, or active. If your numbers stay above normal most of the time, you're at risk for health problems. The risk grows as blood pressure numbers rise. "Prehypertension" means you may end up with HBP, unless you take steps to prevent it.

If you're being treated for HBP and have repeat readings in the normal range, your blood pressure is under control. However, you still have the condition. You should see your doctor and follow your treatment plan to keep your blood pressure under control.

Your systolic and diastolic numbers may not be in the same blood pressure category. In this case, the more severe category is the one you're in. For example, if your systolic number is 160 and your diastolic number is 80, you have stage 2 HBP. If your systolic number is 120 and your diastolic number is 95, you have stage 1 HBP.

If you have diabetes or chronic kidney disease, HBP is defined as 130/80 mmHg or higher. HBP numbers also differ for children and teens.

Outlook

Blood pressure tends to rise with age. Following a healthy lifestyle helps some people delay or prevent this rise in blood pressure.

People who have HBP can take steps to control it and reduce their risk for related health problems. Key steps include following a healthy lifestyle, having ongoing medical care, and following your treatment plan.

How Is High Blood Pressure Treated?

High blood pressure (HBP) is treated with lifestyle changes and medicines.

Most people who have HBP will need lifelong treatment. Sticking to your treatment plan is important. It can help prevent or delay problems related to HBP and help you live and stay active longer.

Goals of Treatment

The treatment goal for most adults is to get and keep blood pressure below 140/90 mmHg. For adults who have diabetes or chronic kidney disease, the goal is to get and keep blood pressure below 130/80 mmHg.

Lifestyle Changes

Healthy lifestyle habits can help you control HBP. These habits include the following:

- Following a healthy diet
- Being physically active
- Maintaining a healthy weight
- Quitting smoking
- Managing your stress and learning to cope with stress

If you combine healthy lifestyle habits, you can achieve even better results than taking single steps.

You may find it hard to make lifestyle changes. Start by making one healthy lifestyle change and then adopt others.

Some people can control their blood pressure with lifestyle changes alone, but many people can't. Keep in mind that the main goal is blood pressure control.

If your doctor prescribes medicines as a part of your treatment plan, keep up your healthy lifestyle habits. They will help you better control your blood pressure.

Following a healthy diet: Your doctor may recommend the DASH (Dietary Approaches to Stop Hypertension) eating plan if you have HBP. The DASH eating plan focuses on fruits, vegetables, whole grains, and other foods that are heart healthy and low in fat, cholesterol, and sodium (salt).

DASH also focuses on fat-free or low-fat dairy products, fish, poultry, and nuts. The DASH eating plan is reduced in red meats (including lean red meats), sweets, added sugars, and sugar-containing beverages. It's rich in nutrients, protein, and fiber.

To help control HBP, you should limit the amount of salt that you eat. This means choosing low-sodium and no-added-salt foods and seasonings at the table and while cooking. The nutrition facts label on food packaging shows the amount of sodium in an item. You should eat no more than about one teaspoon of salt a day.

Also, try to limit alcoholic drinks. Too much alcohol will raise your blood pressure. Men should have no more than two alcoholic drinks a day. Women should have no more than one alcoholic drink a day. One drink is a glass of wine, beer, or a small amount of hard liquor.

Being physically active: Routine physical activity can lower HBP and reduce your risk for other health problems. Talk with your doctor before you start a new exercise plan. Ask him or her how much and what kinds of physical activity are safe for you.

People gain health benefits from as little as sixty minutes of moderate-intensity aerobic activity per week. The more active you are, the more you will benefit.

Maintaining a healthy weight: Maintaining a healthy weight can help you control HBP and reduce your risk for other health problems.

If you're overweight or obese, aim to reduce your weight by 5 to 10 percent during your first year of treatment. This amount of weight loss can lower your risk for health problems related to HBP.

To lose weight, cut back your calorie intake and do more physical activity. Eat smaller portions and choose lower-calorie foods. Don't feel that you have to finish the entrees served at restaurants. Many restaurant portions are oversized and have too many calories for the average person.

After your first year of treatment, you may have to continue to lose weight so you can lower your body mass index (BMI) to less than 25. BMI measures your weight in relation to your height and gives an estimate of your total body fat.

A BMI between 25 and 29.9 is considered overweight. A BMI of 30 or more is considered obese. A BMI of less than 25 is the goal for controlling blood pressure.

Quit smoking: If you smoke or use tobacco, quit. Smoking can damage your blood vessels and raise your risk for HBP. Smoking also can worsen health problems related to HBP.

Talk with your doctor about programs and products that can help you quit smoking. Also, try to avoid secondhand smoke.

If you have trouble quitting smoking on your own, consider joining a support group. Many hospitals, workplaces, and community groups offer classes to help people quit smoking.

Managing stress: Learning how to manage stress, relax, and cope with problems can improve your emotional and physical health.

Physical activity helps some people cope with stress. Other people listen to music or focus on something calm or peaceful to reduce stress. Some people learn yoga, tai chi, or how to meditate.

Medicines

Today's blood pressure medicines can safely help most people control their blood pressure. These medicines are easy to take. The side effects, if any, tend to be minor.

If you have side effects from your medicines, talk with your doctor. He or she might adjust the doses or prescribe other medicines. You shouldn't decide on your own to stop taking your medicines.

Blood pressure medicines work in different ways to lower blood pressure. Some remove extra fluid and salt from the body to lower blood pressure. Others slow down the heartbeat or relax and widen blood vessels. Often, two or more medicines work better than one.

Diuretics: Diuretics sometimes are called water pills. They help your kidneys flush excess water and salt from your body. This reduces the amount of fluid in your blood, and your blood pressure goes down.

Diuretics often are used with other HBP medicines and sometimes combined into one pill.

Beta blockers: Beta blockers help your heart beat slower and with less force. As a result, your heart pumps less blood through your blood vessels. This causes your blood pressure to go down.

Angiotensin-converting enzyme (ACE) inhibitors: ACE inhibitors keep your body from making a hormone called angiotensin II. This hormone normally causes blood vessels to narrow. ACE inhibitors prevent this, so your blood pressure goes down.

Angiotensin II receptor blockers: Angiotensin II receptor blockers are newer blood pressure medicines that protect your blood vessels from the angiotensin II hormone. As a result, blood vessels relax and widen, and your blood pressure goes down.

Calcium channel blockers: Calcium channel blockers keep calcium from entering the muscle cells of your heart and blood vessels. This allows blood vessels to relax, and your blood pressure goes down.

Alpha blockers: Alpha blockers reduce nerve impulses that tighten blood vessels. This allows blood to flow more freely, causing blood pressure to go down.

Alpha-beta blockers: Alpha-beta blockers reduce nerve impulses the same way alpha blockers do. However, they also slow the heartbeat like beta blockers. As a result, blood pressure goes down.

Nervous system inhibitors: Nervous system inhibitors increase nerve impulses from the brain to relax and widen blood vessels. This causes blood pressure to go down.

Vasodilators: Vasodilators relax the muscles in blood vessel walls. This causes blood pressure to go down.

Chapter 60

Treating High Cholesterol

What Is Cholesterol?

To understand high blood cholesterol, it helps to learn about cholesterol. Cholesterol is a waxy, fat-like substance that's found in all cells of the body.

Your body needs some cholesterol to make hormones, vitamin D, and substances that help you digest foods. Your body makes all the cholesterol it needs. However, cholesterol also is found in some of the foods you eat.

Cholesterol travels through your bloodstream in small packages called lipoproteins. These packages are made of fat (lipid) on the inside and proteins on the outside.

Two kinds of lipoproteins carry cholesterol throughout your body: low-density lipoproteins (LDL) and high-density lipoproteins (HDL). Having healthy levels of both types of lipoproteins is important.

LDL cholesterol sometimes is called "bad" cholesterol. A high LDL level leads to a buildup of cholesterol in your arteries. (Arteries are blood vessels that carry blood from your heart to your body.)

HDL cholesterol sometimes is called "good" cholesterol. This is because it carries cholesterol from other parts of your body back to your liver. Your liver removes the cholesterol from your body.

Excerpted from "What Is Cholesterol?" and "How Is High Blood Cholesterol Treated?" National Heart, Lung, and Blood Institute, September 19, 2012.

What Is High Blood Cholesterol?

High blood cholesterol is a condition in which you have too much cholesterol in your blood. By itself, the condition usually has no signs or symptoms. Thus, many people don't know that their cholesterol levels are too high.

People who have high blood cholesterol have a greater chance of getting coronary heart disease, also called coronary artery disease.

The higher the level of LDL cholesterol in your blood, the *greater* your chance is of getting heart disease. The higher the level of HDL cholesterol in your blood, the *lower* your chance is of getting heart disease.

Coronary heart disease is a condition in which plaque builds up inside the coronary (heart) arteries. Plaque is made up of cholesterol, fat, calcium, and other substances found in the blood. When plaque builds up in the arteries, the condition is called atherosclerosis.

Over time, plaque hardens and narrows your coronary arteries. This limits the flow of oxygen-rich blood to the heart.

Eventually, an area of plaque can rupture (break open). This causes a blood clot to form on the surface of the plaque. If the clot becomes large enough, it can mostly or completely block blood flow through a coronary artery.

If the flow of oxygen-rich blood to your heart muscle is reduced or blocked, angina or a heart attack may occur.

Angina is chest pain or discomfort. It may feel like pressure or squeezing in your chest. The pain also may occur in your shoulders, arms, neck, jaw, or back. Angina pain may even feel like indigestion.

A heart attack occurs if the flow of oxygen-rich blood to a section of heart muscle is cut off. If blood flow isn't restored quickly, the section of heart muscle begins to die. Without quick treatment, a heart attack can lead to serious problems or death.

Plaque also can build up in other arteries in your body, such as the arteries that bring oxygen-rich blood to your brain and limbs. This can lead to problems such as carotid artery disease, stroke, and peripheral arterial disease (P.A.D.).

Outlook

Lowering your cholesterol may slow, reduce, or even stop the build-up of plaque in your arteries. It also may reduce the risk of plaque rupturing and causing dangerous blood clots.

How Is High Blood Cholesterol Treated?

High blood cholesterol is treated with lifestyle changes and medicines. The main goal of treatment is to lower your low-density lipoprotein (LDL) cholesterol level enough to reduce your risk for coronary heart disease, heart attack, and other related health problems.

Your risk for heart disease and heart attack goes up as your LDL cholesterol level rises and your number of heart disease risk factors increases.

Some people are at high risk for heart attacks because they already have heart disease. Other people are at high risk for heart disease because they have diabetes or more than one heart disease risk factor.

Talk with your doctor about lowering your cholesterol and your risk for heart disease. Also, check the list to find out whether you have risk factors that affect your LDL cholesterol goal:

- Cigarette smoking

- High blood pressure (140/90 mmHg or higher), or you're on medicine to treat high blood pressure

- Low high-density lipoprotein (HDL) cholesterol (less than 40 mg/dL)

- Family history of early heart disease (heart disease in father or brother before age fifty-five; heart disease in mother or sister before age sixty-five)

- Age (men forty-five years or older; women fifty-five years or older)

The two main ways to lower your cholesterol (and, thus, your heart disease risk) are as follows:

- **Therapeutic Lifestyle Changes (TLC):** TLC is a three-part program that includes a healthy diet, weight management, and physical activity. TLC is for anyone whose LDL cholesterol level is above goal.

- **Medicines:** If cholesterol-lowering medicines are needed, they're used with the TLC program to help lower your LDL cholesterol level.

Lowering Cholesterol Using Therapeutic Lifestyle Changes

TLC is a set of lifestyle changes that can help you lower your LDL cholesterol. The main parts of the TLC program are a healthy diet, weight management, and physical activity.

The TLC diet: With the TLC diet, less than 7 percent of your daily calories should come from saturated fat. This kind of fat is found in some meats, dairy products, chocolate, baked goods, and deep-fried and processed foods.

No more than 25 to 35 percent of your daily calories should come from all fats, including saturated, trans, monounsaturated, and polyunsaturated fats.

You also should have less than 200 mg a day of cholesterol. The amounts of cholesterol and the types of fat in prepared foods can be found on the foods' nutrition facts labels.

Foods high in soluble fiber also are part of the TLC diet. They help prevent the digestive tract from absorbing cholesterol. These foods include the following:

- Whole-grain cereals such as oatmeal and oat bran

- Fruits such as apples, bananas, oranges, pears, and prunes

- Legumes such as kidney beans, lentils, chick peas, black-eyed peas, and lima beans

A diet rich in fruits and vegetables can increase important cholesterol-lowering compounds in your diet. These compounds, called plant stanols or sterols, work like soluble fiber.

A healthy diet also includes some types of fish, such as salmon, tuna (canned or fresh), and mackerel. These fish are a good source of omega-3 fatty acids. These acids may help protect the heart from blood clots and inflammation and reduce the risk of heart attack. Try to have about two fish meals every week.

You also should try to limit the amount of sodium (salt) that you eat. This means choosing low-salt and "no-added-salt" foods and seasonings at the table or while cooking. The nutrition facts label on food packaging shows the amount of sodium in the item.

Try to limit drinks with alcohol. Too much alcohol will raise your blood pressure and triglyceride level. (Triglycerides are a type of fat found in the blood.) Alcohol also adds extra calories, which will cause weight gain.

Men should have no more than two drinks containing alcohol a day. Women should have no more than one drink containing alcohol a day. One drink is a glass of wine or beer, or a small amount of hard liquor.

Weight management: If you're overweight or obese, losing weight can help lower LDL cholesterol. Maintaining a healthy weight is especially important if you have a condition called metabolic syndrome.

Metabolic syndrome is the name for a group of risk factors that raise your risk for heart disease and other health problems, such as diabetes and stroke.

The five metabolic risk factors are a large waistline (abdominal obesity), a high triglyceride level, a low HDL cholesterol level, high blood pressure, and high blood sugar. Metabolic syndrome is diagnosed if you have at least three of these metabolic risk factors.

Physical activity: Routine physical activity can lower LDL cholesterol and triglycerides and raise your HDL cholesterol level.

People gain health benefits from as little as sixty minutes of moderate-intensity aerobic activity per week. The more active you are, the more you will benefit.

Cholesterol-Lowering Medicines

In addition to lifestyle changes, your doctor may prescribe medicines to help lower your cholesterol. Even with medicines, you should continue the TLC program.

Medicines can help control high blood cholesterol, but they don't cure it. Thus, you must continue taking your medicine to keep your cholesterol level in the recommended range.

The five major types of cholesterol-lowering medicines are statins, bile acid sequestrants, nicotinic acid, fibrates, and ezetimibe:

- Statins work well at lowering LDL cholesterol. These medicines are safe for most people. Rare side effects include muscle and liver problems.

- Bile acid sequestrants also help lower LDL cholesterol. These medicines usually aren't prescribed as the only medicine to lower cholesterol. Sometimes they're prescribed with statins.

- Nicotinic acid lowers LDL cholesterol and triglycerides and raises HDL cholesterol. You should only use this type of medicine with a doctor's supervision.

- Fibrates lower triglycerides, and they may raise HDL cholesterol. When used with statins, fibrates may increase the risk of muscle problems.

- Ezetimibe lowers LDL cholesterol. This medicine works by blocking the intestine from absorbing cholesterol.

While you're being treated for high blood cholesterol, you'll need ongoing care. Your doctor will want to make sure your cholesterol

577

levels are controlled. He or she also will want to check for other health problems.

If needed, your doctor may prescribe medicines for other health problems. Take all medicines exactly as your doctor prescribes. The combination of medicines may lower your risk for heart disease and heart attack.

While trying to manage your cholesterol, take steps to manage other heart disease risk factors too. For example, if you have high blood pressure, work with your doctor to lower it.

If you smoke, quit. Talk with your doctor about programs and products that can help you quit smoking. Also, try to avoid secondhand smoke. If you're overweight or obese, try to lose weight. Your doctor can help you create a reasonable weight-loss plan.

Chapter 61

Steps to Control Diabetes

Step 1: Learn about Diabetes

Diabetes means that your blood glucose (blood sugar) is too high. There are two main types of diabetes.

Type 1 diabetes: The body does not make insulin. Insulin helps the body use glucose from food for energy. People with type 1 need to take insulin every day.

Type 2 diabetes: The body does not make or use insulin well. People with type 2 often need to take pills or insulin. Type 2 is the most common form of diabetes.

Gestational diabetes: Occurs in some women when they become pregnant. It raises a woman's future risk of developing diabetes, mostly type 2. It may raise her child's risk of being overweight and developing type 2 diabetes.

All people with diabetes need to make healthy food choices, stay at a healthy weight, and move more every day.

Taking good care of yourself and your diabetes can help you feel better. It may help you avoid health problems caused by diabetes such as the following:

- Heart attack and stroke.

- Eye problems that can lead to trouble seeing or going blind.

Excerpted from "Four Steps to Control Your Diabetes for Life," National Diabetes Education Program, National Institutes of Health, June 2013.

- Nerve damage that can cause your hands and feet to hurt, tingle, or feel numb. Some people may even lose a foot or a leg.

- Kidney problems that can cause your kidneys to stop working.

- Gum disease and loss of teeth

Step 2: Know Your Diabetes ABCs

Talk to your health care team about how to manage your A1C, blood pressure, and cholesterol. This can help lower your chances of having a heart attack, stroke, or other diabetes problems. Here's what the ABCs of diabetes stand for.

A for the A1C Test (A-one-C)

It shows what your blood glucose has been over the last three months. The A1C goal for many people is below 7. High blood glucose can harm your heart and blood vessels, kidneys, feet, and eyes.

B for Blood Pressure

The goal for most people with diabetes is below 130/80.

High blood pressure makes your heart work too hard. It can cause heart attack, stroke, and kidney disease.

C for Cholesterol

The LDL goal for people with diabetes is below 100.

The HDL goal for men with diabetes is above 40.

The HDL goal for women with diabetes is about 50.

LDL or "bad" cholesterol can build up and clog your blood vessels. It can cause a heart attack or a stroke. HDL or "good" cholesterol helps remove cholesterol from your blood vessels.

Ask your health care team the following things:

- What your A1C, blood pressure, and cholesterol numbers are

- What your A1C1, blood pressure, and cholesterol numbers should be

- What you can do to reach your targets

Step 3: Manage Your Diabetes

Many people avoid the long-term problems of diabetes by taking good care of themselves. Work with your health care team to reach your ABC target. Use this self-care plan:

- Follow your diabetes meal plan. If you do not have one, ask your health care team to help you develop a meal plan.

- Get thirty to sixty minutes of physical activity on most days of the week. Brisk walking is a great way to move more.

- Stay at a healthy weight by using your meal plan and moving more.

- Ask for help if you feel down. A mental health counselor, support group, member of the clergy, friend, or family member who will listen to your concerns may help you feel better.

- Learn to cope with stress. Stress can raise your blood glucose. While it is hard to remove stress from your life, you can learn to handle it.

- Stop smoking. Ask for help to quit.

- Take medicines even when you feel good. Ask your doctor if you need aspirin to prevent a heart attack or stroke. Tell your doctor if you cannot afford your medicines or if you have any side effects.

- Check your feet every day for cuts, blisters, red spots, and swelling. Call your health care team right away about any sores that do not go away.

- Brush your teeth and floss every day to avoid problems with your mouth, teeth, or gums.

- Check your blood glucose. You may want to test it one or more times a day. Keep a record of your blood glucose numbers. Be sure to show it to your health care team.

- Check your blood pressure if your doctor advises.

- Report any changes in your eyesight to your health care team.

Talk with your health care team about your blood glucose targets. Ask how and when to test your blood glucose and how to use the results to manage your diabetes.

Step 4: Get Routine Care

See your health care team at least twice a year to find and treat any problems early.

At each visit be sure you have the following things:

- A blood pressure check

- A foot check

- A weight check
- A review of your self-care plan shown in Step 3

Two times each year have the following:

- An A1C test (it may be checked more often if it is over 7)

Once each year be sure you have the following:

- A cholesterol test
- A triglyceride test (a type of blood fat)
- A complete foot exam
- A dental exam to check teeth and gums
- A dilated eye exam to check for eye problems
- A flu shot
- A urine and a blood test to check for kidney problems

At least once get the following:

- A pneumonia shot
- A hepatitis B shot

Ask your health care team about these and other tests you may need. Ask what yours results mean.

Note

1. An A1C of less than 7 is the goal for many people but not for everyone. Talk to your health care team about what A1C target is right for you.

Chapter 62

Heart-Healthy Eating

Why do I need to be concerned about heart healthy eating?

What you eat affects your risk for having heart disease and poor blood circulation, which can lead to a heart attack or stroke. Heart disease is the number one killer and stroke is the number three killer of American women and men.

In the main type of heart disease, a fatty substance called plaque builds up in the arteries that bring oxygen-rich blood to the heart. Over time, this buildup causes the arteries to narrow and harden. When this happens, the heart does not get all the blood it needs to work properly. The result can be chest pain or a heart attack.

Most cases of stroke occur when a blood vessel bringing blood to the brain becomes blocked. The underlying condition for this type of blockage is having fatty deposits lining the vessel walls.

What foods should I eat to help prevent heart disease and stroke?

You should eat mainly the following things:

- Fruits and vegetables

"Heart Healthy Eating Fact Sheet," U.S. Department of Health and Human Services, Office on Women's Health, January 1, 2008. Reviewed by David A. Cooke, M.D., FACP, October 2013.

- Grains (at least half of your grains should be whole grains, such as whole wheat, whole oats, oatmeal, whole-grain corn, brown rice, wild rice, whole rye, whole-grain barley, buckwheat, bulgur, millet, quinoa, and sorghum)

- Fat-free or low-fat versions of milk, cheese, yogurt, and other milk products

- Fish, skinless poultry, lean meats, dry beans, eggs, and nuts

- Polyunsaturated and monounsaturated fats (found in fish, nuts, and vegetable oils)

Also, you should limit the amount of foods you eat that contain the following things:

- Saturated fat (found in foods such as fatty cuts of meat, whole milk, cheese made from whole milk, ice cream, sherbet, frozen yogurt, butter, lard, cakes, cookies, doughnuts, sausage, regular mayonnaise, coconut, palm oil)

- Trans fat (found mainly in processed foods such as cakes, cookies, crackers, pies, stick or hard margarine, potato chips, corn chips)

- Cholesterol (found in foods such as liver, chicken and turkey giblets, pork, sausage, whole milk, cheese made from whole milk, ice cream, sherbet, frozen yogurt)

- Sodium (found in salt and baking soda)

- Added sugars (such as corn syrup, corn sweetener, fructose, glucose, sucrose, dextrose, lactose, maltose, honey, molasses, raw sugar, invert sugar, malt syrup, syrup, caramel, and fruit juice concentrates)

Eating lots of saturated fat, trans fat, and cholesterol may cause plaque buildup in your arteries. Eating lots of sodium may cause you to develop high blood pressure, also called hypertension. Eating lots of added sugars may cause you to develop type 2 diabetes. Both hypertension and diabetes increase your risk of heart disease and stroke.

How can I tell how much saturated fat, trans fat, and other substances are in the foods I eat?

Prepared foods that come in packages—such as breads, cereals, canned and frozen foods, snacks, desserts, and drinks—have a Nutrition Facts label on the package. The label states how many calories and how much saturated fat, trans fat, and other substances are in each serving.

For food that does not have a Nutrition Facts label, such as fresh salmon or a raw apple, you can use the U.S. Department of Agriculture (USDA) National Nutrient Database. This is a bit harder than using the Nutrition Facts label, but by comparing different foods you can get an idea if a food is high or low in saturated fat, sodium, and other substances.

What is a calorie?

When talking about a calorie in food, it is a measure of the energy that the food supplies to your body. When talking about burning calories during physical activity, a calorie is a measure of the energy used by your body. To maintain the same body weight, the number of food calories you eat during the day should be about the same as the number of calories your body uses.

The number of calories you should eat each day depends on your age, sex, body size, how physically active you are, and other conditions. For instance, a woman between the ages of thirty-one and fifty who is of normal weight and moderately active should eat about two thousand calories each day.

Are there eating plans that can help me choose foods that are good for my heart?

There are four eating plans that can help you choose heart healthy foods:

- MyPyramid eating plan
- Dietary Approaches to Stop Hypertension (DASH) eating plan
- Heart Healthy Diet
- Therapeutic Lifestyle Changes (TLC) Diet

The MyPyramid eating plan is based on the Dietary Guidelines for Americans. It was developed by the U.S. Department of Agriculture and the U.S. Department of Health and Human Services to help people lower their risk of serious diseases linked to diet, including heart disease. DASH was developed by the National Heart, Lung, and Blood Institute (NHLBI) to help people with hypertension lower their blood pressure but it can also be used to help prevent heart disease. The Heart Healthy Diet was developed by NHLBI to help people keep their blood levels of total cholesterol and low-density lipoprotein (LDL) cholesterol, or "bad" cholesterol, low. The TLC diet was developed by NHLBI to help people with unhealthy blood cholesterol levels.

These eating plans have interactive websites to help you choose foods that meet their guidelines. You type in your age, sex, height, weight, and activity level. Based on this information the websites give you tips on what types of foods to eat and how much of each type.

How do these eating plans work?

The four eating plans are similar. They are all designed to help you eat foods that are good for your heart and avoid foods that are bad for your heart. Table 62.1 compares the main guidelines of the four eating plans.

Notice that all four eating plans limit the amount of sodium you should eat each day to about one teaspoon of salt (two-thirds of a teaspoon for people with hypertension or at risk for hypertension). Most of the salt we eat each day actually comes from processed foods rather than salt that we add to foods that we cook. Make sure to check the sodium content on the Nutrition Facts label when buying food. The sodium content in similar foods can vary a lot. For instance, the sodium content in regular tomato soup may be 700 mg per cup in one brand and 1,100 mg per cup in another brand. Choosing the brands with lower sodium content can be one way to lower the amount of sodium you eat.

Table 62.1. Heart-Healthy Eating Plans: How They Compare

	% of the day's total calories from saturated fat	% of the day's total calories from fat	amount of trans fat	milligrams (mg) of dietary cholesterol per day	milligrams (mg) of dietary sodium per day
MyPyramid	less than 10%	20–35%	as low as possible	less than 300 mg	less than 2,300 mg[a]
DASH[b]	5%	22%	as low as possible	136 mg	less than 2,300 mg[a]
Heart Healthy Diet	8–10%	30% or less	as low as possible	less than 300 mg	less than 2,400 mg
TLC Diet	less than 7%	25–35% or less	as low as possible	less than 200 mg	less than 2,400 mg

Notes: [a]2,300 milligrams of sodium in table salt is about 1 teaspoon of salt. People with hypertension should eat no more than 1,500 milligrams (mg) of sodium a day (about two-thirds of a teaspoon of salt). African Americans and middle-aged and older adults should also eat no more than 1,500 mg of sodium per day. The reason is that these groups have a high risk of developing hypertension.

[b]These DASH guidelines are for someone eating 2,000 calories each day.

Another way to limit sodium is to use spices other than salt. There are plenty of salt-free spice combinations that you can find in your grocery store. It may take a while for you to get used to the taste. But give it time. After a while, you may like them better than salt.

Besides limiting the amount of sodium you eat, it is also a good idea to eat foods rich in potassium. A potassium-rich diet blunts the harmful effects of sodium on blood pressure. Aim to eat 4,700 mg of potassium a day. Foods rich in potassium include fruits and vegetables, especially the following:

- Tomatoes and tomato products

- Orange juice and grapefruit juice

- Raisins, dates, prunes

- White potatoes and sweet potatoes

- Lettuce

- Papayas

I've heard that eating fish is good for my heart. Why is that?

Fish and shellfish contain a type of fat called omega-3 fatty acids. Research suggests that eating omega-3 fatty acids lowers your chances of dying from heart disease. Fish that naturally contain more oil (such as salmon, trout, herring, mackerel, anchovies, and sardines) have more omega-3 fatty acids than lean fish (such as cod, haddock, and catfish). Be careful, though, about eating too much shellfish. Shrimp is a type of shellfish that has a lot of cholesterol.

You can also get omega-3 fatty acids from plant sources, such as the following:

- Canola oil
- Soybean oil
- Walnuts
- Ground flaxseed (linseed) and flaxseed oil

Is drinking alcohol bad for my heart?

Drinking too much alcohol can, over time, damage your heart and raise your blood pressure. If you drink alcohol, you should do so moderately. For women, moderate drinking means one drink per day. For men, it means two drinks per day. One drink counts as the following:

- 5 ounces of wine

- 12 ounces of beer

- 1½ ounces of 80-proof hard liquor

Research suggests that moderate drinkers are less likely to develop heart disease than people who don't drink any alcohol or who drink too much. Red wine drinkers in particular seem to be protected to some degree against heart disease. Red wine contains flavonoids, which are thought to prevent plaque buildup. Flavonoids also are found in the following foods:

- Red grapes
- Apples
- Berries
- Broccoli

On the other hand, drinking more than one drink per day increases the risks of certain cancers, including breast cancer. And if you are pregnant, could become pregnant, or have another health condition that could make alcohol use harmful, you should not drink.

With the help of your doctor, decide whether moderate drinking to lower heart attack risk outweighs the possible increased risk of breast cancer or other medical problems.

I need help working out an eating plan that's right for me. Who can I ask for help?

You may want to talk with a registered dietitian. A dietitian is a nutrition expert who can give you advice about what foods to eat and how much of each type. Ask your doctor to recommend a dietitian. You also can contact the American Dietetic Association.

Besides eating healthy foods, what else can I do to keep my heart healthy?

To reduce your risk of heart disease do the following things:

- Quit smoking. Talk with your doctor or nurse if you need help quitting.
- Get at least two hours and thirty minutes of moderate aerobic physical activity each week.
- Lose weight if you are overweight, and keep a healthy weight.
- Get your blood pressure, cholesterol, and blood sugar levels checked regularly.

Chapter 63

Dietary Supplements
and Heart Health

Chapter Contents

Section 63.1

Homocysteine, Folic Acid, and Cardiovascular Disease Prevention

The American Heart Association has not yet called hyperhomocysteinemia (high homocysteine level in the blood) a major risk factor for cardiovascular disease. We don't recommend widespread use of folic acid and B vitamin supplements to reduce the risk of heart disease and stroke. We advise a healthy, balanced diet that's rich in fruits and vegetables, whole grains, and fat-free or low-fat dairy products. For folic acid, the recommended daily value is 400 micrograms. Citrus fruits, tomatoes, vegetables, and grain products are good sources. Since January 1998, wheat flour has been fortified with folic acid to add an estimated 100 micrograms per day to the average diet. Supplements should only be used when the diet doesn't provide enough.

What is homocysteine, and how is it related to cardiovascular risk?

Homocysteine is an amino acid in the blood. Too much of it is related to a higher risk of coronary heart disease, stroke, and peripheral vascular disease (fatty deposits in peripheral arteries).

Evidence suggests that homocysteine may promote atherosclerosis (fatty deposits in blood vessels) by damaging the inner lining of arteries and promoting blood clots. However, a causal link hasn't been established.

How do folic acid and other B vitamins affect homocysteine levels?

Folic acid and other B vitamins help break down homocysteine in the body. Homocysteine levels in the blood are strongly influenced by diet and genetic factors. Dietary folic acid and vitamins B-6 and B-12 have the greatest effects. Several studies found that higher blood levels of B vitamins are related, at least in part, to lower concentrations of homocysteine. Other evidence shows that low blood levels of folic acid are linked with a higher risk of fatal coronary heart disease and stroke.

So far, no controlled treatment study has shown that folic acid supplements reduce the risk of atherosclerosis or that taking these vitamins affects the development or recurrence of cardiovascular disease. Researchers are trying to find out how much folic acid, B-6 and/ or B-12 are needed to lower homocysteine levels. Screening for homocysteine levels in the blood may be useful in patients with a personal or family history of cardiovascular disease but who don't have the well-established risk factors (smoking, high blood cholesterol, high blood pressure, physical inactivity, obesity, and diabetes).

Although evidence for the benefit of lowering homocysteine levels is lacking, patients at high risk should be strongly advised to be sure to get enough folic acid and vitamins B-6 and B-12 in their diet. They should eat fruits and green, leafy vegetables daily.

This is just one possible risk factor. A physician taking any type of nutritional approach to reducing risk should consider a person's overall risk factor profile and total diet.

Section 63.2

Omega-3 Fatty Acids for Prevention of Heart Disease

"5 Things to Know about Omega-3s for Heart Disease,"
National Center for Complementary and Alternative Medicine,
National Institutes of Health, December 21, 2012.

Omega-3 fatty acids are a group of polyunsaturated fatty acids that are important for a number of functions in the body. They are found in foods such as fatty fish and certain vegetable oils and are also available as dietary supplements. While experts agree that fish rich in omega-3 fatty acids should be included in a heart-healthy diet, there isn't conclusive evidence that shows omega-3s have a protective effect against heart disease.

1. Experts agree that fish rich in omega-3 fatty acids should be included in a heart-healthy diet. Much research has been done on fish and heart disease, and the results provide strong, though not conclusive, evidence that people who eat fish at least once a week are less likely to die of heart disease than those who rarely or never eat fish.

2. Omega-3s in supplement form have not been shown to protect against heart disease. While there has been a substantial amount of research on omega-3 supplements and heart disease, the findings of individual studies have been inconsistent. In 2012, two combined analyses of the results of these studies did not find convincing evidence that omega-3s protect against heart disease.

3. Omega-3 supplements may interact with drugs that affect blood clotting. Omega-3 supplements may extend the time it takes for a cut to stop bleeding. People who take drugs such as anticoagulants ("blood thinners") or nonsteroidal anti-inflammatory drugs should discuss the use of omega-3 fatty acid supplements with a health care provider.

4. Fish liver oils (which are not the same as fish oils) contain vitamins A and D as well as omega-3 fatty acids; these vitamins can be toxic in high doses. The amounts of vitamins in fish liver oil supplements vary from one product to another.

5. Talk to your health care provider before using omega-3 supplements. If you are pregnant or nursing a child, if you take medicine that affects blood clotting, if you are allergic to fish or shellfish, or if you are considering giving a child an omega-3 supplement, it is especially important to consult your (or your child's) health care provider.

Section 63.3

Phytochemicals and Cardiovascular Disease

What Are Phytochemicals?

Phytochemicals are chemicals found in plants. Plant sterols, flavonoids (FLAV'oh-noidz), and sulfur-containing compounds are three classes of micronutrients found in fruits and vegetables. These compounds may be important in reducing the risk of atherosclerosis (ath"er-o-skleh-RO'sis), which is the buildup of fatty deposits in artery walls. Within these categories are many possible compounds, most of which aren't well described and whose modes of action aren't established. Many other plant products may also be linked to the atherosclerotic process, such as antioxidant vitamins, phytoestrogens, and trace minerals. These plant micronutrients will clearly be the topic of future research. As work continues on all these compounds, other unrecognized components in plants will be identified that may have promise in reducing risk of cardiovascular disease.

American Heart Association (AHA) Recommendation

More research on phytochemicals is needed in these areas:

- Nutritional databases must include better information on micronutrients.

- Large population-based studies with collected dietary data should then be reanalyzed to quantify intakes of plant sterols, flavonoids, and sulfur-containing compounds, and to assess possible relationships with atherosclerosis and other chronic diseases.

- Studies using newer techniques to measure cholesterol absorption and lipoprotein metabolism must be conducted to define the mechanism of action of each of these micronutrients.

- A direct assessment of the influence of micronutrients on lipoprotein profiles, hemostatic factors, and cardiovascular disease must be made. Some micronutrients may not act alone but in concert with other dietary components.

Until more of this information is gathered and fully understood, the American Heart Association recommends eating a balanced diet containing a wide variety of fruits, vegetables, and whole-grain products. Eating a variety of foods is the most prudent way to ensure that you get the optimum amounts of both macronutrients and micronutrients. Use of foods containing plant sterols should be reserved for adults requiring lower total and low-density lipoprotein (LDL) cholesterol levels because they are at high risk of—or have had—a heart attack.

Background

Large population studies have often shown links between the intake of vegetables and fruits and coronary heart disease that aren't clearly attributable to major macronutrients or known vitamins and minerals. This suggests that other components of plants may be important in lowering risk of cardiovascular disease. Although the literature contains studies of numerous possible plant components, many of these studies are based on a small sample of subjects or were poorly controlled. Further, the notion itself has led to claims of "miracle" ingredients with supposed beneficial effects on cardiovascular diseases and other chronic diseases.

Substantial evidence exists in three areas: plant sterols, flavonoids, and plant sulfur compounds. Here is a summary of the state of knowledge in these three areas and information about possible future work.

Plant Sterols

The plant kingdom contains a number of sterols that differ from cholesterol by having ethyl or methyl groups or unsaturation in the side chain. The major ones—sitosterol (si"to-STEER'ol), stigmasterol (stig"mah-STEER'ol), and campesterol (kam-PES'ter-ol)—can be present in Western diets in amounts almost equal to dietary cholesterol. The most prominent is sitosterol. In the early 1950s it was noted that adding sitosterol to the diet of cholesterol-fed chickens or rabbits lowered cholesterol levels in both species and inhibited the development of atherosclerosis in rabbits. Sitosterol or mixtures of soy sterols were studied extensively as cholesterol-lowering agents between 1950 and 1960. They lowered cholesterol by about 10 percent. This area merits reinvestigation using newer technologies.

In the 1980s it was demonstrated that sitostanol (si"to-STAN'ol), a saturated sitosterol derivative, reduced the absorption of cholesterol and blood cholesterol more effectively than sitosterol and at doses below those of sitosterol. In a recent study, sitostanol was combined or "interesterified" with margarine. The resultant product reduced plasma cholesterol an average of 10.2 percent in a population with mild hypercholesteremia. The sitostanol wasn't absorbed and didn't seem to interfere with absorption of fat-soluble vitamins. In 1999 several companies began marketing margarine and other products containing either stanol or sterol esters. Studies in Finland suggest these products can help lower cholesterol.

Squalene (SKWAH'leen), a sterol precursor also found in plant products, was originally suggested to have a cholesterol-lowering effect. But earlier studies in animals showed that it had no positive influence on atherosclerosis. Sitosterols and squalene are present in both monounsaturated and polyunsaturated vegetable oils and thus may be responsible for some of the variable cholesterol-lowering effects found in studies using these products. This may explain differences seen between various sources and degrees of refinement of olive oil. There are also cholesterol-lowering alcohols in rice bran oils. Several recent studies suggest that rice bran oil lowers plasma cholesterol levels about 7 to 10 percent in humans.

Finally, cafestol (KAF'es-tol) is a terpene present in coffee. Some studies have suggested that drinking coffee may be linked with changes in plasma cholesterol that may be explained by the presence of this compound. The manner of preparation may influence the effect of coffee; for example, filtering may remove some cholesterol-raising compounds.

Flavonoids

Flavonoids (FLAV'oh-noidz) are compounds with varied chemical structures present in fruits, vegetables, nuts, and seeds. The major flavonoid categories are flavonols (FLAV'oh-nolz), flavones (FLAV'onz), catechins (KAT'eh-kinz), flavanones (FLAV'ah-nonz), and anthocyanins (an"tho-SI'ah-ninz). The main dietary sources of these compounds are tea, onions, soy, and wine. The main flavonoid in onions is quercetin glucoside (KER'seh-tin GLU'ko-syd), and the main flavonoid in tea is quercetin rutinoside (KER'seh-tin roo-TIN'o-syd).

Flavonoid intake has been inversely linked with coronary heart disease in the Zutphen Elderly Study, the Seven Countries Study, and a cohort study in Finland. That is, people with a low intake of flavonoid had a higher death rate from coronary heart disease than did those who consumed more flavonoid (about five to six cups of tea per day). It should be pointed out that some flavonoids have toxic effects (gastrointestinal or allergic), especially if taken in large amounts. Systematic work is needed on the major classes of flavonoids to study their structure, effectiveness, and potential harmful effects.

The link between flavonoids and atherosclerosis is based partly on the evidence that some flavonoids have antioxidant (an"tih-OK'sih-dant) properties. For example, the phenolic (fen-OL'ik) substances in red wine inhibit oxidation of human LDL. Flavonoids also have been shown to inhibit the aggregation and adhesion of platelets in blood, which may be another way they lower the risk of heart disease. Isoflavones (i"so-FLAV'-onz) in soy foods have been reported to lower plasma cholesterol and also to have effects similar to estrogen.

Plant Sulfur Compounds

Naturally occurring sulfur-containing compounds (the allium family) are found especially in garlic, onions, and leeks, the most prominent of these being garlic. In 2000, the Agency for Healthcare Research and Quality (AHRQ) published an evidence-based "Report on Garlic: Effects on Cardiovascular Risks and Disease, Protective Effects Against Cancer, and Clinical Adverse Effects." Here are the main findings:

- Thirty-six randomized trials, all but one in adults, consistently showed that, compared with placebo, various garlic preparations led to small, statistically significant reductions in total cholesterol at one month (range of average pooled reductions 1.1 to 15.8 milligrams per deciliter [mg/dL]) and three months (range of 11.6 to 24.3 mg/dL). Eight trials with outcomes at six months showed no significant reductions of garlic compared with placebo. Changes in low-density lipoprotein levels (LDL) and triglycerides mirrored total cholesterol results; no significant changes in high-density lipoprotein levels (HDL) were found.

- Twenty-six small, randomized, placebo-controlled trials, all but one in adults, reported mixed, but never large, effects of various garlic preparations on blood pressure outcomes.

- Twelve small, randomized trials suggested various garlic preparations had no clinically significant effects on glucose in persons with or without diabetes. Two small short trials reported no statistically significant effects of garlic compared with placebo on serum insulin or C peptide levels.

- Ten small, short-duration trials, all but one in adults, showed effects of various garlic preparations on platelet aggregation and mixed effects on plasma viscosity (vis-KOS'ih-te) and fibrinolytic (fi-brin"o-LIT'ik) activity.

- There were insufficient data to confirm or refute garlic's effects on clinical outcomes such as myocardial infarction and claudication.

- Scant data, primarily from case-control studies, suggest, but do not prove, that dietary garlic consumption is associated with decreased odds of laryngeal, gastric, colorectal, and endometrial cancer and adenomatous (ad-eh-NOM'ah-tus) colorectal polyps.

- Adverse effects of oral ingestion of garlic are "smelly" breath and body odor. Other possible, but not proven, adverse effects include flatulence, esophageal and abdominal pain, small intestinal obstruction, dermatitis, rhinitis, asthma, and bleeding.

What are the conclusions? Trials show several promising, modest, short-term effects of garlic supplements on lipid and antithrombotic factors. Effects on clinical outcomes are not established, and effects on glucose and blood pressure are none to minimal. High dietary intake of garlic may be associated with decreased risks of multiple cancers. Our ability to interpret existing data is limited by marked variability in types of garlic preparations that have been studied and inadequate definition of active constituents in the various preparations.

Chapter 64

Weight Management and Heart Health

Why Is a Healthy Weight Important?

Being overweight or obese increases your risk for many diseases and conditions. The more you weigh, the more likely you are to suffer from heart disease, high blood pressure, diabetes, gallbladder disease, sleep apnea, and certain cancers. On the other hand, a healthy weight has many benefits: It helps you to lower your risk for developing these problems, helps you to feel good about yourself, and gives you more energy to enjoy life.

What Is Your Risk for Weight-Related Diseases?

Body Mass Index (BMI)

Your BMI accurately estimates your total body fat. And, the amount of fat that you carry is a good indicator of your risk for a variety of diseases.

You can check your BMI by using the BMI chart in Table 64.1. First, find your height in the left-hand column. Then, follow it over until you find your weight. The number on the top of that column is your BMI.

"Facts about Healthy Weight," National Heart, Lung, and Blood Institute, National Institutes of Health, 2006. Reviewed by David A. Cooke, M.D., FACP, October 2013.

BMI	Normal						Overweight					Obese										Extreme Obesity														
Height (inches)	19	20	21	22	23	24	25	26	27	28	29	30	31	32	33	34	35	36	37	38	39	40	41	42	43	44	45	46	47	48	49	50	51	52	53	54
58	91	96	100	105	110	115	119	124	129	134	138	143	148	153	158	162	167	172	177	181	186	191	196	201	205	210	215	220	224	229	234	239	244	248	253	258
59	94	99	104	109	114	119	124	128	133	138	143	148	153	158	163	168	173	178	183	188	193	198	203	208	212	217	222	227	232	237	242	247	252	257	262	267
60	97	102	107	112	118	123	128	133	138	143	148	153	158	163	168	174	179	184	189	194	199	204	209	215	220	225	230	235	240	245	250	255	261	266	271	276
61	100	106	111	116	122	127	132	137	143	148	153	158	164	169	174	180	185	190	195	201	206	211	217	222	227	232	238	243	248	254	259	264	269	275	280	285
62	104	109	115	120	126	131	136	142	147	153	158	164	169	175	180	186	191	196	202	207	213	218	224	229	235	240	246	251	256	262	267	273	278	284	289	295
63	107	113	118	124	130	135	141	146	152	158	163	169	175	180	186	191	197	203	208	214	220	225	231	237	242	248	254	259	265	270	278	282	287	293	299	304
64	110	116	122	128	134	140	145	151	157	163	169	174	180	186	192	197	204	209	215	221	227	232	238	244	250	256	262	267	273	279	285	291	296	302	308	314
65	114	120	126	132	138	144	150	156	162	168	174	180	186	192	198	204	210	216	222	228	234	240	246	252	258	264	270	276	282	288	294	300	306	312	318	324
66	118	124	130	136	142	148	155	161	167	173	179	186	192	198	204	210	216	223	229	235	241	247	253	260	266	272	278	284	291	297	303	309	315	322	328	334
67	121	127	134	140	146	153	159	166	172	178	185	191	198	204	211	217	223	230	236	242	249	255	261	268	274	280	287	293	299	306	312	319	325	331	338	344
68	125	131	138	144	151	158	164	171	177	184	190	197	203	210	216	223	230	236	243	249	256	262	269	276	282	289	295	302	308	315	322	328	335	341	348	354
69	128	135	142	149	155	162	169	176	182	189	196	203	209	216	223	230	236	243	250	257	263	270	277	284	291	297	304	311	318	324	331	338	345	351	358	365
70	132	139	146	153	160	167	174	181	188	195	202	209	216	222	229	236	243	250	257	264	271	278	285	292	299	306	313	320	327	334	341	348	355	362	369	376
71	136	143	150	157	165	172	179	186	193	200	208	215	222	229	236	243	250	257	265	272	279	286	293	301	308	315	322	329	338	343	351	358	365	372	379	386
72	140	147	154	162	169	177	184	191	199	206	213	221	228	235	242	250	258	265	272	279	287	294	302	309	316	324	331	338	346	353	361	368	375	383	390	397
73	144	151	159	166	174	182	189	197	204	212	219	227	235	242	250	257	265	272	280	288	295	302	310	318	325	333	340	348	355	363	371	378	386	393	401	408
74	148	155	163	171	179	186	194	202	210	218	225	233	241	249	256	264	272	280	287	295	303	311	319	326	334	342	350	358	365	373	381	389	396	404	412	420
75	152	160	168	176	184	192	200	208	216	224	232	240	248	256	264	272	279	287	295	303	311	319	327	335	343	351	359	367	375	383	391	399	407	415	423	431
76	156	164	172	180	189	197	205	213	221	230	238	246	254	263	271	279	287	295	304	312	320	328	336	344	353	361	369	377	385	394	402	410	418	426	435	443

Source: Adapted from *Clinical Guidelines on the Identification, Evaluation, and Treatment of Overweight and Obesity in Adults: The Evidence Report,* National Institutes of Health, 1998.

Figure 64.1. *Body Mass Index. Weight is measured with underwear but no shoes. (Excerpted from "Insulin Resistance and Pre-Diabetes," National Institute of Diabetes and Digestive and Kidney Diseases, National Institutes of Health, NIH Publication No. 09-4893, October 2008.)*

What Does Your BMI Mean?

Normal weight: BMI = 18.5–24.9. Good for you! Try not to gain weight.

Overweight: BMI = 25–29.9. Do not gain any weight, especially if your waist circumference is high. You need to lose weight if you have two or more risk factors for heart disease and are overweight or have a high waist circumference.

Obese: BMI = 30 or greater. You need to lose weight. Lose weight slowly—about one-half to two pounds a week. See your doctor or a nutritionist if you need help.

Although BMI can be used for most men and women, it does have some limitations:

- It may overestimate body fat in athletes and others who have a muscular build.

- It may underestimate body fat in older persons and others who have lost muscle.

Waist Circumference Measurement

Your waist circumference is also an important measurement to help you figure out your overall health risks. If most of your fat is around your waist, then you are more at risk for heart disease and diabetes. This risk increases with a waist measurement that is as follows:

- Greater than thirty-five inches for women

- Greater than forty inches for men

Other Risk Factors for Heart Disease

Besides being overweight or obese, here are other risk factors to consider:

- Cigarette smoking

- High blood pressure (hypertension)

- High low-density lipoprotein (LDL) cholesterol (bad cholesterol)

- Low high-density lipoprotein (HDL) cholesterol (good cholesterol)

- High triglycerides

- High blood glucose (sugar)

- Family history of premature heart disease

- Physical inactivity

If you have other risk factors for heart disease and are overweight or obese, then you will be at greater risk for health problems. Your doctor will check your BMI, waist circumference, and other risk factors for heart disease:

- If you are overweight (BMI 25–29.9), do not have a high waist circumference, and have less than two risk factors, then it's important that you not gain any more weight.

- If you are overweight (BMI 25–29.9) or have a high waist circumference and have two or more risk factors, then it is important for you to lose weight.

- If you are obese (BMI 30), then it is important for you to lose weight.

Even a small weight loss (just 5 to 10 percent of your current weight) will help to lower your risk of developing weight-related diseases.

How to Lose Weight and Maintain It

Changing the way you approach weight loss can help you be more successful at losing it. Most people who try to lose weight focus on one thing: weight loss. However if you set goals, begin to eat healthy foods, become more physically active, and learn how to change behaviors, then you may be more successful at losing weight. Over time, these changes will become routine and part of your everyday life.

Weight Loss Goals

Setting the right goals is an important first step to losing and maintaining weight:

- Losing just 5 to 10 percent of your current weight over six months will lower your risk for heart disease and other conditions.

- Losing one to two pounds per week is a reasonable and safe weight loss. Losing weight at this rate will help you to keep off the weight. And it will give you the time to make new healthy lifestyle changes.

- Maintaining a modest weight loss over a longer period of time is better than losing a lot of weight and regaining it. You can think about additional weight loss after you've lost 10 percent of your current body weight and have kept it off for six months.

Keeping a Balance

Maintaining a healthy weight calls for keeping a balance . . . a balance of energy. You must balance the calories or energy that you get from food and beverages with the calories that you use to keep your body going and to be physically active:

- The same amount of energy IN and OUT over time = weight stays the same

- More energy IN than OUT over time = weight gain

- More energy OUT than IN over time = weight loss

Your energy IN and OUT doesn't have to balance exactly every day: Balancing energy over time will help you to maintain a healthy weight in the long run.

A Healthy Eating Plan

A healthy eating plan gives your body the nutrients it needs every day and helps you to stay within your daily calorie level. This eating plan will also lower your risk for heart disease and such other conditions as high blood pressure and high blood cholesterol levels.

A healthy eating plan does the following things:

- Emphasizes fruits, vegetables, whole grains, and fat-free or low-fat milk and milk products

- Includes lean meats, poultry, fish, beans, eggs, and nuts

- Is low in saturated fats, trans fat, cholesterol, salt (sodium), and added sugars

- Controls portion sizes

Calories

Cutting back on calories is part of a healthy eating plan to lose weight. Choose foods that are lower in fats, especially saturated and trans fats, cholesterol, and added sugars. Also, pay attention to portion sizes.

To lose one to two pounds a week, daily intake should be reduced by 500 to 1,000 calories. In general, the following is true:

- Eating plans that contain 1,000–1,200 calories each day will help most women to lose weight safely.

- Eating plans that contain 1,200–1,600 calories each day are suitable for men and may also be appropriate for women who weigh 165 pounds or more or who exercise regularly.

If you eat 1,600 calories a day but do not lose weight, then you may want to cut back to 1,200 calories. If you are hungry on either diet, then you may want to boost your calories by 100 to 200 per day. Very low calorie diets of less than 800 calories per day should not be used unless you are being monitored by your doctor.

Physical Activity

Staying physically active and eating fewer calories will help you lose weight and keep the weight off over time. Plus, physical activity has many benefits:

- Lowers the risk of heart disease, diabetes, and cancers such as breast, uterus, and colon

- Strengthens your lungs and helps them to work more efficiently

- Strengthens your muscles and keeps your joints in good condition

- May slow bone loss

- Gives you more energy

- Helps you to relax and cope better with stress

- Builds confidence

- Allows you to fall asleep more quickly and sleep more soundly

- Provides an enjoyable way to share time with friends and family

How Much Physical Activity Should You Aim For?

- For overall health and to reduce the risk of disease, aim for at least thirty minutes of moderate physical activity most days of the week.

- To help manage body weight and prevent gradual weight gain, aim for sixty minutes of moderate-to-vigorous physical activity most days of the week.

- To maintain weight loss, aim for at least sixty to ninety minutes of daily moderate physical activity.

You can break up the amount of time that you do physical activity, such as fifteen minutes at a time. If you haven't been physically active for some time, then don't let that stop you. Start slowly and gradually increase your activity. For example, start walking for ten to fifteen minutes three times a week, then gradually build up to the recommended amount with brisk walking.

Other Weight Loss Options

Weight loss drugs and weight loss surgery may be options for some people who are at high risk from overweight or obesity or who have been unsuccessful at making lifestyle changes. If you think that you may benefit from weight loss drugs or surgery, then talk to your doctor.

Tips to Weight Loss Success

Maintaining long-term weight loss can be difficult. Three keys to success are setting realistic goals, following a healthy diet, and aiming for sixty to ninety minutes of physical activity most days of the week. Other tips for weight loss success include the following:

- Set specific, realistic goals that are forgiving (less than perfect). To start, try walking thirty minutes, three days a week.

- Ask for encouragement from your health care provider(s) via telephone or e-mail; friends and family can help. You can also join a support group.

- Keep a record of your food intake and the amount of physical activity that you do. This is an easy way to track how you are doing. A record can also inspire you. For example, when it shows that you've been more active, you'll be encouraged to keep it up.

- Change your surroundings to avoid overeating. For example, don't eat while watching television. Plan to meet a friend in a nonfood setting.

- Reward your success but not with food. Instead, choose rewards that you'll enjoy, such as a movie, a music CD, an afternoon off from work, a massage, or personal time.

You can feel healthier by doing any of the following activities. For added fun, ask friends or family to join you:

- Walk or ride a bike in your neighborhood.

- Join a walking club at a mall or at work.

- Play golf at a local club.

- Join a dance or yoga class.

- Work in your garden.

- Use local athletic facilities.

- Join a hiking or biking club.

- Join a softball team or play other sports with co-workers, friends, and family.

Portion Distortion: How to Choose Sensible Servings

It's very easy to "eat with your eyes" and misjudge what equals a serving—piling on unwanted pounds. This is especially true when you eat out, because restaurant portions are often supersized and enough for two or more people to share.

To keep portion sizes sensible, do the following things:

- When eating out, choose small portions, share an entrée with a friend, or take some of the food home.

- Check a product's Nutrition Facts label to learn how much food is considered a serving and how many calories, fat grams, and other nutrients are in the item.

- Limit portion sizes of such high-calorie foods as cookies, cakes, and other sweets; French fries; and oils.

- Use smaller plates. We eat most of what is on our plate, no matter what the size. Smaller plates can mean smaller portions.

Chapter 65

Physical Activity Key to a Healthy Heart

Physical Activity: The Heart Connection

Chances are, you already know that physical activity is good for you. "Sure," you may say, "When I get out and move around, I know it helps me to look and feel better." But you may not realize just how important regular physical activity is to your health. Inactive people are nearly twice as likely to develop heart disease as those who are active. Lack of physical activity also leads to more visits to the doctor, more hospitalizations, and more use of medicines for a variety of illnesses. The good news is that physical activity can protect your heart in a number of important ways and keep you healthy overall.

Heart Disease Risk Factors

Risk factors are conditions or habits that make a person more likely to develop a disease. They can also increase the chances that an existing disease will get worse. Certain risk factors for heart disease, such as getting older or having a family history of early heart disease, can't be changed. But physical inactivity is a major risk factor for heart disease that you can control. Other major risk factors for heart disease that you can control are smoking, high blood pressure, high blood cholesterol, overweight, and diabetes. Every risk factor greatly increases

Excerpted from "In Brief: Your Guide to Physical Activity and Your Heart," National Heart, Lung, and Blood Institute, National Institutes of Health, January 2008. Reviewed by David A. Cooke, M.D., FACP, October 2013.

the chances of developing heart disease and having a heart attack. A damaged heart can keep you from doing simple, enjoyable things, such as taking a walk or climbing steps. But it's important to know that you have a lot of power to protect your heart health. Getting regular physical activity is especially important because it directly reduces your heart disease risk and your chances of developing other risk factors for heart disease. Physical activity can also protect your heart by helping to prevent and control diabetes. Finally, physical activity can help you to lose excess weight or to stay at a healthy weight, which will also help to lower your risk of heart disease.

Physical Activity and Your Health

What does it mean to get "regular physical activity?" To reduce the risk of heart disease, adults only need to do about thirty minutes of moderate activity on most, preferably all, days of the week. This level of activity can also lower your chances of having a stroke, colon cancer, high blood pressure, diabetes, and other medical problems. If you're also trying to manage your weight and prevent gradual, unhealthy weight gain, try to get sixty minutes of moderate- to vigorous-intensity activity on most days of the week. At the same time, watch your calories. Take in only enough calories to maintain your weight. If you're trying to keep weight off, aim a bit higher: Try to get sixty to ninety minutes of moderate-intensity activity daily, without taking in extra calories.

Physical Activity: The Calorie Connection

One way that regular physical activity protects against heart disease is by burning extra calories, which can help you to lose excess weight or stay at your healthy weight. To understand how physical activity affects calories, it's helpful to consider the concept of "energy balance." Energy balance is the amount of calories you take in relative to the amount of calories you burn. If you need to lose weight for your health, eating fewer calories and being more active is the best approach. You're more likely to be successful by combining a healthful, lower-calorie diet with physical activity. For example, a two-hundred-pound person who consumes 250 fewer calories per day and walks briskly each day for one-half mile will lose about forty pounds in one year. Most of the energy you burn each day—about three-quarters of it—goes to activities that your body automatically engages in for survival, such as breathing, sleeping, and digesting food. The part of your energy output that you control is daily physical activity. Any activity you take part in beyond your body's automatic activities will burn extra calories. Even seated activities, such as using the computer or watching TV, will burn calories—but only a very small number. That's why it's important to make time each day for moderate-to vigorous-intensity physical activity.

Great Moves

Given the numerous benefits of regular physical activity, you may be ready to get in motion! Three types of activity are important for a complete physical activity program: aerobic activity, resistance training, and flexibility exercises.

Types of Physical Activity

Aerobic activity is any physical activity that uses large muscle groups and causes your body to use more oxygen than it would while resting. Aerobic activity is the type of movement that most benefits the heart. Examples of aerobic activity are brisk walking, jogging, and bicycling. If you're just starting to be active, try brisk walking for short periods such as five or ten minutes, and build up gradually to thirty to sixty minutes at least five days per week. Always start with a five-minute, slower-paced walk to warm up, and end with a five-minute, slower-paced walk to cool down. Resistance training—also called strength training—can firm, strengthen, and tone your muscles, as well as improve bone strength, balance, and coordination. Examples of resistance training are pushups, lunges, and bicep curls using dumbbells. Flexibility exercises stretch and lengthen your muscles. These activities help improve joint flexibility and keep muscles limber, thereby preventing injury. An example of a flexibility exercise is sitting cross-legged on the floor and gently pushing down on the tops of your legs to stretch the inner-thigh muscles.

Family Fitness

When it comes to getting in shape, what's good for you is good for your whole family. Children and teenagers should be physically active for at least sixty minutes per day. A great way to pry kids off the couch—and help you to stay fit as well—is to do enjoyable activities together. Some ideas are as follows:

- **Kick up your heels:** Take turns picking out your favorite music, and dance up a storm in the living room.

609

- **Explore the outdoors:** Hit your local trail on weekends for some biking or hiking. Pack a healthy lunch and let the kids choose the picnic spot.

- **Get classy:** Join family members in an active class, such as martial arts, yoga, or aerobics.

- **Play pupil:** Ask one of your children or grandchildren to teach you an active game or sport. Kids love to be the experts, and you'll get a workout learning a new activity!

Creating Opportunities

It's easier to stay physically active over time if you take advantage of everyday opportunities to move around. For example, do the following:

- Use the stairs—both up and down—instead of the elevator. Start with one flight of stairs and gradually build up to more.

- Park a few blocks from the office or store and walk the rest of the way. If you take public transportation, get off a stop or two early and walk a few blocks.

- While working, take frequent activity breaks. Get up and stretch, walk around, and give your muscles and mind a chance to relax.

- Instead of eating that extra snack, take a brisk stroll around the neighborhood or your office building.

- Do housework, gardening, or yard work at a more vigorous pace.

- When you travel, walk around the train station, bus station, or airport rather than sitting and waiting.

Chapter 66

Managing Stress for a Healthy Heart

The American Heart Association describes a coronary attack (heart attack) as an occurrence that happens when the blood flow to a part of the heart is blocked. This happens because coronary arteries that supply the heart with blood slowly become thicker and harder from a buildup of plaque that consists of fat, cholesterol, and other substances. A heart attack occurs when the plaque breaks open and a blood clot forms to block the blood flow; damage increases the longer an artery stays blocked. Damaged heart muscles supplied by that artery begin to die, resulting in permanent heart damage. Hypertension is commonly known as "high blood pressure" and is a condition in which the force of the blood against your artery walls is high enough that it increases your risk of serious health problems, including heart attack and stroke if it is not controlled. For most individuals, living with a few basic principles to prevent stress can greatly reduce the risk of a heart-related health issue.

Manage Stress

An important piece to heart disease prevention is managing stress. Stress makes the heart beat faster to get the body ready for action. People who are stressed all the time secrete a hormone called cortisol that raises blood pressure and causes the body to retain fluids placing excessive stress on the heart. Prolonged high levels of stress cause:

- high blood pressure;
- irregular heart rhythms;
- damage to arteries;
- higher cholesterol levels;
- the development and progression of coronary artery disease (atherosclerosis);
- a weakened immune system.

Suggestions for managing stress are:

- Take time out each day to relax.
- Maintain a healthy lifestyle through exercising, eating healthy, and getting enough sleep.
- Leave the worksite at lunchtime to take a short walk or relax outside your work environment, taking a five-minute relaxation break for a relaxation exercise.
- Control stress at work by switching from caffeinated to decaffeinated coffee beverages.
- Begin to take note of things that cause you to feel stressed.
- Take control of your schedule and set realistic goals and expectations.
- Prioritize what needs to be done each day.
- Put an emphasis on what was accomplished, and not what failed to be accomplished.
- Take time to praise yourself for a job well done.
- Avoid negative "self-talk." Avoid "what-ifs." Avoid focusing on what you do not know or can't control.
- Accept the fact you may not be able to change certain situations.
- Get answers to questions that may be worrying you (such as your health).

Getting help:

- If you are having a hard time controlling vices, such as cigarettes, alcohol, or drugs to reduce your stress, you may need help from a professional to learn how to control your stress.

- Family counselors can help develop strategies to reduce family stress.

- Work with your doctors and ask for referrals to find the best way to learn stress management.

- A business coach can help you get organized with goals, work plans, and setting priorities.

References

American Heart Association. (2009). What is a Heart attack? (10/07LS1466).

Cleveland Clinic Miller Family Heart & Vascular Institute. Heart and vascular health & prevention. (n.d.). Retrieved from http://my.clevelandclinic.org/heart/prevention/nutrition/antioxidants.aspx.

Mayo Clinic Staff. (2009, January 15). 5 medication free strategies to help prevent heart disease. Retrieved from http://www.mayoclinic.com/health/heart-disease-prevention/WO00041.

Chapter 67

Quitting Smoking: Why It Is Important and How to Do It

Why Should I Quit Now?

Most smokers say they want to quit. So how do you move from wanting to quit to actually quitting? A first step is to find reasons to quit that are important to you. Consider the many good reasons to quit smoking.

Your Health

Your health begins to improve the minute you stop smoking, and you begin to lower your long-term risk of many smoking-related diseases. Smoking causes or can contribute to many serious health problems, including the following:

- Cancers of the lung, throat, mouth, voice box, esophagus, pancreas, kidney, bladder, cervix, uterus, stomach, and blood

- Lung diseases

- Heart disease

- Stroke

- Atherosclerosis, or hardening and narrowing of the arteries

- Gum disease

Excerpted from "Why Should I Quit Now?" and "How to Quit," U.S. Department of Health and Human Services, Office on Women's Health, May 19, 2010.

- Eye diseases that can lead to blindness
- Osteoporosis and the risk of hip fracture

Smoking also does the following things:

- Makes illnesses last longer
- Causes more wound infections after surgery
- Makes it harder to get pregnant

Why Does Birth Weight Matter?

Low-birth-weight babies are more likely to die or have serious health problems. They are also more likely to have long-term disabilities, such as problems seeing or hearing.

Smoking during pregnancy can hurt the mother and baby. It increases the risk of the following things:

- Placenta previa—when the placenta covers part of or the entire cervix inside of the uterus. This can lead to bed rest, early labor, and cesarean section.

- Placental abruption—the placenta separates too early from the wall of the uterus. This can lead to early labor or infant death.

- Early rupture of membranes, or water breaking, before labor starts, so the baby is born too early.

- A baby with a low birth weight.

- Damage to an infant's lungs.

- Sudden infant death syndrome (SIDS).

- Miscarriage.

- Stillbirth.

Your Quality of Life

When you quit, you will never again have to leave your workplace, your home, or other places to smoke. You won't need to worry about whether your smoke is bothering others. The money you would have spent on cigarettes can be saved or used to buy other things. Plus, you will be surprised by how good you feel overall. Over time, here are some of the ways you will look and feel better:

- You will breathe more easily.

- You will have more energy.
- Your lungs will be stronger, making it easier to be active.
- You will be able to smell and taste things better.
- Your hair, breath, and clothes will smell better.
- The stain marks on your fingers will fade.
- Your skin will look healthier.
- Your teeth and gums will be healthier.
- You will feel good about being able to quit!

Other People's Health

When you quit, you no longer create secondhand smoke, which is harmful to the people around you, and especially children. When you quit, you become a role-model to children and other smokers who want to quit. When you quit, your own children are less likely to grow up to become smokers themselves.

How to Quit

Make the Decision to Quit and Feel Great!

If you have made the decision to quit smoking, congratulations! Not only will you improve your own health, you will also protect the health of your loved ones by no longer exposing them to secondhand smoke.

We know how hard it can be to quit smoking. Did you know that many people try to quit two or three times before they give up smoking for good? Nicotine is a very addictive drug—as addictive as heroin and cocaine. The good news is that millions of people have given up smoking for good. It's hard work to quit, but you can do it! Freeing yourself of an expensive habit that threatens your health and the health of others will make you feel great!

Many people who smoke worry that they will gain weight if they quit. In fact, nearly 80 percent of people who quit smoking do gain weight, but the average weight gain is just five pounds. Keep in mind, however, that more than half of people who keep smoking will gain weight too. Plus, the health benefits of quitting far exceed any risks from the weight gain related to quitting.

How to Quit

Research has shown that the following steps will help you to quit for good.

Pick a date to stop smoking. Before that day, get rid of all cigarettes, ashtrays, and lighters everywhere you smoke. Do not allow anyone to smoke in your home. List the reasons why you want to quit and keep this list with you, so you can refer to it if you have an urge to light up. It will remind you why you want to stop.

Talk to your doctor or nurse about medicines to help you quit. Many people have withdrawal symptoms when they quit smoking. These symptoms can include depression, trouble sleeping, feeling irritable or restless, and trouble thinking clearly. Medicines work well at relieving these symptoms and can boost your chances of quitting for good. Your chances of quitting are even better when medicine and counseling are used together. Most medicines help you quit smoking by giving you small, steady doses of nicotine, the drug in cigarettes that causes addiction. Also, for some people, certain combinations of medicine work better than using one medicine alone. Talk to your doctor or nurse to see if one of these medicines may be right for you:

- *Nicotine patch:* Worn on the skin and supplies a steady amount of nicotine to the body through the skin

- *Nicotine gum or lozenge:* Releases nicotine into the bloodstream through the lining in your mouth

- *Nicotine nasal spray:* Inhaled through your nose and passes into your bloodstream

- *Nicotine inhaler:* Inhaled through the mouth and absorbed in the mouth and throat

- *Bupropion (Zyban):* A medicine that reduces nicotine withdrawal symptoms and the urge to smoke

- *Varenicline (Chantix):* a medicine that reduces nicotine withdrawal symptoms and the pleasurable effects of smoking

Seek counseling. You can improve your chances of quitting for good with professional help. Counseling can provide you with practical skills to overcome nicotine addiction, as well as support and encouragement. Many forms of counseling and support can help, whether alone, in a group, or through a telephone "quit line." Your chances of success are best with in-person, intense counseling and when all forms are used. Seeking frequent counseling, at least once a week, especially in the first months after quitting, also will boost your chances of success.

Get support from your family, friends, and coworkers. You will be more likely to quit for good if you have help. Let the people important to you know the date you will be quitting and ask them for their support. Ask them not to smoke around you or leave cigarettes out.

Find substitutes for smoking and vary your routine. When you get the urge to smoke, do something to take your mind off smoking. Talk to a friend, go for a walk, or go to the movies. Find ways other than smoking to reduce stress, such as exercise, meditation, hot baths, or reading. Try sugar-free gum or candy to help handle your cravings. Drink lots of water. You might want to try changing your daily routine as well. Try drinking tea instead of coffee, eating your breakfast in a different place, or taking a different route to work.

Be prepared for relapse. Most people relapse, or start smoking again, within the first three months after quitting. Don't get discouraged if you relapse. Remember, many people try to quit several times before quitting for good. Think of what helped and didn't help the last time you tried to quit. Figuring these out before you try to quit again will increase your chances for success. Certain situations can increase your chances of smoking. These include drinking alcohol, being around other smokers, gaining weight, stress, or becoming depressed. Talk to your doctor or nurse to learn ways to cope with these situations.

Where to Get Help

Get more help if you need it. Join a quit-smoking program or support group to help you quit. These programs can help you handle withdrawal and stress and teach you skills to resist the urge to smoke. Contact your local hospital, health center, or health department for information about quit-smoking programs and support groups in your area.

Chapter 68

Other Interventions to Help Reduce Risk of Cardiovascular Disease

Chapter Contents

Section 68.1

Aspirin for Reducing Your Risk of Heart Attack and Stroke

"Aspirin for Reducing Your Risk of Heart Attack and Stroke:
Know the Facts," U.S. Food and Drug Administration, April 27, 2012.

You can walk into any pharmacy, grocery, or convenience store and buy aspirin without a prescription. The Drug Facts label on medication products, will help you choose aspirin for relieving headache, pain, swelling, or fever. The Drug Facts label also gives directions that will help you use the aspirin so that it is safe and effective.

But what about using aspirin for a different use, time period, or in a manner that is not listed on the label? For example, using aspirin to lower the risk of heart attack and clot-related strokes. In these cases, the labeling information is not there to help you with how to choose and how to use the medicine safely. Since you don't have the labeling directions to help you, you need the medical knowledge of your doctor, nurse practitioner, or other health professional.

You can increase the chance of getting the good effects and decrease the chance of getting the bad effects of any medicine by choosing and using it wisely. When it comes to using aspirin to lower the risk of heart attack and stroke, choosing and using wisely means knowing the facts and working with your health professional.

Fact: Daily Use of Aspirin Is Not Right for Everyone

Aspirin has been shown to be helpful when used daily to lower the risk of heart attack, clot-related strokes, and other blood flow problems. Many medical professionals prescribe aspirin for these uses. There may be a benefit to daily aspirin use for you if you have some kind of heart or blood vessel disease, or if you have evidence of poor blood flow to the brain. However, the risks of long-term aspirin use may be greater than the benefits if there are no signs of or risk factors for heart or blood vessel disease.

Every prescription and over-the-counter medicine has benefits and risks—even such a common and familiar medicine as aspirin. Aspirin use can result in serious side effects, such as stomach bleeding, bleeding in the brain, kidney failure, and some kinds of strokes. No medicine is completely safe. By carefully reviewing many different factors, your health professional can help you make the best choice for you.

When you don't have the labeling directions to guide you, you need the medical knowledge of your doctor, nurse practitioner, or other health professional.

Fact: Daily Aspirin Can Be Safest When Prescribed by a Medical Health Professional

Before deciding if daily aspirin use is right for you, your health professional will need to consider the following things:

- Your medical history and the history of your family members

- Your use of other medicines, including prescription and over-the-counter

- Your use of other products, such as dietary supplements, including vitamins and herbals

- Your allergies or sensitivities, and anything that affects your ability to use the medicine

- What you have to gain, or the benefits, from the use of the medicine

- Other options and their risks and benefits

- What side effects you may experience

- What dose, and what directions for use are best for you

- How to know when the medicine is working or not working for this use

Make sure to tell your health professional all the medicines (prescription and over-the-counter) and dietary supplements, including vitamins and herbals, that you use—even if only occasionally.

Fact: Aspirin Is a Drug

If you are at risk for heart attack or stroke, your doctor may prescribe aspirin to increase blood flow to the heart and brain. But any drug—including aspirin—can have harmful side effects, especially when mixed with other products. In fact, the chance of side effects increases with each new product you use.

New products include prescription and other over-the-counter medicines, dietary supplements (including vitamins and herbals), and sometimes foods and beverages. For instance, people who already use a prescribed medication to thin the blood should not use aspirin unless recommended by a health professional. There are also dietary supplements known to thin the blood. Using aspirin with alcohol or with another product that also contains aspirin, such as a cough-sinus drug, can increase the chance of side effects.

Your health professional will consider your current state of health. Some medical conditions, such as pregnancy, uncontrolled high blood pressure, bleeding disorders, asthma, peptic (stomach) ulcers, liver and kidney disease, could make aspirin a bad choice for you.

Make sure that all your health professionals are aware that you are using aspirin to reduce your risk of heart attack and clot-related strokes.

Fact: Once Your Doctor Decides That Daily Use of Aspirin Is For You, Safe Use Depends on Following Your Doctor's Directions

There are no directions on the label for using aspirin to reduce the risk of heart attack or clot-related stroke. You may rely on your health professional to provide the correct information on dose and directions for use. Using aspirin correctly gives you the best chance of getting the greatest benefits with the fewest unwanted side effects. Discuss with your health professional the different forms of aspirin products that might be best suited for you.

Aspirin has been shown to lower the risk of heart attack and stroke, but not all over-the-counter pain and fever reducers do that. Even though the directions on the aspirin label do not apply to this use of aspirin, you still need to read the label to confirm that the product you buy and use contains aspirin at the correct dose. Check the Drug Facts label for "active ingredients: aspirin" or "acetylsalicylic acid" at the dose that your health professional has prescribed.

Remember, if you are using aspirin every day for weeks, months, or years to prevent a heart attack, stroke, or for any use not listed on the label—without the guidance from your health professional—you could be doing your body more harm than good.

Section 68.2

Influenza Vaccine May Reduce Cardiovascular Disease Risk

A new study from researchers at the University of Iowa suggests that the flu vaccine may provide protection against heart attacks in older adults, particularly those over age eighty.

Scientists have long recognized that deaths due to influenza and deaths from other non-influenza-related diseases follow a similar seasonal pattern. This has lead researchers to suspect that acute infection caused by influenza may trigger events leading to heart attacks and strokes.

To determine if heart attacks and strokes are associated with influenza activity, the UI researchers built a set of time-series models using inpatient data from a national sample of more than one thousand hospitals.

Across all models, the researchers found consistent significant associations between heart attacks and influenza activity. The study was published online January 3, 2013, in the journal *Epidemiology and Infection*.

In these models, the research team, led by Eric Foster, Ph.D., visiting assistant professor of biostatistics in the UI College of Public Health, used influenza activity to predict the incidence of heart attack and stroke. The team produced national models as well as models based on four geographical regions and five age groups.

"We found that associations between influenza and heart attack increased with age, were greatest in those more than eighty years old, and were found in all geographical regions," says Foster. "Our findings, in conjunction with findings in other countries, provide another reason for annual influenza vaccination."

In addition, the second wave of the H1N1 pandemic in autumn 2009 provided further evidence of the relationship between influenza and heart attack, because both series peaked in the same nonwinter month.

The researchers did not find an association between influenza and strokes.

"We were surprised," says Foster, citing a recent German study that found influenza virus infection to be a risk factor for triggering strokes.

While there are a number of possible reasons for this discrepancy, the researchers write that "there are still many reasons for patients at risk for strokes to undergo annual vaccination against influenza."

Part Eight

Additional Help and Information

Chapter 69

Glossary of Terms Related to Cardiovascular Disease

aerobic (say: air-oh-bik) activity: Aerobic activity is any kind of movement that makes your muscles use oxygen. It gets your heart pumping, too. Swimming, dancing, and soccer are all types of aerobic activity, so hit that pool, dance floor, or soccer field and get moving!

anesthesia (say: ah-nes-thee-zhuh): Special medicine that causes sleepiness and prevents pain during surgery.

angina (say: an-jy-nuh): People with angina feel a pain in the chest that means the heart isn't getting enough oxygen.

angioplasty (say: an-jee-uh-plas-tee): This operation opens a blocked blood vessel by using a balloon-like device at an artery's narrowest point. The doctor also may insert a stent, which is a tiny tube that props the vessel open and makes sure blood flows freely.

aorta (say: ay-or-tah): The aorta is the major blood vessel that carries blood away from the heart to the rest of the body.

aortic stenosis (say: ay-or-tick steh-noh-sis): In aortic stenosis, the aortic valve is stiffened and has a narrowed opening (a condition called stenosis). It does not open properly, which increases strain on the heart because the left ventricle has to pump harder to send blood out to the body.

aortic valve: The aortic valve is one of two valves in charge of controlling the flow of blood as it leaves the heart. The other is the pulmonary valve. These valves work to keep the blood flowing forward. They open up to let the blood move ahead, then close quickly to keep the blood from flowing backward.

arrhythmia (say: uh-rith-mee-uh): An arrhythmia is an abnormal heartbeat usually caused by an electrical "short circuit" in the heart. It can cause the heart to pump too fast, too slow, or irregularly, which may lead to shortness of breath, dizziness, and chest pain.

arteries (say: ar-tuh-reez) and veins (say: vayns): If you've ever seen a road map, you probably saw many roads going here, there, and everywhere. Your body has a highway system all its own that sends blood to and from your body parts. It's called the circulatory system and the roads are called arteries and veins. Arteries, which usually look red, carry blood away from the heart. Veins, which usually look blue, return blood to the heart.

arteriosclerosis (say: ar-teer-ee-oh-skluh-roh-sus): Also called hardening of the arteries, arteriosclerosis means the arteries become thickened and less flexible.

atria (say: ay-tree-yuh): The two chambers at the top of the heart are called the atria. The atria are the chambers that fill with the blood returning to the heart from the body and lungs. The heart has a left atrium and a right atrium.

atrial septal (say: ay-tree-uhl sep-tuhl) defect (ASD): ASD is a hole in the heart wall (called the septum) that separates the left atrium and the right atrium.

atrioventricular canal (say: ay-tree-oh-ven-trick-yoo-lar cah-nal) defect: This defect—also known as endocardial cushion defect or atrioventricular septal defect—is caused by a poorly formed central area of the heart. Typically there is a large hole between the upper chambers of the heart (the atria) and, often, an additional hole between the lower chambers of the heart (the ventricles). Instead of two separate valves allowing flow into the heart, there is one large common valve that might be quite malformed.

atrium (say: ay-tree-uhm): The two upper chambers of the heart are called the atria. They are the chambers that fill with the blood returning to the heart from the body and lungs. The heart has a left atrium and a right atrium.

bacterial endocarditis (say: bak-teer-ee-ul en-doh-kar-dye-tus): If bacteria travel through the blood and get stuck on a heart valve, this can cause this infection in the heart. People with congenital heart disease or heart valve problems are most at risk of getting bacterial endocarditis.

blood pressure: Check your blood pressure! When you go to the doctor, a nurse might put a band (called a blood pressure cuff) around part of your arm and pump air into the cuff, blowing it up like a balloon. Your arm might feel a little squished, but don't worry—that's how a nurse checks your blood pressure. This test shows how hard your heart is pumping to move blood through your body. Blood pressure can be too high or too low.

blood vessels: Blood moves through many tubes called arteries and veins, which together are called blood vessels. The blood vessels that carry blood away from the heart are called arteries. The ones that carry blood back to the heart are called veins.

capillary (say: kap-uh-ler-ee): A capillary is an extremely small, thin blood vessel that allows oxygen to pass from the blood into the tissues of the body. Waste products like carbon dioxide pass from the tissues to the blood through the capillaries.

cardiac catheterization (say: kar-dee-ak ka-thuh-ter-uh-zay-shun): A cardiac catheterization is a medical procedure that provides information about the heart structures and function. Doctors can measure pressure and blood oxygen levels within the heart chambers.

cardiologist (say: kar-dee-ah-luh-jist): This kind of doctor knows all about the heart and how it works. A kid who has a heart problem will visit a pediatric cardiologist, who mainly treats kids. Cardiologists treat all kinds of heart problems, from heart murmurs to high blood pressure.

cardiovascular (say: kar-dee-oh-vas-kyuh-ler) disease: Cardiovascular disease is a group of problems that occur when the heart and blood vessels aren't working the way they should.

cardiovascular system: The heart and circulatory system (also called the cardiovascular system) make up the network that delivers blood to the body's tissues. With each heartbeat, blood is sent throughout our bodies, carrying oxygen and nutrients to all of our cells. The cardiovascular system is composed of the heart and blood vessels, including arteries, veins, and capillaries.

carotid (say: kuh-rah-tid) artery: The carotid arteries are the two large blood vessels in the neck that supply blood to the brain.

catheter (say: ka-thuh-ter): A catheter is a thin, flexible tube. It can be inserted into a blood vessel in the leg, arm, or neck and threaded to the heart during a cardiac catheterization.

catheterization (say: ka-thuh-tuh-ruh-zay-shun): In this procedure, a long, thin tube is inserted into the patient's body to inject a special dye, which can show narrowed areas in arteries due to plaque buildup and find other heart problems.

chambers (say: chaym-berz): The heart has four different sections, or chambers. These chambers are connected to each other by valves that control how much blood enters each chamber at any one time.

circulation (say: ser-kyuh-lay-shun): The movement of the blood through the heart and around the body is called circulation. Your heart is really good at it—it takes less than sixty seconds to pump blood to every cell in your body.

circulatory (say: ser-kyuh-luh-tor-ee) system: The circulatory system is composed of the heart and blood vessels, including arteries, veins, and capillaries. Our bodies actually have two circulatory systems: The pulmonary circulation is a short loop from the heart to the lungs and back again, and the systemic circulation (the system we usually think of as our circulatory system) sends blood from the heart to all the other parts of our bodies and back again.

coarctation (say: coh-ark-tay-shun) of the aorta (COA): Coarctation of the aorta is a narrowing of a portion of the aorta, and often seriously decreases the blood flow from the heart out to the lower portion of the body.

congenital (say: kuhn-jen-ih-tuhl) heart defects: Congenital heart defects are abnormalities in the heart's structure that are present at birth. Congenital heart defects happen because of incomplete or abnormal development of the fetus's heart during the very early weeks of pregnancy. Some are known to be associated with genetic disorders, such as Down syndrome, but the cause of most congenital heart defects is unknown. While they can't be prevented, there are many treatments for the defects and related health problems.

contraction (say: kuhn-trak-shun): You'll know that you've found your pulse when you can feel a small beat under your skin. Each beat is caused by the contraction (squeezing) of your heart.

echocardiogram (say: eh-ko-kar-dee-uh-gram): An echocardiogram test uses sound waves to diagnose heart problems. These waves are bounced off the parts of the heart, creating a picture of the heart that is displayed on a monitor. Getting an echocardiogram doesn't hurt at all.

electrocardiogram (say: eh-lek-tro-kar-dee-uh-gram): An electrocardiogram (or EKG) test records the heart's electrical activity. Sticky pads (electrodes) are placed on the chest and hooked up to a machine that records the heart activity onto paper or a monitor. A doctor can interpret the EKG to see the heart beating and determine if it's normal. Getting an EKG doesn't hurt at all.

endocarditis (say: en-doh-car-dye-tis): An infection of the inner lining of the heart and heart valves.

heart: The heart is a strong muscle about the size of your fist. It pumps blood through blood vessels around the body and sits inside the chest, protected by the ribcage. The blood carries oxygen and other nutrients your body needs.

heart and circulatory system: The heart and circulatory system (also called the cardiovascular system) make up the network that delivers blood to the body's tissues. With each heartbeat, blood is sent throughout our bodies, carrying oxygen and nutrients to all of our cells. The circulatory system is composed of the heart and blood vessels, including arteries, veins, and capillaries.

heart attack: A heart attack happens when a blood clot or other blockage cuts blood flow to a part of the heart.

heart murmur (say: mer-mer): You know the sound of your heartbeat: lub-dub, lub-dub. In some people, there's an extra noise that the blood makes as it flows through the heart. This sound is called a murmur. They're commonly heard in healthy kids with normal hearts, but an abnormal heart murmur can mean a person has a heart defect or heart valve problem.

hypertension: This is another word for high blood pressure.

hypoplastic (say: hi-poh-plas-tik) left heart syndrome: When the structures of the left side of the heart (the left ventricle, the mitral valve, and the aortic valve) are underdeveloped, they're unable to pump blood adequately to the entire body. This condition is usually diagnosed within the first few days of life.

involuntary (say: in-vah-lun-tair-ee) muscle: You don't have any say over what this kind of muscle does and when. It just does its thing and works without you even thinking about it. Your heart is an involuntary muscle, which is how it keeps beating all day and night. Other involuntary muscles help digest food and are found in your stomach and intestines.

left atrium: The left atrium is one of the four chambers of the heart. It receives oxygen-rich blood from the lungs and then empties the blood into the left ventricle through the mitral valve.

left ventricle: The left ventricle is one of the four chambers of the heart. It pumps oxygen-rich blood out to the rest of the body. Blood leaves the left ventricle through the aortic valve and enters the aorta, the largest artery in the body. Blood then flows from the aorta into the branches of many smaller arteries, providing the body's organs and tissues with the oxygen and nutrients they need.

mitral (say: my-truhl) valve: The mitral valve lets blood flow from the left atrium to the left ventricles.

mitral valve prolapse: In someone with mitral valve prolapse (MVP), one or both of the valve's flaps don't close smoothly and collapse (or prolapse) back into the atrium.

murmur: See heart murmur.

patent ductus arteriosus (say: duck-tuss ar-tee-ree-oh-sis) (PDA): The ductus arteriosus (DA) is a normal blood vessel in a fetus (a baby before it is born) that diverts blood flow away from the lungs. (The lungs are not used until a baby is born—the fetus gets oxygen directly from the mother's placenta.) The DA usually closes on its own shortly after birth because the newborn can breathe on his or her own. If the DA doesn't close, this is called patent ductus arteriosus (PDA), which can result in too much blood flow to a newborn's lungs. PDA is common in premature babies.

pediatric cardiologist: This kind of doctor knows all about children's hearts and how they work. A kid with a heart problem will visit a pediatric cardiologist. Cardiologists treat all kinds of heart problems, from heart murmurs to high blood pressure.

pulmonary (say: pull-muh-nair-ee): Pulmonary is word that means lungs or related to breathing.

pulmonary artery: a blood vessel that carries blood from the heart to the lungs, where the blood picks up oxygen and then returns to the heart.

pulmonary vein: one of four veins that carry oxygen-rich blood from the lungs to the heart.

pulmonary atresia (say: uh-tree-szhuh): With pulmonary atresia, the pulmonic valve does not open at all and may indeed be completely absent. The main blood vessel that runs between the right ventricle and the lungs also may be malformed and the right ventricle can be abnormally small.

pulmonary stenosis (say: steh-noh-sis): In pulmonary stenosis, the pulmonic valve is stiffened and has a narrowed opening. It does not open properly, which increases strain on the right side of the heart because the right ventricle has to pump harder to send blood out to the lungs.

pulmonary (pulmonic) valve: One of two valves in charge of controlling the flow as the blood leaves the heart. The other one is the aortic valve. These valves all work to keep the blood flowing forward. They open up to let the blood move ahead, then they close quickly to keep the blood from flowing backward.

pulse (say: pulss): Your beating heart creates a pulse. Your heart has to push so much blood through your body that you can feel a little thump in your arteries each time the heart beats. Wow! The most common places to feel a pulse are on your wrist and your neck. So try to find your pulse and feel the beat!

red blood cells: Red blood cells have the important job of carrying oxygen. These cells, which float in your blood, begin their journey in the lungs, where they pick up oxygen from the air you breathe. Then they travel to the heart, which pumps out the blood, delivering oxygen to all parts of your body.

right atrium: The right atrium is one of the four chambers of the heart. After oxygen in the blood is released to the tissues, the now deoxygenated (oxygen-poor) blood returns to the heart through veins, the blood vessels that carry deoxygenated blood. This blood, which appears blue, enters the right atrium of the heart and then travels across the tricuspid valve into the right ventricle.

right ventricle: The right ventricle is one of the four chambers of the heart. It pumps deoxygenated blood through the pulmonic valve into the lungs. The oxygen in the air we breathe binds to red blood cells that are being pumped through the lungs. The oxygen-rich blood, which appears red, then returns to the left atrium and enters the left ventricle, where it is pumped out to the body once again.

septum (say: sep-tum): The septum is a thick wall of muscle that divides the heart. It separates the left and right sides of the heart.

stent: A tiny tube that props a blood vessel open and makes sure blood flows freely.

stethoscope (say: steth-eh-skope): A doctor uses a stethoscope to hear your heartbeat and other sounds that the inside of your body makes. By listening to your heart, lungs, and belly, the doctor gets information about how things are working inside.

stress test: For this test, the person exercises (usually on a treadmill) while the doctor checks breathing, heart rate, blood pressure, and electrocardiogram to see how the heart muscle reacts.

stroke: A stroke can happen when part of the brain doesn't get enough blood due to a clot or a burst blood vessel.

tricuspid (say: try-kus-pid) atresia: Blood normally flows from the right atrium to the right ventricle through the tricuspid valve. In tricuspid atresia, the valve is replaced by a plate or membrane that does not open. The right ventricle therefore does not receive blood normally and is often small.

tricuspid valve: The tricuspid valve lets blood flow from the right atria to the right ventricle.

truncus arteriosus (say: trun-kuss ar-tee-ree-oh-sis): In an embryo, the aorta and the pulmonary artery are initially a single vessel. During normal development, that vessel splits to form the two major arteries. If that split does not occur, the child is born with a single blood vessel called the truncus arteriosus. There is usually a hole between the ventricles associated with this defect.

valve: Your heart has four valves. A valve lets something in and keeps it there by closing, like a door. The door shuts behind you and keeps you from going backward. Heart valves ensure that blood flows properly in and out of the heart.

veins and arteries: Your body has a highway system all its own that sends blood to and from your body parts. It's called the circulatory system, and the roads are arteries and veins. Arteries, which usually look red, carry blood away from the heart. Veins, which usually look blue, return blood to the heart.

ventricles (say: ven-trih-kuhls): The two chambers at the bottom of the heart are called the ventricles. The heart has a left ventricle and a right ventricle. Their job is to pump the blood to the body and lungs.

ventricular (say: ven-trih-kyuh-ler) septal defect (VSD): One of the most common congenital heart defects, VSD is a hole in the wall (septum) between the heart's left and right ventricles. These can occur at different locations and vary in size from very small to very large. Smaller defects may gradually close on their own.

white blood cells: White blood cells are part of the germ-fighting immune system. They are like little warriors floating around in your blood waiting to attack invaders, like viruses and bacteria. You have several types of white blood cells and each has its own special role in fighting off the different kinds of germs that make people sick.

Chapter 70

Directory of Resources Providing Information about Cardiovascular Disease

General

AboutKidsHealth
The Hospital for Sick Children
(SickKids)
555 University Avenue
Toronto, ON
M5G 1X8
Canada
Website: http://www.aboutkids
health.ca

American Academy of Family Physicians
P.O. Box 11210
Shawnee Mission,
KS 66207-1210
Toll-Free: 800-274-2237
Phone: 913-906-6000
Fax: 913-906-6075
Website: http://www.aafp.org

American Academy of Pediatrics
141 Northwest Point Boulevard
Elk Grove Village,
IL 60007-1098
Toll-Free: 800-433-9016
Phone: 847-434-4000
Fax: 847-434-8000
Website: http://www.aap.org
E-mail: kidsdocs@aap.org

American Association for Clinical Chemistry
1850 K Street NW, Suite 625
Washington, DC 20006
Toll-Free: 800-892-1400
Fax: 202-887-5093
Website: http://www.aacc.org
E-mail: custserv@aacc.org

Resources in this chapter were compiled from several sources deemed reliable. All contact information was verified and updated in September 2013.

**American Association
of Cardiovascular and
Pulmonary Rehabilitation**
330 North Michigan Avenue
Suite 2000
Chicago, IL 60611
Phone: 312-321-5146
Fax: 312-673-6924
Website: http://www.aacvpr.org
E-mail: aacvpr@aacvpr.org

**American College of
Cardiology**
Heart House
2400 N Street NW
Washington, DC 20037
Toll-Free: 800-253-4636 x 5603
Phone: 202-375-6000
Fax: 202-375-7000
Website: http://www.acc.org
E-mail: resource@aac.org

**American College of Chest
Physicians**
3300 Dundee Road
Northbrook, IL 60062-2348
Toll-Free: 800-343-2227
Phone: 847-498-1400
Fax: 847-498-5460
Website:
http://www.chestnet.org

**American College of
Emergency Physicians**
P.O. Box 619911
Dallas, TX 75261-9911
Toll-Free: 800-798-1822
Phone: 972-550-0911
Fax: 972-580-2816
Website: http://www.acep.org
E-mail: membership@acep.org

**American College of
Rheumatology**
2200 Lake Boulevard NE
Atlanta, GA 30319
Phone: 404-633-3777
Fax: 404-633-1870
Website:
http://www.rheumatology.org
E-mail: acr@rheumatology.org

**American Heart
Association**
7272 Greenville Avenue
Dallas, TX 75231
Toll-Free: 800-AHA-USA-1
(800-242-8721)
Phone: 214-570-5978
Website: http://www.heart.org
E-mail: info@heart.org

**American Society of
Echocardiography**
2100 Gateway Centre Boulevard
Suite 310
Morrisville, NC 27560
Phone: 919-861-5574
Fax: 919-882-9900
Website: http://www.asecho.org
E-mail: ase@asecho.org

**American Society of
Hypertension**
45 Main Street, Suite 712
Brooklyn, NY 11202
Phone: 212-696-9099
Fax: 347-916-0267
Website: http://www.ash-us.org
E-mail: ash@ash-us.org

American Stroke Association
7272 Greenville Avenue
Dallas, TX 75231
Toll-Free: 888-4-STROKE
(888-478-7653)
Website:
http://www.strokeassociation.org

Brain Aneurysm Foundation
269 Hanover Street
Building 3
Hanover, MA 02339
Toll-Free: 888-272-4602
Phone: 781-826-5556
Website:
http://www.bafound.org
E-mail: office@bafound.org

Cardiovascular Research Foundation
111 East 59th Street
New York, NY 10022-1202
Phone: 646-434-4500
Website: http://www.crf.org
E-mail: info@crf.org

Center for Prevention of Heart and Vascular Disease
535 Mission Bay Boulevard South
San Francisco, CA 94143
Phone: 415-353-2873
Fax: 415-353-2528
Website:
http://www.healthyheart.ucsf.edu
E-mail:
info@healthyheart.ucsf.edu

Centers for Disease Control and Prevention
1600 Clifton Road
Atlanta, GA 30333
Toll-Free: 800-CDC-INFO
(800-232-4636)
Toll-Free TTY: 888-232-6348
Fax: 770-488-8151
Website: http://www.cdc.gov
E-mail: cdcinfo@cdc.gov

Children's Cardiomyopathy Foundation
P.O. Box 547
Tenafly, NJ 07670
Phone: 866-808-CURE
(866-808-2873)
Fax: 201-227-7016
Website: http://www.childrens
cardiomyopathy.org
E-mail: info@
childrenscardiomyopathy.org

Children's Hemiplegia and Stroke Association (CHASA)
4101 West Green Oaks
Suite 305 #149
Arlington, TX 76016
Phone: 817-492-4325
Website: http://www.chasa.org

Cleveland Clinic
9500 Euclid Avenue
Cleveland, OH 44195
Toll-Free: 800-223-2273
Phone: 216-444-2200
TTY: 216-444-0261
Website:
http://www.clevelandclinic.org

Heart and Stroke Foundation of Canada
222 Queen Street
Suite 1402
Ottawa, ON
K1P 5V9
Canada
Phone: 613-569-4361
Fax: 613-569-3278
Website:
http://www.heartandstroke.com

Heart Failure Society of America
5425 Wisconsin Avenue
Suite 600
Chevy Chase, MD 20815
Phone: 301-718-4800
Fax: 301-968-2431
Website: http://www.hfsa.org
E-mail: info@hfsa.org

Heart Rhythm Society
1400 K Street NW
Suite 500
Washington, DC 20005
Phone: 202-464-3400
Fax: 202-464-3401
Website:
http://www.hrsonline.org
E-mail: info@HRSonline.org

Hypertrophic Cardiomyopathy Association
P.O. Box 306
Hibernia, NJ 07842
Phone: 973-983-7429
Fax: 973-983-7870
Website: http://www.4hcm.org
E-mail: support@4hcm.org

The Mended Hearts, Inc.
8150 North Central Expressway
M2248
Dallas, TX 75206
Toll-Free: 888-HEART99
(888-432-7899)
Phone: 214-206-9259
Fax: 214-295-9552
Website:
http://www.mendedhearts.org
E-mail: info@mendedhearts.org

Minneapolis Heart Institute Foundation
920 East 28th Street
Suite 100
Minneapolis, MN 55407
Toll-Free: 877-800-2729
Phone: 612-863-3833
Fax: 612-863-3801
Website:
http://www.mplsheart.org
E-mail: info@mhif.org

National Center for Complementary and Alternative Medicine
9000 Rockville Pike
Bethesda, MD 20892
Toll-free: 888-644-6226
Toll-Free TTY: 866-464-3615
Website:
http://www.nccam.nih.gov

National Heart, Lung, and Blood Institute

NHLBI Health Information
Center
P.O. Box 30105
Bethesda, MD 20824-0105
Phone: 301-592-8573
Fax: 240-629-3246
Website:
http://www.nhlbi.nih.gov
E-mail:
nhlbiinfo@nhlbi.nih.gov

National Human Genome Research Institute

National Institutes of Health
Building 31, Room 4B09
31 Center Drive, MSC 2152
9000 Rockville Pike
Bethesda, MD 20892-2152
Phone: 301-402-0911
Fax: 301-402-2218
Website:
http://www.genome.gov

National Institute of Arthritis and Musculoskeletal and Skin Diseases

National Institutes of Health
1 AMS Circle
Bethesda, MD 20892-3675
Toll-Free: 877-22-NIAMS
(877-226-4267)
TTY: 301-565-2966
Phone: 301-495-4484
Fax: 301-718-6366
Website:
http://www.niams.nih.gov
E-mail:
NIAMSinfo@mail.nih.gov

National Institute of Diabetes, Digestive, and Kidney Diseases

Building 31, Room 9A06
31 Center Drive, MSC 2560
Bethesda, MD 20892-2560
Phone: 301-496-3583
Website: http://www.niddk.nih.gov

National Institute of Neurological Disorders and Stroke

National Institutes of Health
(NIH) Neurological Institute
P.O. Box 5801
Bethesda, MD 20824
Toll-Free: 800-352-9424
Phone: 301-496-5751
TTY: 301-468-5981
Website: http://www.ninds.nih.gov
E-mail: braininfo@ninds.nih.gov

National Institute on Aging

Building 31, Room 5C27
31 Center Drive, MSC 2292
Bethesda, MD 20892
Toll-Free: 800-222-2225
Toll-Free TTY: 800-222-4225
Phone: 301-496-1752
Fax: 301-496-1072
Website: http://www.nia.nih.gov
E-mail: niaic@nia.nih.gov

National Institutes of Health

9000 Rockville Pike
Bethesda, MD 20892
Phone: 301-496-4000
TTY: 301-402-9612
Website: http://www.nih.gov
E-mail: NIHinfo@od.nih.gov

National Stroke Association
9707 East Easter Lane, Suite B
Centennial, CO 80112
Toll-Free: 800-STROKES
(800-787-6537)
Fax: 303-649-1328
Website: http://www.stroke.org
E-mail: info@stroke.org

Nemours Foundation
Website: http://kidshealth.org

Office of Minority Health
Resource Center
P.O. Box 37337
Washington, DC 20103-7337
Toll-Free: 800-444-6472
Fax: 301-251-2160
Website:
https://minorityhealth.hhs.gov
E-mail: info@
minorityhealth.hhs.gov

**Society for
Vascular Surgery**
633 North Saint Clair
22nd Floor
Chicago, IL 60611
Toll-Free: 800-258-7188
Phone: 312-334-2300
Fax: 312-334-2320
Website:
http://www.vascularsociety.org
E-mail: vascular@
vascularsociety.org

**The Society of Thoracic
Surgeons**
Phone: 312-202-5800
Fax: 312-202-5801
Website: http://www.sts.org

Texas Heart Institute
MC 3-116
P.O. Box 20345
Houston, TX 77225-0345
Phone: 832-355-4011
Website:
http://www.texasheart.org

Office on Women's Health
Department of Health
and Human Services
200 Independence Avenue SW
Room 712E
Washington, DC 20201
Toll-Free: 800-994-9662
Phone: 202-690-7650
Fax: 202-205-2631
Website: http://womenshealth.gov

**U.S. Food and Drug
Administration**
10903 New Hampshire Avenue
Silver Spring, MD 20993-0002
Toll-Free: 888-INFO-FDA
(888-463-6332)
Website: http://www.fda.gov

**Vascular Disease
Foundation**
550 M Ritchie Highway
PMB-281
Severna Park, MD 21146
Phone: 443-261-5564
Website: http://www.vdf.org
E-mail: info@vdf.org

Women's Heart Foundation
P.O. Box 7827
West Trenton, NJ 08628
Phone: 609-771-9600
Website:
http://www.womensheart.org

World Heart Federation
7, rue des Battoirs
Case postale 155
1211 Geneva 4
Switzerland
Website: http://
www.world-heart-federation.org

Arrhythmias

Heart Rhythm Society
1400 K Street NW, Suite 500
Washington, DC 20005
Phone: 202-464-3400
Fax: 202-464-3401
Website: http://www.hrsonline.org
E-mail: info@HRSonline.org

Washington Heart Rhythm Associates, LLC
10230 New Hampshire Avenue
Suite 204
Silver Spring, MD 20903
Phone: 301-408-7890
Fax: 301-408-7892
Website:
http://www.washingtonhra.com

Congenital Disorders

Congenital Heart Information Network
P.O. Box 3397
Margate City, NJ 08402-0397
Phone: 609-823-4507
Website: http://www.tchin.org

March of Dimes Foundation
1275 Mamaroneck Avenue
White Plains, NY 10605
Phone: 914-997-4488
Website:
http://www.marchofdimes.com

Myocarditis

Myocarditis Foundation
100 West Main Street
Utica, MN 55979
Toll Free: 866-846-1600
Phone: 732-295-3700
Fax: 732-295-3701
Website: http://www.myocarditis
foundation.org

Peripheral Arterial Disorders

Erythromelalgia Association
200 Old Castle Lane
Wallingford, PA 19086
Phone: 610-566-0797
Website:
http://www.erythromelalgia.org
E-mail: memberservices@
burningfeet.org

Fibromuscular Dysplasia Society of America
20325 Center Ridge Road
Suite 620
Rocky River, OH 44116
Toll-Free: 888-709-7089
Phone: 216-834-2410
Website: http://www.fmdsa.org
E-mail: admin@fmdsa.org

Sudden Cardiac Arrest

Sudden Cardiac Arrest Association
12100 Sunset Hills Road
Suite 130
Reston, VA 20190
Toll-Free: 866-972-SCAA
(866-972-7222)
Website: http://www.sudden
cardiacarrest.org
E-mail: info@
suddencardiacarrest.org

Sudden Cardiac Arrest Foundation
7500 Brooktree Road
Suite 207
Wexford, PA 15090
Toll Free: 877-722-8641
Website: http://
www.sca-aware.org

Valvular Disorders

The Howard Gilman Institute for Heart Valve Disease
635 Madison Avenue
Third Floor
New York, NY 10022
Phone: 212-289-7777
Website:
http://www.gilmanheartvalve.us
E-mail:
info@gilmanheartvalve.us

Vasculitis

Vasculitis Foundation
P.O. Box 28660
Kansas City, MO 64188
Toll-Free: 800-277-9474
Phone: 816-436-8211
Fax: 816-436-8211
Website: http://www.vasculitis
foundation.org

Vasculitis Foundation Canada
425 Hespeler Road
Suite 446
Cambridge, ON
N1R 8J6
Canada
Phone: 877-572-9474
Website:
http://www.vasculitis.ca
E-mail: contact@vasculitis.ca

Index

Index

Page numbers followed by 'n' indicate a footnote. Page numbers in *italics* indicate a table or illustration.

Health Reference Series